Evidence-Based
Geriatric Medicine

Website: Evidence-Based Medicine Series

The Evidence-Based Medicine Series has a website at:

www.evidencebasedseries.com

Where you can find:

- Links to companion websites with additional resources and updates for books in the series

- Details of all new and forthcoming titles

- Links to more Evidence-Based products: including the Cochrane Library, Essential Evidence Plus, and EBM Guidelines.

How to access the companion sites with additional resources and updates:

- Go to the Evidence-Based Series site: **www.evidencebasedseries.com**

- Select your book from the list of titles shown on the site

- If your book has a website with supplementary material, it will show an icon [Companion Website] next to the title

- Click on the icon to access the website

Evidence-Based Geriatric Medicine

A Practical Clinical Guide

Edited by

Jayna M. Holroyd-Leduc, MD FRCPC

Associate Professor
Departments of Medicine and Community Health Sciences
Division of Geriatrics
University of Calgary
Calgary, AB
Canada

Madhuri Reddy, MD MSc

Hebrew Senior Life
Boston, MA
USA

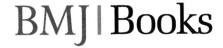

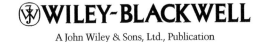

A John Wiley & Sons, Ltd., Publication

Library of Congress Cataloging-in-Publication Data

Evidence-based geriatric medicine : a practical clinical guide / edited by Jayna M. Holroyd-Leduc and Madhuri Reddy.
    p. ; cm.
  Includes bibliographical references and index.
  ISBN 978-1-4443-3718-1 (pbk. : alk. paper)
  I. Holroyd-Leduc, Jayna M., 1970–   II. Reddy, Madhuri, 1972–
  DNLM: 1. Geriatrics–methods.   2. Aged.   3. Aging–physiology.   4. Evidence-Based Medicine.
5. Geriatric Assessment.   WT 100]
  618.97–dc23

                                                                    2011049726

A catalogue record for this book is available from the British Library.

Wiley also publishes its books in a variety of electronic formats. Some content that appears in print may not be available in electronic books.

Set in 9.5/12 pt Minion by Aptara® Inc., New Delhi, India

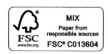

Contents

Evidence-Based Medicine Series

The Evidence-Based Medicine Series has a website at:

www.evidencebasedseries.com

v

List of Contributors

Ranjani Aiyar
Fellow
General Internal Medicine
Division of General Internal Medicine
Department of Medicine
University of Calgary
Calgary, AB, Canada

Shabbir M.H. Alibhai
Associate Professor
Departments of Medicine and Health Policy,
    Management, and Evaluation
University of Toronto
Toronto, ON, Canada;
Consultant Geriatrician
Toronto Rehabilitation Institute
Toronto, ON, Canada;
Staff Physician
Internal Medicine and Geriatrics
University Health Network
Toronto, ON, Canada

Anita Asgar
Director
Transcatheter Valve Therapy Clinic
Institut de Cardiologie de Montréal
Montréal, Quebec, Canada;
Assistant Professor
Université de Montréal
Montréal, Quebec, Canada

Stuart Carney
Deputy National Director
UK Foundation Programme Office
Cardiff Bay, UK

Dov Gandell
Resident, Geriatric Medicine
Department of Medicine
Division of Geriatrics
University of Toronto
Toronto, ON, Canada

Sudeep S. Gill
Associate Professor
Department of Medicine
Division of Geriatric Medicine
Queen's University
Kingston, ON, Canada

Mary K. Goldstein
Director
Geriatrics Research Education and Clinical Center (GRECC)
VA Palo Alto Health Care System
Palo Alto, CA, USA;
Professor of Medicine (Center for Primary Care &
    Outcomes Research)
Stanford University School of Medicine
Stanford, CA, USA

Jayna M. Holroyd-Leduc
QI Lead
Department of Medicine
University of Calgary and Alberta Health Services
Calgary, AB, Canada;
Medical Coordinator of Clinical Informatics
Department of Medicine
Alberta Health Services
Calgary, AB, Canada;

Associate Professor
Departments of Medicine and Community Health Sciences
Director, Geriatric Medicine Training Program
Division of Geriatrics
University of Calgary
Calgary, AB, Canada

Landon D. Hough

Resident Physician
Department of Family and Community Medicine
University of Missouri
Columbia, MO, USA

Sunila R. Kalkar

Research Coordinator
Women's College Research Institute
Women's College Hospital
Toronto, ON, Canada

Jean S. Kutner

Professor of Medicine
University of Colorado
Denver School of Medicine
Aurora, CO, USA

Emily Kwan

Resident, Geriatric Medicine
Department of Medicine
Division of Geriatrics
University of Toronto
Toronto, ON, Canada

Philip E. Lee

Assistant Professor
Division of Geriatric Medicine
University of British Columbia
Vancouver, BC, Canada

Cari Levy

Associate Professor of Medicine
University of Colorado Denver School of Medicine
Denver, CO, USA;
Denver VA Medical Center
Denver, CO, USA

Erik J. Lindbloom

Associate Professor
Department of Family and Community Medicine
University of Missouri
Columbia, MO, USA

Salahaddin Mahmudi-Azer

Clinical Fellow
Department of Critical Care Medicine
Foothills Hospital
University of Calgary
Calgary, AB, Canada

Marina Martin

Clinical Instructor of Medicine (General Internal Medicine)
Stanford University
Stanford, CA, USA

Paige K. Moorhouse

Assistant Professor
Geriatric Medicine
Dalhousie University
Halifax, NS, Canada

Jane Pearce

Consultant Old Age Psychiatrist and Honorary Senior
    Clinical Lecturer in Psychiatry
University of Oxford
Oxford, UK;
Fulbrook Centre
Churchill Hospital
Oxford, UK

Madhuri Reddy

Hebrew Senior Life
Boston, MA, USA

Paula A. Rochon

Vice President, Research
Women's College Research Institute
Women's College Hospital
Toronto, ON, Canada;
Senior Scientist
Institute for Clinical Evaluative Sciences
Toronto, ON, Canada;
Professor
Department of Medicine
University of Toronto
Toronto, ON, Canada

Kenneth Rockwood

Professor
Geriatric Medicine
Dalhousie University
Halifax, NS, Canada;

Kathryn Allen Weldon Professor of Alzheimer Research
Dalhousie University
Halifax, NS, Canada;
Consultant Physician
Queen Elizabeth II Health Sciences Centre
Halifax, NS, Canada

Dallas P. Seitz
Assistant Professor
Department of Psychiatry
Division of Geriatric Psychiatry
Queen's University
Kingston, ON, Canada;
Fellow
Women's College Research Institute
Toronto, ON, Canada

Sharon Straus
Professor
Department of Medicine
Director, Division of Geriatrics
University of Toronto
Toronto, ON, Canada;
Director, Knowledge Translation Program
Li Ka Shing Knowledge Institute of St. Michael's
Toronto, ON, Canada

Cara Tannenbaum
Associate Professor
Faculties of Medicine and Pharmacy
Université de Montréal
Montréal, QC, Canada;
Director
Geriatric Incontinence Clinic
Institut Universitaire de Gériatrie
Université de Montréal
Montréal, QC, Canada

Karli R.E. Urban
Resident Physician
Department of Family and Community Medicine
University of Missouri
Columbia, MO, USA

Wei Wu
Statistical Analyst
Women's College Research Institute
Women's College Hospital
Toronto, ON, Canada

Foreword

Worldwide a major change in the population demographic is posing challenges to health care systems. In many countries the baby boom, that followed World War II and extended to the 1960s, will soon result in a substantial increase in the number of people over 65 years of age. Moreover, most countries including Canada, the United States and the United Kingdom have experienced a continuing increase in life expectancy, with an increase of approximately 1 year occurring every 5 years. These factors translate into a growing proportion of people aged 65 and older and these people will have many more years of life after attaining age 65. This situation is not unique to western countries; many developing countries will grow old before they get rich. For example, in 2000, 7% of China's population was $\geq$ 65 years old; by 2030 this will increase to 16%. As the proportion of older people increases, there is an increasing need for services targeted to care for older people, in particular to optimize the independence and vitality of those living in the community. There is an urgent need for health care professionals from all disciplines (aside from paediatrics!) to become comfortable with caring for this population. This book will address this demand and provide a resource for health care professionals to provide evidence-based care for older patients.

Evidence-Based Geriatric Medicine, a Practical Guide focuses on bringing together 2 critically important issues in health care – evidence-based practice (EBP) and care of the older patient. Interest in EBP has grown exponentially since the coining of the term in 1992, from 1 MEDLINE citation in that year to more than 75000 hits in January 2012. Training in EBP has become a component of educational curricula for health care disciplines, patients and policy makers amongst others[1]. This growing interest arose from a number of realisations including: our inability to afford more than a few seconds per patient for finding and assimilating evidence[2] or to set aside more than half an hour per week for general reading and study[3]; and the finding that the gaps between evidence and practice (including underuse and overuse of evidence) lead to variations in practice and quality of care[4, 5].

To meet these challenges, this book focuses on providing an approach to care for older patients that is based on the best available evidence. An ideal evidence-based resource should use rigorous and transparent methods for seeking and appraising the evidence, and provide the evidence in a clinically useful format. The format of each chapter in this book includes questions that have been generated by clinicians while the content focuses on a systematic review of the evidence and provides the reader with the bottom line for their clinical practice. Finally, the book highlights the gaps in the evidence, which are targets for future research (we hope!).

Topics addressed in the book include assessing and managing the geriatric giants such as delirium, dementia, urinary incontinence and falls. The authors also tackle issues, such as elder abuse, that are often underappreciated in clinical care. And, the book includes discussion of the management of chronic diseases in the complex older patient which is useful information for any generalist clinician.

This book will be a resource for trainees and clinicians from various disciplines, worldwide. It addresses issues of global importance – promoting healthy aging and building capacity to care for older persons.

References

1. Straus SE, Richardson WS, Glasziou P, Haynes RB (2011) Evidence-based Medicine: How to practice and teach it. Fourth Edition. Elsevier; Edinburgh.
2. Sackett DL, Straus SE (1998) Finding and applying evidence during clinical rounds: the 'evidence cart'. *JAMA* 280: 1336–8.
3. Sackett DL (1997) Using evidence-based medicine to help physicians keep up-to-date. *Serials* 9: 178–81.
4. Shah BR, Mamdani M, Jaakkimainen L, Hux JE (2004) Risk modification for diabetic patients. *Can J Clin Pharmacol* 11: 239–44.
5. Pimlott NJ, Hux JE, Wilson LM, et al. (2003) Educating physicians to reduce benzodiazepine use by elderly patients. *CMAJ* 168: 835–9.

Sharon Straus
February 2012

CHAPTER 1

Function and frailty: the cornerstones of geriatric assessment

Paige K. Moorhouse[1,2] & Kenneth Rockwood[1,2]
[1]*Department of Geriatric Medicine, Dalhousie University, Halifax, NS, Canada*
[2]*Queen Elizabeth II Health Sciences Centre, Halifax, NS, Canada*

Introduction

Older people are more likely to be ill than younger people, and most of the older people who are ill have more than one illness. Yet this is generally not what we teach medical students. Instead, reflecting the scientific tradition of reductionism from which real progress has been possible, medicine is generally taught on a "one thing wrong at once" basis, often with younger patients as prototype [1]. Consequently, many physicians have an ambivalent understanding about medicine and aging.

We discuss two main topics in this chapter. The first is frailty. Frail older adults often behave as complex systems that are close to failure. One aspect of acting in a complex system is that when the system fails, it will fail in its highest order functions first. For humans, these high order functions are divided attention, upright bipedal ambulation, opposable thumbs, and social interaction. Their failures are delirium, mobility impairment and falls, impaired function, and social withdrawal/abandonment. Another essential aspect of acting in a complex system is that any single act is likely to have multiple consequences. For example, the medication given in an evidence-based way to treat inflammatory arthritis to allow mobilization, so as to comply with evidence-based exercises and to improve cardiac conditioning, might decrease heart function in a frail patient through fluid retention that precipitates heart failure. That is why the specialty of geriatrics has evolved dicta such as "start low, go slow". This is not simply codified common sense, but a rational response to the patients' complexity.

The second main topic that we discuss in this chapter is function. Functional impairment in an older adult is often characterized as a "sensitive but nonspecific" sign of illness. While true, it is an inadequate account of why it should have the iconic status of a "geriatric giant" [2], because medicine is replete with other sensitive but nonspecific signs, from chest pain to chapped lips. Intact functioning requires a lot to be right; compromised function can reflect a single cause (e.g., a catastrophic stroke), but commonly, in older adults, it reflects problems in more than one area. It is this "more than one thing wrong" aspect of functional impairment that makes it so useful as an overall sign of a patient's state of health.

Search strategy

Frailty

We searched PubMed for systematic reviews, meta-analyses, and practice guidelines published in the last 5 years in English for those aged 65 and older using the following search terms: "frailty," "frailty index," and "frailty phenotype." This yielded 144 articles, 25 of which were narrative reviews and 21 of which were systematic reviews.

Evidence-Based Geriatric Medicine: A Practical Clinical Guide, First Edition. Edited by Jayna M. Holroyd-Leduc and Madhuri Reddy.
© 2012 Blackwell Publishing Ltd. Published 2012 by Blackwell Publishing Ltd.

Table 1.1 Contrasting the frailty phenotype and the frailty index

	Frailty Phenotype	Frailty Index
General	Five items: (1) weakness, (2) exhaustion, (3) reduced activity, (4) motor slowing, and (5) weight loss	Any set of items that are age associated, associated with adverse outcomes, do not saturate at some young age, and have <5% missing data.
Data collection	Usually must be prospective	Can be operationalized in many existing data sets
Number of items	5	Can be as few as 30, as many as 100; most often about 40–50
Is supported by a theory of frailty	Yes	Yes
Uses performance measures	Yes	Usually not
Uses disability items	No	Usually
Uses comorbidity items	No	Yes
Cross-validated	Extensively (>100 groups)	Somewhat (about a dozen groups)
Samples other than physical domains	Possibly (feeling of exhaustion)	Yes
Most common criticism	Covers too few domains	Includes too many items, especially disability and comorbidity
Animal model	Yes	Yes

Functional assessment

We searched PubMed for systematic reviews, meta-analyses, and practice guidelines published in English with subjects 65 and older in the last 24 months using the following search terms: "activities of daily living" (ADL), "ADL," "evaluation," "measurement," "assessment," and "functional." This yielded 50 articles, 13 of which were pertinent to the topic. Expanding the search to articles published in the last 5 years yielded 138 new articles, 15 of which were pertinent to the topic. We then searched related citations of the 28 articles selected. This yielded four additional items. A total of 32 articles were reviewed in detail.

For this chapter, we graded relevant clinical studies using the US Preventative Task Force levels of evidence.

What is frailty?

Frailty is the variable susceptibility to adverse health outcomes, including death, of people of the same chronological age. Controversy in the definition of frailty arises in how frailty is best operationalized. Pending the results of an ongoing large meta-analysis [3], two frailty operationalization camps have arisen (Table 1.1). One group emphasizes a frailty phenotype [4]. Another emphasizes a frailty index, and states that susceptibility to adverse outcomes arises as a consequence of the accumulation and interaction of deficits, for which various phenotypes might exist [5, 6].

The frailty phenotype

The frailty phenotype specifies five characteristics: (1) slowness, (2) weight loss, (3) impaired strength, (4) exhaustion, and (5) low physical activity/energy expenditure. A person is said to be frail if they have any three of these five characteristics. People who have only one or two of the characteristics, while still at an increased risk compared to people with none of the phenotypic characteristics, are said to be "prefrail." People with none of the characteristics are said to be "robust." A strength of this approach is that at least four of the items are measurable by performance and in that way, objective. It also offers some prospect of finding mechanisms that might be associated with development and progression of frailty. The phenotype definition has been extensively validated and is reliably associated with an increased risk of death and with other adverse health outcomes.

The phenotypic view is well accepted, in that over a hundred separate groups have conducted studies which show that for almost any adverse outcomes and for many physiological ones, such as levels of proinflammatory molecules [7], hemoglobin [8], or sex hormones [9], female robust people have, on an average, the most favorable profile, frail people the least favorable, and "prefrail" people an intermediate profile.

Despite widespread use and consistency of results, the frailty phenotype has been criticized for misclassifying people who are clinically recognizable as frail [10]. In particular, some critics argue that the frailty phenotype includes *too few* items, and suggest the inclusion of some or all of the subjective perceptions of health status, cognitive performance, sensory or physical impairments, current health status needs, or appearance (as consistent or not with age) [11–13]. Some evidence supports the inclusion of cognitive performance, just short of dementia, to improve the predictive validity of the phenotypic approach [14, 15].

Among people who criticize the frailty phenotype for including *too many* items, there is recent evidence to support the primacy of slow mobility among the five potential markers of frailty [16]. On the other hand, gait speed correlates only modestly with adverse health outcomes [17]. Moreover, a frailty definition based on only three items ((1) weight loss, (2) inability to rise from a chair, and (3) low energy) has been tested against the five-item phenotypic definition and found to perform comparably with respect to risk classification [18, 19]. It is also established that obese people can be frail, even if they have not had weight loss [20].

Many authors hold that any operational definition of frailty should not include disability [21–23], although it is recognized empirically that the large majority of disabled older adults will be frail in the sense of either meeting the frailty phenotype [24] or in having an increased risk of adverse health outcomes [25]. Short of that, phenotypes other than the classic five-item phenotype are studied [18, 19, 26–28].

The frailty index

A contrasting view of frailty more broadly considers the items that could be counted to define someone as frail [6, 29]. Typically, a large number of items (40 or more) are counted and combined in a so-called frailty index [30]. The only restriction on the items is that they should count as health deficits (i.e., be associated with adverse health outcomes), and increase in prevalence with age, at least into the ninth decade. For an individual, their frailty index score is the number of deficits that they have, divided by the total number of deficits considered (e.g., a person with 10 deficits out of 40 considered would have a frailty index score of $10/40 = 0.25$). The frailty index shows many consistent properties, independent of its make up. Various frailty indexes have been constructed with as few as 31 items to as many as 100, including many ADLs or none, or using self-reported data or observer assessed/test/clinic data. Notwithstanding this variability in how the frailty index is constructed, in Western community-dwelling samples, the index generally increases at about 0.03 points per year, is highly correlated with mortality, and shows a characteristic pattern of change that can be modeled stochastically with the output conforming to a Poisson distribution [29]. There appears to be a limit to frailty, i.e., a proportion of deficits beyond which survival is not possible. That limit is at a frailty index value of approximately 0.7 [31–35]. Whether that limit can be used to guide decisions about a patient's suitability for an elective procedure or therapeutic regimen has not been established yet.

The frailty index has been criticized as being too labor intensive for clinical use compared with the five-item frailty phenotype [36]. Although the few head-to-head comparisons of the value of the frailty index versus the frailty phenotype in predicting vulnerability to adverse outcomes appear to favor the former [34, 37, 38], more widespread testing within clinical settings is required.

As with the frailty phenotype, there is no uniformity of the frailty index yet. Some reports employ simple three- or five-item frailty indexes. These simpler indexes have ceiling effects and therefore, do not allow the potential property of a limit to be tested, nor can they show the same relationship with age as the more complex indexes [18, 19].

Between the operational propositions of frailty, as three or five carefully defined "phenotypic" items and a frailty index that takes 30 or more items into account, are a large number of scales that classify risk based on ten or more items [39–41]. Nevertheless, scales that include age (however well they might characterize risk) [42–44] should be excluded as measures of frailty because frailty refers to differential susceptibility to adverse outcomes among people of the same age.

The frailty state is clearly dynamic, and while people can improve, the greater tendency is for frailty to worsen over time, especially as adverse outcomes accumulate [45, 46]. The dynamics of frailty further complicates clinical decision-making.

Clinical bottom line

Frailty can be thought of in terms of a phenotype or as an index. The frailty phenotype specifies five characteristics: (1) slowness, (2) weight loss, (3) impaired strength, (4) exhaustion, and (5) low physical activity/ energy expenditure. For a frailty index, typically a large number of items (40 or more) are counted and combined into a score. An individual's frailty index score is the number of deficits that they have divided by the total number of deficits considered.

Is this person frail?

The quickest answer to the question "Is this person frail?" is the response "What do you mean by frail?" The evidence suggests that a person will be susceptible to adverse outcomes if they conform to the frailty phenotype of slow, weak, thin, and exhausted, with reduced physical activity, especially if they have all five of these characteristics. Equally, a person will be frail if they have many things wrong with them, with a frailty index score of about 0.25 or higher. In both cases, the likelihood of susceptibility to adverse outcomes is empirically the case in presence of functional disability, and worsens as the extent of disability increases.

The fewest things that a person can have wrong with them, and be considered frail has not been established yet. The leading candidate appears to be motor-slowing in the absence of a single specific lesion to cause it [16], although risk can be classified without considering motor slowing [18, 19]. Notably, low handgrip strength more than measures frailty or function predicted risk of treatment toxicity from cancer chemotherapy [47]. Low mood, or at the very least poor self-rated health, also seem to be important in defining frailty among people who otherwise might meet more restrictive criteria [28, 48]. Although people who have dementia will meet many frailty criteria, it is not evident that their risk is better understood by also calling them frail, as compared with staging their dementia [49, 50].

Clinical bottom line

A person will be susceptible to adverse outcomes if they conform to the frailty phenotype. Equally, a person will be frail if they have a frailty index score of 0.25 or higher. In both cases, the likelihood of susceptibility to adverse outcomes is related to the presence of functional disability, with the greater the extent of disability, the higher the susceptibility.

What are ADLs?

Functional assessment allows goal setting and provides important information for measuring progress and estimating prognosis. Assessment of ADLs forms the cornerstone of functional assessment in older adults, because it offers a broad view of the impact of disability and disease on the patient and caregiver [51]. ADLs can be divided into two levels (Table 1.2): (1) Basic Activities of Daily Living (BADLs) refer to the tasks of self-maintenance (dressing, bathing, toileting, feeding, management of continence, and ability to transfer from a bed to chair and back), while (2) Instrumental Activities of Daily Living (IADLs) refer to those activities that foster independence in the community (managing finances and medications, shopping, housekeeping, meal preparation, and transportation). Impaired function is highly associated with but distinguishable from so-called geriatric conditions, such as dizziness and somatosensory impairment, with which it can exist in the absence of disabling chronic illness [52].

How do I assess ADLs?

Functional assessment generally relies on self-reported questionnaire, informant-based questionnaire, or direct observation. Self-reported questionnaires are of limited utility in dementia where insight is commonly affected, while direct observation scales are time consuming. Therefore, informant-based or team-assessed questionnaires are most often used in the assessment of function (Table 1.3). One assessment seldom fits

Table 1.2 Basic and instrumental activities of daily living

Basic Activities of Daily Living (BADL)	Instrumental Activities of Daily Living (IADL)
Feeding: Ability to consume food safely and with reasonable hygiene, including the ability to use utensils appropriately	Banking: Ability to carry out personal transactions and keep track of income and bills
Bathing: Ability to initiate and complete personal bathing, with or without the use of assistive aids	Transportation: Driving
Dressing: Ability to choose and don appropriate clothing	Cooking: Ability to prepare nutritionally appropriate meals
Toileting: Ability to initiate and complete mechanics of toileting with proper hygiene and manage any incontinence of bowel or bladder	Cleaning: Ability to maintain acceptable standard of cleanliness in own home.
Ambulation: Ability to transport with or without use of assistive aids including the ability to transfer self	Managing medications
	Shopping: Ability to select appropriate household needs

all, therefore, a variety of functional assessment tools have evolved and have been adapted for use in specific patient populations.

Functional assessment in people with dementia

Functional assessment is central to the evaluation of cognitive impairment. Functional decline is a core feature of all dementias (DSM-IV), is widely used as an outcome for treatment in dementia drug trials, and is an important prognostic marker for caregiver burden and institutionalization [53]. Consensus is lacking on how broad the functional assessment should be, and how to distinguish cognitive from noncognitive causes of functional impairment [54].

Functional assessment tools commonly used in dementia

Several functional assessment tools have been validated in Alzheimer dementia. The Lawton Brody Physical Self-Maintenance Scale (PSMS) and Activities of Daily Living Scale (IADL) are two subscales that assess BADLs and IADLs respectively, with descriptors for each domain that range from independence to complete dependence with resistive behaviors [55]. The subscales were originally validated together, but are often used separately in clinical practice. The subscales have several limitations. First, although the descriptors of function in each domain reflect degrees of functional impairment seen in dementia, neither scale allows the user to distinguish noncognitive reasons for the impairment. Further, although the source of information provided has been shown to have a significant effect on the overall score [56], neither scale stipulates standards for the source of information.

The Lawton Brody IADL scale does not take into consideration the tasks that were not performed by the individual at baseline (traditionally women were scored on all eight areas of IADL function; while food preparation, housekeeping, and laundering were excluded for men). Despite these limitations, the Lawton Brody IADL scale is the most commonly applied questionnaire for dementia patients[57].

The Lawton Brody PSMS subscale evaluates the same six domains of BADL as the Katz index of independence in ADLs [58]. While the PSMS is most often used in dementia, the Katz has been used in a wide variety of chronic illnesses. The Katz provides a dichotomous rating (dependent/independent) on a three-point scale of independence for BADL functions arranged in a hierarchical order (bathing being the highest). The PSMS includes a five-point rating scale for each of the same BADL domains. Two scoring methods have been described for the PSMS: one involves counting the number of items with any degree of impairment, while the other involves summing the severity score (1–5) of the impairment in each domain for an overall score of 6–30.

Functional assessment tools developed specifically for dementia

Most functional scales for dementia were developed for Alzheimer's disease, although some have been used in other cognitive syndromes such as Mild Cognitive

Table 1.3 Some commonly used, nondisease specific, disability assessment tools

Scale Name	Scoring	Items	Clinical Setting
Barthel Index	0 (complete dependence) to 100 (independence in all items) (higher score is better)	Ten items measuring bowel and bladder function, transfers, mobility, and stairs (15-item versions also available)	– Well suited to patients who may begin bed-bound and improve from there – Comparatively more detailed mobility information aids responsiveness in hospital setting – Both floor and ceiling effects are notable
Physical Self-Maintenance Scale (PSMS)	Items scored 1–4 or 1–5 (higher score is worse)	Basic activities of daily living (BADL) items	– Commonly used in clinical geriatric settings – Especially helpful in dementia
Lawton Brody Instrumental Activities of Daily Living (IADL) Scale	Items scored 1–4 or 1–5 (higher score is worse)	IADL items	– Commonly used in conjunction with the PSMS
Disability Assessment in Dementia (DAD)	Items scored one point each for initiation, planning and performance (higher score is better)	40 items including IADLs, BADLs and leisure activities	– Used to assess function in patients with dementia
Functional Independence Measure (FIM)	Items scored on a seven-point scale (total scores range from 18 to 126) (higher score is worse)	18 items (5 measure cognition; 13 measure motor performance)	– Widely used in rehabilitation settings

Impairment (MCI) or Vascular Cognitive Impairment (VCI). A more detailed review of functional assessment scales that are used in clinical trials for dementia is presented elsewhere [53].

A recent systematic review evaluated the measurement properties of IADL scales in dementia [57]. The authors compared the content validity, construct validity, criterion validity, internal consistency, reproducibility, responsiveness, floor and ceiling effects, and interpretability of 12 scales for assessing function using IADLs. The authors found that the validation studies for most scales did not include sufficient information through which to assess and compare measurement properties, and none of the 12 scales included information for all measurement properties. Based on the limited information available, the Disability Assessment for Dementia (DAD) and the Bristol ADL (a scale that assesses 20 ADLs in dementia [59]) scales received the best ratings, but further studies are required in order to make definitive recommendations about whether one scale is recommended for general use in dementia and the circumstances in which particular scales should be used (Level C evidence).

The DAD [60] was designed to assess treatment response and follow disease progression in community-dwelling patients with Alzheimer's dementia. The 40-item DAD includes IADLs, BADLs, and leisure activities and uses the characteristic hierarchical pattern of functional decline described in observational studies. The scale is unique in that it takes into account the proxy's perceived reason for the functional impairment, for example initiation, planning and organization, or ineffective performance. The DAD was developed and validated in English and French, and is not affected by age, education, or gender.

Function assessment in rehabilitation settings

In addition to providing information about progression, treatment response, and prognosis in dementia, functional assessment can be used in chronic disease and rehabilitation settings such as poststroke rehabilitation. Two commonly used scales include the Barthel Index and the Functional Independence Measure (FIM).

The Barthel Index [61] was originally developed as a ten-item ordinal scale, measuring function in the domains of ADLs, bowel and bladder function, transfers, mobility, and stairs. It has been modified to 15-item versions [62, 63], which includes domains of cognition, socialization, and vision/visual neglect. The Barthel index has demonstrated good reliability and validity and has been shown to predict care needs, length of stay, and mortality [64]. The scale is most often administered by clinical observation but has also been scored using self-report, which tends to result in higher scores in cases of cognitive impairment, acute illness, or older patients [65].

The FIM [66] is an 18-item ordinal scale (13 items measure motor function, while 5 items measure cognitive function) for measuring progress in rehabilitative programs. The scale is based on the Barthel Index. Each item is scored on a seven-point ordinal scale such that total scores range from 18 to 126, with higher scores denoting more functional independence. The FIM is proprietary (Uniform Data System for Medical Rehabilitation) and is used to report rehabilitation outcomes as part of large-scale data aggregation services.

Functional assessment in oncology

The majority of older cancer patients have some degree of frailty, functional impairment, and comorbid disease [67]. The interplay of these factors and the cancer may affect treatment tolerance and survival. A major challenge in the emerging field of geriatric oncology is determining the most appropriate treatment, with the best therapeutic ratio of survival/palliation and toxicity, taking into account the relative frailty of the individual. Scales to assess functional status have been developed for use in oncology, but these have not routinely taken frailty into account.

At present, the most consistent predictive clinical factor for treatment tolerance and survival is performance status (PS). PS is an ordinal scale that describes the overall functional limitations and severity of symptoms in relation to cancer. The two most commonly used scales for PS are the Karnofsky Performance Scale (KPS) [68, 69] and the Eastern Cooperative Oncology Group (ECOG) scale [70]. The KPS is an ordinal scale to describe global function. The score is reported in increments of 10 with total scores ranging from 0 to 100, a score of 100 being the best and a score of less than 50 denoting inability to perform self-care. The ECOG or Zubrod scale ranges from 0 to 4, with 0 indicating better function (corresponding to 90–100 on the KPS). Although the predictive validity for both scales has been consistently demonstrated, there is emerging evidence that a more comprehensive assessment, using tools such as the comprehensive geriatric assessment, and consideration of degree of frailty may help clinicians make better therapeutic decisions by providing insights into the interaction between aspects of fitness, frailty, and chemotherapeutic toxicity [71–73].

Clinical bottom line

There are a variety of functional assessment tools, all of which are designed to measure a patient's dependence in ADLs. The tool to be used depends on the purpose for collecting the information.

How can I prevent this frail older adult from declining in ADLs?

Prevention of functional decline in frail older adults is a priority area for research and public health, and the absence of disability has demonstrated consistent association with successful aging [74]. In 2004, the Interventions on Frailty Working Group published consensus recommendations on the design of randomized controlled trials for the prevention of functional decline and disability in frail older adults [75].

Systematic reviews addressing prevention of functional decline are limited and most are conducted on studies examining outcomes in particular patient settings.

Interventions for older hospital inpatients

Hospital admission is often a sentinel event in the natural history of frailty. Thirty to sixty percent of older adults develop new dependency in ADLs, following admission to hospital that can translate into increased mortality, prolonged hospital stay and readmission, poor quality of life, and need for institutionalization or increased care at home [76]. Factors influencing functional decline after hospital admission may be related to baseline health status or events that occur after admission [77].

An important component of any program designed to prevent functional decline is screening for those individuals at most risk. A recent systematic review found that older age, depressive symptoms, cognitive impairment, preadmission dependency in ADLs, and length of hospital stay were each predictive of functional decline following hospital admission [76].

The same review evaluated three screening instruments for postdischarge functional decline, the Hospital Admission Risk Profile (HARP) [78], the Identification of Seniors at Risk (ISAR) [79], and the Care Complexity Prediction Instrument (COMPRI) [80]. All three instruments have been tested in large populations, but their reliability, sensitivity, specificity, and predictive value were not described in the original studies, and they have not been compared with existing frailty measures. The specific items and outcome measures for each assessment tool varied, but components of successful assessments generally included the domains of comprehensive geriatric assessment (Level B evidence). A randomized controlled trial that evaluated the effectiveness of an intervention designed to reduce functional decline in frail hospitalized patients, screened using the ISAR, resulted in reduced rates of functional decline but no effect on satisfaction, caregiver health, or depressive symptoms [81] (Level C evidence).

A second systematic review [82] evaluating six studies of five screening instruments (including the HARP and the ISAR) for identifying those at a risk of functional decline, 3–6 months after presentation to the emergency department, found considerable overlap in the domains and items of assessment in the screening instruments. The Inouye screening tool [83] had the highest sensitivity (88%), but the lowest specificity (54%) of all five instruments. The SHERPA (Score Hospitalier d'Evaluation du Risque de Perte d'Autonomie) [84] was the most accurate tool (AUC 0.734), but it has not been prospectively validated. The utility of the ISAR was limited by its reliance on self-report, with many participants unable to complete the

screen independently. The Inouye tool was limited by the clinical expertise required to complete the items.

The most recent systematic review of screening tools for prediction of functional decline [85] is consistent with previous studies in its conclusion that further research is needed to overcome the lack of published data on reliability and validity of existing screening instruments in order to allow direct comparisons (Level C evidence).

Geriatric Evaluation and Management Units (GEMU) are specialized inpatient wards that provide multidisciplinary assessment, review, and therapy for frail older adults [86]. The GEMU model combines comprehensive geriatric assessment with management strategies including individualized care planning, rehabilitation, and discharge planning. A recent systematic review and meta-analysis [87] examined seven randomized controlled studies evaluating the effectiveness of the GEMU for mortality, institutionalization, length of stay, functional decline, and readmission. All studies used comprehensive geriatric assessment and multidisciplinary team models. GEMUs differed in their admission processes (direct admission from home or emergency department or transfer from another hospital unit), definition of frailty, and ambulatory follow-up. Meta-analysis showed significant reductions in institutionalization at 12 months (relative risk (RR) 0.78; 95% confidence interval (CI) 0.66–0.92) and functional decline at discharge (RR 0.87; 95% CI 0.77–0.99), with a trend toward a reduction in 12-month functional decline (RR 0.84; 95% CI 0.69–1.03) but no reduction in mortality, readmission, length of stay, or institutionalization at 3 or 6 months (Level C evidence). The small number of studies evaluated precluded analysis of which patient characteristics had the most favorable effect on outcomes.

Interventions for community-dwelling older adults

Multicomponent interventions designed to prevent functional decline in community-dwelling older adults may be useful for short-term prevention of some adverse outcomes (Level B evidence).

Beswick et al recently evaluated the effectiveness of community-based complex interventions designed to preserve physical function and independence in older adults [88]. Studies ($n = 89$) were analyzed according to type of intervention (geriatric assessment of older people, geriatric assessment of frail older adults, community based care after hospital discharge, fall prevention, education, and counseling) and the outcomes examined included hospital and nursing home admission, physical function, and falls. Geriatric assessment of elderly people without selection for frailty ($n = 28$) increased physical function (RR −0.12; 95% CI −0.16 to −0.08) and decreased nursing home admission (RR 0.86, 95% CI 0.83–0.90), and falls (RR 0.76; 95% CI 0.67–0.86). When applied to populations selected as frail ($n = 24$), geriatric assessment reduced the risk of hospital admission (RR 0.90; 95% CI 0.84–0.98) and improved physical function (RR −0.05; 95% CI −0.06 to −0.04). Interventions involving community-based care after discharge from hospital ($n = 21$) reduced the risk of nursing home admission (RR 0.77; 95% CI 0.64–0.91), but had no effect on hospital readmission. Interventions directed at fall prevention ($n = 13$) reduced the risk of falls (RR 0.92; 95% CI 0.87–0.97) and improved physical function (RR −0.25; 95% CI −0.36 to −0.13). This was the only intervention group that resulted in reduced mortality (RR 0.79; 95% CI 0.66–0.96). Interventions that focused on counseling and education ($n = 3$) increased the likelihood of improved physical function (RR −0.08; 95% CI −0.11 to −0.06).

A systematic review by Daniels et al [89] evaluated two nutritional interventions and eight physical exercise interventions designed to prevent disability in community-dwelling frail older adults. Nutritional interventions and single component physical exercise programs were not associated with reductions in disability. Three trials using multicomponent long lasting high intensity physical exercise programs were associated with reductions in disability, expressed as less difficulty with BADLs and IADLs, with effects persisting at 9 and 12 months in two of the three trials. Subgroup analysis suggests that those with severe frailty did not benefit from intervention as compared to those with mild or moderate frailty. These conclusions are congruent with a contemporary systematic review of physical exercise training in frail older adults [90].

Home visitation programs may provide an effective model by which to deliver multidisciplinary care for the prevention of functional decline in older adults (Level B evidence). A meta-analysis evaluating 18 randomized controlled trials of home-visit programs [91] found a reduction in nursing home admission (RR 0.66; 95% CI 0.48–0.92) in trials involving nine or more visits. Reductions in functional decline were noted in trials that used multidimensional assessment and follow-up (RR 0.76; 95% CI 0.64–0.91), and trials that were directed toward healthier populations (RR 0.78; 95% CI 0.64–0.95). A mortality benefit was evident in patients >77.5 years (RR 0.76; 95% CI 0.65–0.88).

Interventions for long-term care residents

Although most research has been focused on community-dwelling older adults living at home or during acute hospital admission, a recent systematic review examined the effectiveness of physical rehabilitation for frail adults in long-term care [92]. Forty-nine trials were identified, most of which involved 30 minutes of intervention (usually exercise) for 12 weeks. Residents with cognitive impairment were excluded from 34 of the studies. Twelve of the 49 studies assessed longer term outcomes. Nine studies showed functional improvements, while 34 studies showed reduction in activity restriction, most commonly related to improvement in walking (Level B evidence).

Clinical bottom line

Prevention of functional decline in frail older adults should be a priority for hospitals, long-term care facilities, and in the community. It is important to screen an older patient's risk for decline at the time of admission to hospital. Multicomponent preventative interventions appear to be of variable effectiveness

Chapter summary

Frailty can be thought of in terms of a phenotype or as an index. The frailty phenotype specifies five characteristics: (1) slowness, (2) weight loss, (3) impaired strength, (4) exhaustion, and (5) low physical activity/ energy expenditure. For a frailty index, typically a large number of items (40 or more) are counted and combined into a score. An individual's frailty index score is the number of deficits that they have, divided by the total number of deficits considered. A person will be susceptible to adverse outcomes if they conform to the frailty phenotype. Equally, a person will be frail if they have a frailty index score of 0.25 or higher. In both cases, the likelihood of susceptibility to adverse outcomes is related to the presence of functional disability, with the greater the extent of disability, the higher the susceptibility.

There is a variety of functional assessment tools designed to measure a patient's dependence in ADLs. Different tools may be appropriate in differing clinical settings, and can be used to assess prognosis, along with rehabilitation potential and progress.

Prevention of functional decline in frail older adults should be a priority for hospitals, long-term care facilities, and in the community. It is important to screen an older patient's risk for decline at the time of admission to hospital. Multicomponent preventative interventions appear to be of variable effectiveness.

References

1. Gordon J, Powell C, Rockwood K (2000) Current awareness in geriatric psychiatry. *Int J Geriatr Psychiatry* 15: 669–676.
2. Isaacs B (1992) *The Challenge of Geriatric Medicine*. Oxford: Oxford University Press.
3. Karunananthan S, Wolfson C, Bergman H, Béland F, Hogan DB (2009) A multidisciplinary systematic literature review on frailty: overview of the methodology used by the Canadian Initiative on Frailty and Aging. *BMC Med Res Methodol* 9: 68.
4. Fried LP, Tangen CM, Walston J, Newman AB, Hirsch C, Gottdiener J, Seeman T, Tracy R, Kop WJ, Burke G, McBurnie MA (2001) Frailty in older adults: evidence for a phenotype. *J Gerontol A Biol Sci Med Sci* 56(3): M134–M135.
5. Rockwood K, Fox RA, Stolee P, Robertson D, Beattie BL (1994) Frailty in elderly people: an evolving concept. *CMAJ* 150(4): 489–495.
6. Mitnitski AB, Mogilner AJ, Rockwood K (2001) Accumulation of deficits as a proxy measure of aging. *ScientificWorldJournal* 1: 323–336.
7. Hubbard RE, O'Mahony MS, Savva GM, Calver BL, Woodhouse KW (2009a) Inflammation and frailty measures in older people. *J Cell Mol Med* 13(9B): 3103–3109.
8. Chaves PH, Semba RD, Leng SX, Woodman RC, Ferrucci L, Guralnik JM, Fried LP (2005) Impact of anemia and cardiovascular disease on frailty status of community-dwelling older women: the Women's Health and Aging Studies I and II. *J Gerontol A Biol Sci Med Sci* 60(6): 729–735.
9. Travison TG, Shackelton R, Araujo AB, Morley JE, Williams RE, Clark RV, McKinlay JB (2010) Frailty, serum androgens, and the CAG repeat polymorphism: results from the Massachusetts Male Aging Study. *J Clin Endocrinol Metab* 95: 2746–2754.
10. Whitson HE, Purser JL, Cohen HJ (2007) Frailty they name is . . . phrailty? *J Gerontol A Biol Sci Med Sci* 62(7): 728–730.
11. Bergman H, Ferrucci L, Guralnik J, Hogan DB, Hummel S, Karunananthan S, Wolfson C (2007) Frailty: an emerging research and clinical paradigm–issues and controversies. *J Gerontol A Biol Sci Med Sci* 62(7): 731–737.
12. Abellan van Kan G, Rolland Y, Bergman H, Morley JE, Kritchevsky SB, Vellas B (2008) The I.A.N.A Task Force on frailty assessment of older people in clinical practice. *J Nutr Health Aging* 12(1): 29–37.
13. Lang PO, Michel JP, Zekry D (2009) Frailty syndrome: a transitional state in a dynamic process. *Gerontology* 55(5): 539–549.
14. Sarkisian CA, Gruenewald TL, John Boscardin W, Seeman TE (2008) Preliminary evidence for subdimensions of geriatric frailty: the MacArthur study of successful aging. *J Am Geriatr Soc* 56(12): 2292–2297.
15. Avila-Funes JA, Amieva H, Barberger-Gateau P, Le Goff M, Raoux N, Ritchie K, Carrière I, Tavernier B, Tzourio C, Gutiérrez-Robledo LM, Dartigues JF (2009) Cognitive impairment improves the predictive validity of the phenotype of frailty for adverse health outcomes: the three-city study. *J Am Geriatr Soc* 57(3): 453–461.
16. Rothman MD, Leo-Summers L, Gill TM (2008) Prognostic significance of potential frailty criteria. *J Am Geriatr Soc* 56(12): 2211–2116.
17. Tiedemann A, Shimada H, Sherrington C, Murray S, Lord S (2008) The comparative ability of eight functional mobility tests for predicting falls in community-dwelling older people. *Age Ageing* 37(4): 430–435.
18. Ensrud KE, et al (2008) Comparison of 2 frailty indexes for prediction of falls, disability, fractures, and death in older women. *Arch Intern Med* 168(4): 382–389.
19. Ensrud KE, et al (2009) A comparison of frailty indexes for the prediction of falls, disability, fractures, and mortality in older men. *J Am Geriatr Soc* 57(3): 492–498.
20. Blaum CS, Xue QL, Michelon E, Semba RD, Fried LP (2005) The association between obesity and the frailty syndrome in older women: the Women's Health and Aging Studies. *J Am Geriatr Soc* 53(6): 927–934.
21. Fried LP, Ferrucci L, Darer J, Williamson JD, Anderson G (2004) Untangling the concepts of disability, frailty, and comorbidity: implications for improved targeting and care. *J Gerontol Med Sco* 59A: 255–263.
22. Abellan van Kan G, Rolland Y, Houles M, Gillette-Guyonnet S, Soto M, Vellas B (2010) The assessment of frailty in older adults. *Clin Geriatr Med* 26(2): 275–286.
23. Inouye SK, Studenski S, Tinetti ME, Kuchel GA (2007) Geriatric syndromes: clinical, research, and policy implications of a core geriatric concept. *J Am Geriatr Soc* 55(5): 780–791.
24. Wong CH, Weiss D, Sourial N, Karunananthan S, Quail JM, Wolfson C, Bergman H (2010) Frailty and its association with disability and comorbidity in a community-dwelling sample of seniors in Montreal: a cross-sectional study. *Aging Clin Exp Res* 22: 54–62.
25. Rockwood K, Song X, MacKnight C, Bergman H, Hogan D, McDowell I, Mitnitski A (2005) A Global clinical measure of fitness and frailty in elderly people. *Canadian Medical Association Journal* 175: 488–495.
26. Passarino G, et al (2007) A cluster analysis to define human aging phenotypes. *Biogerontology* 8(3): 283–290.
27. Sarkisian CA, Gruenewald TL, John Boscardin W, Seeman TE (2008) Preliminary evidence for subdimenstions of

geriatric frailty: the MacArthur study of successful aging. *J Am Geriatr Soc* 56(12): 2292–2297.

28. Hyde Z, et al (2011) Low free testosterone predicts mortality from cardiovascular disease but not other causes: The Health in Men Study. *J Clin Endocrinol Metab* [Epub ahead of print]

29. Rockwood K, and Mitnitksi A (2007) Frailty in relation to the accumulation of deficits: a review. *J Gerontol: Med Sci* 62A: 722–727.

30. Searle SD, Mitnitski A, Gahbauer EA, Gill TM, Rockwood K (2008) A standard procedure for creating a frailty index. *BMC Geriatr* 8: 24.

31. Rockwood K, Mitnitski A (2006) Limits to deficit accumulation in elderly people. *Mech Ageing Dev* 127(5): 494–496.

32. Jones DM, Song X, Rockwood K (2004) Operationalizing a frailty index from a standardized comprehensive geriatric assessment. *J Am Geriatr Soc* 52(11): 1929–1933.

33. Rockwood K, Rockwood MR, Andrew MK, Mitnitski A (2008) Reliability of the hierarchical assessment of balance and mobility in frail older adults. *J Am Geriatr Soc* 56(7): 1213–1217.

34. Hubbard RE, O'Mahony MS, Woodhouse KW (2009b) Characterising frailty in the clinical setting–a comparison of different approaches. *Age Ageing* 38(1): 115–119.

35. Rockwood K, Rockwood MR, Mitnitski A (2010) Physiological redundancy in older adults in relation to the change with age in the slope of a frailty index. *J Am Geriatr Soc* 58(2): 318–323.

36. Martin FC, Brighton P (2008) Frailty: different tools for different purposes? *Age Ageing* 37(2): 129–131.

37. Rockwood K, Andrew M, Mitnitski A (2007) A comparison of two approaches to measuring frailty in elderly people. *J Gerontol A Biol Sci Med Sci* 62(7): 738–743.

38. Kulminski AM, Ukraintseva SV, Kulminskaya IV, Arbeev KG, Land K, Yashin AI (2008) Cumulative deficits better characterize susceptibility to death in elderly people than phenotypic frailty: lessons from the cardiovascular health study. *J Am Geriatr Soc* 56(5): 898–903.

39. Rolfson DB, Majumdar SR, Tsuyuki RT, Tahir A, Rockwood K (2006) Validity and reliability of the edmonton frail scale. *Age Ageing* 35(5): 526–529.

40. Hilmer SN, et al (2009) The assessment of frailty in older people in acute care. *Australas J Ageing* 28(4): 182–188.

41. Andela RM, Dijkstra A, Slaets JP, Sanderman R (2010) Prevalence of frailty on clinical wards: description and implications. *Int J Nurs Pract* 16(1): 14–19.

42. Lee SJ, Lindquist K, Segal MR, Covinsky KE (2006) Development and validation of a prognostic index for 4-year mortality in older adults. *JAMA* 295(7): 801–808. Erratum in: *JAMA* 2006; 295(16): 1900.

43. Ravaglia G, Forti P, Lucicesare A, Pisacane N, Rietti E, Patterson C (2008) Development of an easy prognostic score for frailty outcomes in the aged. *Age Ageing* 37(2): 161–166.

44. Pijpers E, Ferreira I, van de Laar RJ, Stehouwer CD, Nieuwenhuijzen Kruseman AC (2009) Predicting mortality of psychogeriatric patients: a simple prognostic frailty risk score. *Postgrad Med J* 85(1007): 464–469.

45. Mitnitski A, Bao L, Rockwood K (2006) Going from bad to worse: a stochastic model of transitions in deficit accumulation, in relation to mortality. *Mech Ageing Dev* 127(5): 490–493.

46. Gill TM, Gahbauer EA, Han L, Allore HG (2010) Trajectories of disability in the last year of life. *N Engl J Med* 362: 1173–1180.

47. Puts MT, et al (2011) Are frailty markers useful for predicting treatment toxicity and mortality in older newly diagnosed cancer patients? Results from a prospective pilot study. *Crit Rev Oncol Hematol* 78: 138–149.

48. Lucicesare A, et al (2010) Comparison of two frailty measures in the Conselice Study of Brain Ageing. *J Nutr Health Aging* 14: 278–281.

49. Reisberg B (1988) Functional assessment staging (FAST). *Psychopharmacol Bull* 24: 653–659.

50. Morris JC (1997) Clinical assessment of Alzheimer's disease. *Neurology* 49(3 Suppl 3): S7–S10.

51. World Health Organization (1980) *International Classification of Impairments, Disabilities and Handicaps*. Geneva: WHO.

52. Cigolle CT, Langa KM, Kabeto MU, Tian Z, Blaum CS (2007) Geriatric conditions and disability: the Health and Retirement Study. *Ann Intern Med* 147(3): 156–164.

53. Massoud F (2007) The role of functional assessment as an outcome measure in antidementia treatment. *Can J Neurol Sci* 34(Suppl 1): S47–S51.

54. Rockwood K (2007) The measuring, meaning and importance of activities of daily living (ADLs) as an outcome. *Int Psychogeriatr* 19: 467–482.

55. Lawton MP, Brody EM (1969) Assessment of older people: self-maintaining and instrumental activities of daily living. *Gerontologist* 9: 179–186.

56. Rubenstein LZ, Schairer C, Wieland GD, Kane R (1984) Systematic biases in functional status assessment of elderly adults: effects of different data sources. *J Gerontol* 39: 686–691.

57. Sikkes SA, de Lange-de Klerk ES, Pijnenburg YA, Scheltens P, Uitdehaag BM (2009) A systematic review of Instrumental Activities of Daily Living scales in dementia: room for improvement. *J Neurol Neurosurg Psychiatry* 80: 7–12.

58. Katz S, Ford AB, Moskowitz RW, Jackson BA, Jaffe MW (1963) Studies of illness in the aged. the index of ADL: a standardized measure of biological and psychosocial function. *JAMA* 185: 914–919.

59. Bucks RS, Ashworth DI, Wilcock GK (1996) Assessment of activities of daily living in dementia: development of the Bristol Activities of Daily Living scales. *Age Ageing* 25: 113–120

60. Gélinas I, Gauthier L, McIntyre M, Gauthier S (1999) Development of a functional measure for persons with Alzheimer's disease: the disability assessment for dementia. *Am J Occup Ther* 53: 471–481.

61. Mahoney FI, Barthel DW (1965) Functional evaluation: the Barthel Index. *Maryland State Medical Journal* 14–62.

62. Granger CV, Dewis LS, Peters NC, Sherwood CC, Barrett JE (1979) Stroke rehabilitation: analysis of repeated Barthel Index measures. *Arch Phys Med Rehabil* 60: 14–17.

63. Fortinsky RH, Granger CV, Seltzer GB (1981) The use of functional assessment in understanding home care needs. *Med Care* 19: 489–497.

64. Wylie CM, White BK (1964) A measure of disability. *Arch Eviron Health* 8: 834–839.

65. Sinoff G, Ore L (1997) The Barthel activities of daily living index: self-reporting versus actual performance in the old-old (> or = 75 years). *J Am Geriatr Soc* 45: 832–836.

66. Keith RA, Granger CV, Hamilton BB, Sherwin FS (1987) The functional independence measure: a new tool for rehabilitation. *Adv Clin Rehabil* 1: 6–18.

67. Stafford RS, Cyr PL (1997) The impact of cancer on the physical function of the elderly and their utilization of health care. *Cancer* 80: 1973–1980.

68. Karnofsky DA, Abelmann WH, Craver LF, Burchenal JH (1948) The use of nitrogen mustards in the palliative treatment of cancer. *Cancer* 1: 634–656.

69. Schag CC, Heinrich RL, Ganz PA (1984) Karnofsky performance status revisited: reliability, validity, and guidelines. *J Clin Oncol* 2: 187–193.

70. Zubrod CG, Schneiderman M, Frei E (1960) Appraisal of methods for the study of chemotherapy of cancer in man: comparative therapeutic trial of nitrogen mustard and thriethylene thiophosphoramide. *J Chron Dis* 11: 7–33.

71. Extermann M (2005) Geriatric assessment with focus on instrument selectivity for outcomes. *Cancer J* 11: 474–480.

72. Extermann M, Hurria A (2007) Comprehensive geriatric assessment for older patients with cancer. *J Clin Oncol* 25: 1824–1831.

73. Repetto L, et al (2002) Comprehensive geriatric assessment adds information to Eastern Cooperative Oncology Group performance status in elderly cancer patients: an Italian Group for Geriatric Oncology Study. *J Clin Oncol* 20: 494–502.

74. Depp CA, Jeste DV (2006) Definitions and predictors of successful aging: a comprehensive review of larger quantitative studies. *Am J Geriatr Psychiatry* 14: 6–20.

75. Ferrucci L, Guralnik JM, Studenski S, Fried LP, Cutler GBJ, Walston JD (2004) Designing randomized, controlled trials aimed at preventing or delaying functional decline and disability in frail, older persons: a consensus report. *J Am Geriatr Soc* 52: 625–634.

76. Hoogerduijn JG, Schuurmans MJ, Duijnstee MS, de Rooij SE, Grypdonck MF (2007) A systematic review of predictors and screening instruments to identify older hospitalized patients at risk for functional decline. *J Clin Nurs* 16: 46–57.

77. Gillick MR, Serrell NA, Gillick LS (1982) Adverse consequences of hospitalization in the elderly. *Soc Sci Med* 16: 1033–1038.

78. Sager MA, et al (1996) Hospital admission risk profile (HARP): identifying older patients at risk for functional decline following acute medical illness and hospitalization. *J Am Geriatr Soc* 44: 251–257.

79. McCusker J, Bellavance F, Cardin S, Trepanier S, Verdon J, Ardman O (1999) Detection of older people at increased risk of adverse health outcomes after an emergency visit: the ISAR screening tool. *J Am Geriatr Soc* 47: 1229–1237.

80. Huyse FJ, et al (2001) COMPRI–an instrument to detect patients with complex care needs: results from a European study. *Psychosomatics* 42: 222–228.

81. McCusker J, Verdon J, Tousignant P, de Courval LP, Dendukuri N, Belzile E (2001) Rapid emergency department intervention for older people reduces risk of functional decline: results of a multicenter randomized trial. *J Am Geriatr Soc* 49: 1272–1281.

82. Sutton M, Grimmer-Somers K, Jeffries L (2008) Screening tools to identify hospitalised elderly patients at risk of functional decline: a systematic review. *Int J Clin Pract* 62: 1900–1909.

83. Inouye SK, et al (1993) A predictive index for functional decline in hospitalized elderly medical patients. *J Gen Intern Med* 8: 645–652.

84. Cornette P, Swine C, Malhomme B, Gillet JB, Meert P, D'Hoore W (2006) Early evaluation of the risk of functional decline following hospitalization of older patients: development of a predictive tool. *Eur J Public Health* 16: 203–208.

85. De Saint-Hubert M, Schoevaerdts D, Cornette P, D'Hoore W, Boland B, Swine C (2010) Predicting functional adverse outcomes in hospitalized older patients: a systematic review of screening tools. *J Nutr Health Aging* 14: 394–399.

86. Ellis G, Langhorne P (2004) Comprehensive geriatric assessment for older hospital patients. *Br Med Bull* 71: 45–59.

87. Van Craen K, et al (2010) The effectiveness of inpatient geriatric evaluation and management units: a systematic review and meta-analysis. *J Am Geriatr Soc* 58: 83–92.

88. Beswick AD, et al (2008) Complex interventions to improve physical function and maintain independent living in elderly people: a systematic review and meta-analysis. *Lancet* 371: 725–735.

89. Daniels R, van Rossum E, de Witte L, Kempen GI, van den Heuvel W (2008) Interventions to prevent disability in frail community-dwelling elderly: a systematic review. *BMC Health Serv Res* 8: 278.

90. Chin APMJ, van Uffelen JG, Riphagen I, van Mechelen W (2008) The functional effects of physical exercise training in frail older people : a systematic review. *Sports Med* 38: 781–793.

91. Stuck AE, Egger M, Hammer A, Minder CE, Beck JC (2002) Home visits to prevent nursing home admission and functional decline in elderly people: systematic review and meta-regression analysis. *JAMA* 287: 1022–1028.

92. Forster A, Lambley R, Young JB (2010) Is physical rehabilitation for older people in long-term care effective? Findings from a systematic review. *Age Ageing* 39: 169–175.

CHAPTER 2

Computer-based clinical decision support systems in the care of older patients

Marina Martin[1,2] & Mary K. Goldstein[2,3]
[1]*Department of General Internal Medicine, Stanford University School of Medicine, Stanford, CA, USA*
[2]*Center for Primary Care Outcomes Research, Stanford University, Stanford, CA, USA*
[3]*Geriatrics Research Education and Clinical Center (GRECC), VA Palo Alto Health Care System, Palo Alto, CA, USA*

Introduction

Providing quality care to older adults is complex [1, 2]. Many older patients have multiple comorbid conditions, long lists of medications, frequent encounters with a variety of healthcare professionals, and extensive test result data [1]. They may also receive care in a variety of clinical settings, from outpatient clinics to emergency rooms, inpatient hospital units, and long-term care facilities [1]. Consolidating and accessing these patients' health information is made easier by electronic health records (EHR) [1], but utilizing these data in effective ways for individual medical decision-making remains an important challenge [3]. It can be especially challenging to incorporate all of the special clinical recommendations for older patients into decision-making, including guidelines for drug choice and dosing, or screening for and management of "geriatric syndromes," for example, urinary incontinence and falls [2].

Computer-based clinical decision support (CDS) can be defined as, "the use of the computer to bring relevant knowledge to bear on the health care and well being of a patient" [4]. CDS systems include tools such as clinical reminders or alerts, order sets tailored to conditions, or templates that support the healthcare provider in making appropriate clinical decisions for the individual patient, [3] as well as more elaborate systems that encode clinical guidelines into computer-interpretable formats. Many CDS tools have been incorporated into computerized physician order entry (CPOE) within EHRs, for example, drug allergy alerts or drug interaction warnings [5]. CDS tools integrated into EHRs can process an individual's health information, including age, diagnoses, drug allergies, and medication lists, to generate personalized recommendations to the provider.

Studies of CDS tools to improve dosage selection when prescribing [6] and to remind providers to perform tests or procedures [7] have been systematically reviewed. These reviews concluded that there is at least a modest benefit of CDS use in increasing provider adherence to recommended clinical processes [7] and in improving some clinical outcomes, such as reducing rates of toxic drug levels and decreasing length of hospital stay [6]. However, CDS has been implemented in a relatively small number of institutions with well-established EHRs, and there remains a great deal of work ahead to bring both full EHRs and CDS tools into widespread use [3, 8]. CDS systems hold great potential for improving quality of care and optimizing the benefits of EHRs, and clinicians will increasingly be exposed to these tools as EHRs develop and spread [1, 3]. The components of an effective CDS tool include [9]:

1 Automatic provision of CDS as part of clinician workflow

2 Provision of recommendations rather than just assessments

Evidence-Based Geriatric Medicine: A Practical Clinical Guide, First Edition. Edited by Jayna M. Holroyd-Leduc and Madhuri Reddy.
© 2012 Blackwell Publishing Ltd. Published 2012 by Blackwell Publishing Ltd.

3 Provision of CDS at the time and location of decision-making

4 Computer-based CDS

Because geriatric care can require adjustments to the conventional clinical practice used in adults, and not all providers may be cognizant of best clinical practices for geriatric patients, CDS holds special promise for improving care of older patients. The purpose of this chapter is to systematically review the literature investigating the effects of computerized CDS use on processes and outcomes of care in older patients, focusing specifically on CDS for (1) improving prescribing practices for the older patient, and (2) improving management of hypertension, which is diagnosed in approximately 65% of adults ≥60 years old [10].

Search strategy

We employed a systematic literature search and selection process in order to identify the available articles investigating the effects of computerized CDS tools, on processes and outcomes of care in the two areas of focus: (1) medication prescribing and (2) hypertension.

The articles were then reviewed for quality according to the criteria developed by the Oxford Centre for Evidence-Based Medicine (CEBM) and the data abstracted and analyzed. It is generally not possible to blind providers in trials of CDS interventions, and often difficult to blind the patients to CDS use during a clinical encounter. Therefore, to differentiate higher from lower quality randomized controlled trials (RCTs) of CDS, we determined whether (1) the units of study were truly randomized, (2) allocation was concealed from the research team, and (3) the unit of analysis was the same as the unit of allocation/randomization, or adjustment was made in the analysis for clustering. Trials that met all three of these quality criteria were given the highest evidence ratings.

Relevant articles were obtained by searching PubMed, Scopus (which includes the Cochrane Database), and ISI Web of Science for the period 1990 to May 1, 2010, chosen to include the years in which wider use of EHRs emerged. Multiple searches were conducted, beginning with the Medical Subject Heading (MeSH) term "Decision Support Systems, Clinical" alone as the major topic in PubMed, limited to English-language articles and ages 19+ years. Further searches

paired "Decision Support Systems, Clinical" with the MeSH terms "Aged" or "Medication Errors" or "Disease Management" or "Medication Therapy Management" or "Nursing Homes" or "Hypertension." Further studies were identified by citation tracking from collected articles. Initial searches found 325 citations, of which 10 met inclusion criteria for CDS trials of medication prescribing in older patients, and 4 met inclusion criteria for CDS trials in hypertension management.

Studies were included in the review if they were a clinical trial or pre- and postintervention study of a computerized EHR- or CPOE-based CDS tool to improve care in the two categories of interest: (1) medication prescribing in older patients and (2) hypertension management. To maximize the number of included studies while retaining applicability to geriatric populations, studies of medication prescribing were included only if the patients studied were ≥65 years old, but studies of hypertension were included for adult patients of any age. To be included, the study had to present data for either performance of a clinical process or change in a clinical outcome targeted by the CDS. Studies of CDS for diagnostic purposes, studies of computerized interventions tailored to patients or caregivers instead of providers, and studies of system usability/design features were excluded.

Do CDS tools improve healthcare providers' performance of tasks or clinical outcomes related to appropriate medication prescribing for older patients?

A large proportion of computerized CDS systems target improved prescribing behavior. This is to be expected, with rapid increases in medical knowledge and number of available medications to prescribe in recent years, and the increasingly common use of CPOE systems and EHRs [6, 11–15]. Adverse drug events (ADEs) are very common in medical practice, and while not all are preventable, one study estimated that 28% of ADEs are due to medication prescribing errors and that 56% of these errors occurred at the time of ordering [16]. Therefore, CDS integrated into CPOE has been particularly emphasized and well studied [6, 11–15].

A systematic review of controlled trials investigating the impact of CDS on dosing of medications with narrow therapeutic window, such as warfarin, found some benefits in increasing initial doses and serum drug concentrations, reducing time to therapeutic stabilization, reducing toxic drug levels, and shortening length of hospital stay, but no decrease in ADEs (Level 1a evidence) [6]. Systematic reviews of studies specifically investigating ADEs in general populations have found mixed results, with half or fewer of reviewed studies finding benefits for CDS interventions (Level 1a evidence) [12, 15].

Despite relatively modest success in general populations, computerized CDS may be more likely to show benefit toward appropriate prescribing in geriatric subpopulations [17]. Appropriate use of medications in care of older patients is made particularly complicated by multiple comorbidities, polypharmacy, altered pharmacology with aging and disease, and increased frequency of adverse reactions with age [18]. ADEs are common in geriatric populations, affecting approximately one-third of the ambulatory older population in a 1-year period [19], and potentially causing hospitalization, falls, hip fractures, constipation, depression, and altered mental status in these patients [18]. To help decrease rates of ADEs in older patients, the Beers Criteria were developed in the 1990s by an expert consensus panel to identify medications likely to be ineffective or cause ADEs in any older patient, as well as medications contraindicated in those with specific medical conditions [18].

The Beers Criteria [18, 20, 21] and similar guidelines have subsequently formed the clinical basis for a number of CDS tools, while others have been developed around geriatric pharmacology recommendations of expert panels at the study site. These criteria have not been universally accepted or endorsed, and might vary somewhat from one CDS tool to another. A systematic review of studies published between 1980 and July, 2007 investigating CDS to improve medication prescribing in older patients found that eight out of ten reviewed studies showed at least modest improvement in prescribing (Level 1a evidence) [17]. The majority of these studies, excluding the ones that did not meet inclusion criteria for this review, are discussed later and in Table 2.1. Several more recently published studies are also reviewed.

All trials reviewed here investigating computerized CDS to improve medication prescribing in the older patient have shown some benefit of the intervention in at least one of the study outcomes (Table 2.1) [22–31]. These studies were performed in a variety of settings, including inpatient academic medical centers [22, 25, 26], outpatient primary care clinics of various affiliations [23, 27, 28, 30, 31], long-term care [24], and the emergency department [29]. Most of the CDS interventions studied sought to reduce prescription of psychoactive medications, particularly long-acting benzodiazepines and tertiary amine tricyclic antidepressants, which are not recommended for use in older patients according to the Beers Criteria [18, 20, 21].

Most studies measured provider behavior, but two studies looked at patient outcomes. One investigated the impact of a CDS system on psychoactive medication prescriptions in older inpatients, and found decreased falls but no impact of hospital length of stay or rates of altered mental status [25]. The second investigated a CDS system to reduce polypharmacy in older patients on at least four medications with at least one psychoactive medication, who were considered at high risk for falls [30]. This intervention resulted in a decrease in medical encounters for falls, but not in total falls as measured by medical encounters and patient self-report.

Clinical bottom line

Based on the results of a number of moderate quality controlled trials, it appears that CPOE- or EHR-based CDS has positive impacts on providers' medication choice in older patients, particularly in reducing prescription of nonrecommended psychoactive medications.

Data on clinical outcomes are scant, and further studies should investigate whether improved prescribing behavior translates to decreased ADEs or improved patient outcomes.

Use of fewer medications considered inappropriate for use in older populations according to the Beers Criteria has been associated with fewer diagnoses of medication-related problems [32]. CDS systems that target these medications may indeed improve patient outcomes, but this question requires investigation in well-conducted controlled trials.

Table 2.1 Summary of trials investigating computerized Clinical Decision Support (CDS) interventions to improve medication choice and decrease adverse events in older patients

Study Reference	Study Setting	Study Design (Number of Participants)	Intervention	Main Outcomes	Evidence Rating[a]
Agostini et al [22]	Inpatient, academic medical center, the United States	Prospective pre- and postintervention study (12,356 patient visits in preintervention year and 12,153 patient visits in the year following start of intervention, all patients ≥65 years)	Alerts within computerized physician order entry (CPOE) to increase use of nonpharmacologic and pharmacologic alternatives to nonpreferred sedative hypnotics	1 There is an 18% risk reduction in total orders for the four sedative hypnotics studied (OR 0.82; 95% CI 0.76–0.87) 2 Significant reduction in prescriptions for preferred agent lorazepam and nonpreferred agent diphenhydramine, significant increase in prescriptions for preferred agent trazodone, no change in prescriptions for nonpreferred agent diazepam	2b
Feldstein et al [23]	Outpatient primary care clinics, health maintenance organization, the United States	Randomized controlled trial (RCT) (311 female patients with fracture in 1-year period but no bone mineral density (BMD) measurement or osteoporosis medication: 109 computerized support plus patient letter, 101 computerized support alone, 101 usual care, mean age 73 years)	Electronic medical record reminder to provider plus letter mailed to patient vs. electronic medical record reminder alone vs. usual care to increase proportion of patients with pharmacologic intervention or BMD testing	1 Increase in probability of BMD measurement or medication by 47% (95% CI 35–59) in electronic medical record reminder group vs. usual care 2 The patient letter had no significant additional effect over the electronic medical record reminder	1b
Judge et al [24]	Adult long-term care units, academic medical center, the United States	Cluster RCT (three intervention long-term care units, four control long-term care units, 47,997 medication orders evaluated over 12 months, mean age not reported)	41 different alerts within CPOE system to improve providers' prescribing behavior of medications with potentially significant risks to patients	Increase in probability of provider taking appropriate action (RR 1.11; 95% CI 1.00–1.22), primarily to decrease central nervous system side effects (RR 1.4 (1.0–1.9)) and improve warfarin prescribing (RR 3.5 (2.1–5.7))	1b

Table 2.1 *Continued*

Study Reference	Study Setting	Study Design (Number of Participants)	Intervention	Main Outcomes	Evidence Rating[a]
Peterson et al [25]	Inpatient, academic medical center, the United States	Prospective trial, four consecutive 6-week study periods: (1) no intervention; (2) intervention; (3) no intervention; (4) intervention (3718 patients, mean age 75 years)	During intervention, CPOE system adjusted default dose and frequency for benzodiazepines, neuroleptics, opiates for patients ≥65 years, alerted providers ordering nonpreferred psychotropic medications, to increase adherence to expert recommendations, and decrease length of stay, rates of altered mental status, and falls	**1** Increased adherence to recommended dose and frequency of psychotropic drugs during intervention (29% vs. 19%, $p < 0.001$) **2** Significant decrease in number of falls during intervention periods (0.28 vs. 0.64 falls per 100 patient-days, $p = 0.09$) **3** No change in average length of stay or rates of altered mental status	2b
Peterson et al [26]	Inpatient, academic medical center, the United States	Cluster RCT (randomization strategy not further described, 778 providers generated 9111 orders for 2981 patients >65 years)	Alerts within CPOE to increase use of geriatric dosing and decrease use of Beers Criteria nonrecommended medications	**1** Intervention physicians prescribed recommended doses more often than controls (28.6% vs. 24.1%, p < 0.001) **2** No difference in prescription of Beers Criteria medications	1b
Smith et al [27]	Outpatient primary care clinics, health maintenance organization, the United States	Retrospective pre- and postintervention study with interrupted time series analysis (15 primary care practices, 209 providers, all adult patients for 12 months before intervention, 27 months after)	Alerts within CPOE to decrease the use of seven nonpreferred psychoactive medications for older adults and recommend alternatives	Decreased prescription of nonpreferred agents in patients ≥65 years (21.9 to 16.8 per 10,000, $p < 0.01$) but not patients ≤65 years	2b
Tamblyn et al [28]	Outpatient primary care clinics, national health program, Canada	Cluster RCT (107 physicians, 12,560 patients >65 years: 6284 intervention, 6276 control, mean age 75)	Alerts within electronic medical record to decrease initiation and increase discontinuation of prescriptions contraindicated by age, drug interaction, drug–disease interaction, therapeutic duplication, or duration of therapy	**1** Decreased initiation of inappropriate prescriptions in intervention group (RR 0.82; 95% CI 0.69–0.98) **2** No effect on discontinuation of preexisting inappropriate prescriptions	1b

Continued

Table 2.1 *Continued*

Study Reference	Study Setting	Study Design (Number of Participants)	Intervention	Main Outcomes	Evidence Rating[a]
Terrell et al [29]	Emergency department, academic medical center, the United States	Cluster RCT (63 physicians, 5162 visits of patients ≥65 years discharged from emergency department: 2647 intervention, 2515 control, mean age 74)	Alerts within CPOE to decrease the use of nine commonly used nonpreferred medications for older adults and recommend alternatives	Decreased proportion of discharges given inappropriate prescription in intervention group (2.6% vs. 3.9%, OR 0.55 (0.34–0.89), $p = 0.02$)	1b
Weber et al [30]	Outpatient primary care clinics, large healthcare system, the United States	Cluster RCT (18 clinics, 620 patients ≥70 years with 4 medications and ≥1 psychoactive medication: 413 intervention, 207 control, mean age 77)	Expert reviewed electronic medical record for inappropriate prescriptions, then sent electronic medical record alert to provider to reduce total medications and initiation of medications, and reduce medical encounters for fall and patient-reported falls	1 No change in number of total medications patients used 2 Decreased medications initiated (beta coefficient -0.199, $p < 0.01$) 3 Decreased medical encounters for fall (OR 0.38, $p < 0.01$) 4 No change in falls when including both medical encounters and patient-reported falls	2b
Zillich et al [31]	Outpatient primary care clinics, Veterans Affairs, the United States	Prospective pre- and postintervention cohort study (2753 patients ≥65 years old prescribed ≥1 of 5 Beers Criteria high-risk psychotropic medications, mean age 72)	Alerts within CPOE to decrease use of five high-risk medications (three tricyclic antidepressants and two benzodiazepines)	Decreased number of patients with prescription for ≥1 of five high-risk psychotropic medications by 42% ($p < 0.001$)	2b

[a]Evidence ratings according to Oxford Centre for Evidence-Based Medicine's Levels of Evidence.

Do CDS tools improve healthcare providers' performance of tasks or clinical outcomes in adult patients with hypertension, the most common ambulatory diagnosis among older patients?

According to the National Health and Nutrition Examination Survey (NHANES) data from 2005 to 2006, approximately 65% of Americans over 60 years old have hypertension, defined as either a systolic blood pressure ≥140 mmHg or diastolic blood pressure ≥90 mmHg, or currently taking medication for hypertension [10]. Treating hypertension with antihypertensive medication, even in patients over 80 years old, has been shown to decrease rates of stroke, heart failure, and overall cardiovascular events [33].

CDS trials for improvement of hypertension management are among the earliest trials of computerized systems to assist healthcare providers, with many trials predating the common use of CPOE systems or full EHRs [34]. A systematic review of trials published between 1976 and 1990 found improved documentation of blood pressure in four out of five trials and improved blood pressure control in two out of six trials (Level 1a evidence) [34]. Other older trials have focused on changing prescribing patterns of antihypertensives to adhere more closely to national guidelines. One of these trials examined use of a computer-generated reminder placed in the paper charts of patients receiving calcium channel blockers (CCBs) for hypertension, encouraging use of alternative agents in accordance with US Joint National Committee on Prevention, Detection, Evaluation, and Treatment of High Blood Pressure V (JNC V) guidelines, and effectively resulted in intervention physicians switching medications for 11.3% of patients, while control physicians only switched <1.0% of patients ($p < 0.0001$) (Level 1b evidence) [35]. A more recent randomized trial of computer-generated, paper-delivered reminders for providers to improve adherence to JNC VI guidelines found that reminders that were individualized according to the patient's EHR data led to an 11% increase in concordance with blood pressure guidelines compared to general reminders, which led to a 4% increase in concordance ($p = 0.008$) (Level 1b evidence) [36].

As the use of CPOEs and EHRs has increased, more trials have begun investigating computerized CDS for chronic disease management. Several trials of integrated CDS have looked specifically at management of hypertension. Recent RCTs of EHR-based CDS to improve management and control of hypertension have mostly yielded negative results (Table 2.2) [37–40]. The intervention protocols varied significantly between studies, from simple EHR-based reminders for providers [37] to combinations of CDS and non-EHR-based provider/patient education, [38, 40] or protocols that involved both providers and pharmacists [39]. Although these trials were not intended to specifically examine treatment of hypertension in older patients, the mean age of participants in three of the four trials was >60 years old [37,38, 40]. None of the four trials showed improvements in clinical outcomes, such as blood pressure control. One good quality RCT found improved provider adherence to JNC VII guideline recommended pharmacotherapy for hypertension with use of an EHR-based electronic reminder (adjusted OR (odds ratio) 1.32 (1.09–1.61) [37]. A Swedish study

found that if providers adhered to all recommendations for hypertension generated by a CDS tool, a significant number of patients would be switched from CCBs to thiazide diuretics, with a cost reduction of 33%–40% [41].

Clinical bottom line

EHR-based CDS systems have not been shown to improve blood pressure control in moderate-quality cluster RCTs, although the study protocols are quite variable and therefore difficult to compare.

The greatest strength of CDS for hypertension may be in changing physicians' prescribing behavior to favor guideline-preferred and lower cost medications.

Research is ongoing to see if developing effective CDS tools for chronic disease management improves clinical outcomes, which may be quite a bit more complicated than CDS for medication prescribing or other provider performance measures [7, 11, 42].

It is probably too soon to conclude that CDS tools will be ineffective at improving blood pressure control, as many are in the early-development stage [43].

Summary

As clinical knowledge and treatment options have increased dramatically over the past century, and individuals live much longer with chronic illnesses, the practice of healthcare has become much more complex. Parallel to these societal and technological developments, information technology tools have been created with the goal of improving the quality, safety, efficiency, and cost-effectiveness of modern healthcare [3, 44]. In fact, a 2009 report by the National Research Council concludes that intensive use of information technology will be increasingly necessary to manage the stream of healthcare data [44].

CDS systems are a class of information technology tools intended to guide and facilitate decision-making and clinical action by the user, with the ultimate goal of making the clinical process safer, more efficient, personalized, and thorough. The fundamental CDS structure interfaces individual patient data with algorithms to generate an individualized output, most commonly a clinical recommendation. CDS systems have been in development for several decades, but have been increasingly used in clinical practice over the past decade with the advent of CPOE and EHRs. These tools take

Table 2.2 Summary of trials investigating computerized Clinical Decision Support (CDS) interventions to improve hypertension management and control in adult patients

Study Reference	Study Setting	Study Design (Number of Participants)	Intervention	Main Outcomes	Evidence Rating[a]
Hicks et al [37]	Outpatient primary care clinics, academic medical center, the United States	Cluster randomized controlled trial (RCT) (14 clinics randomized, 2027 hypertensive patients: 1168 usual care, 859 intervention, mean age 62 years)	Electronic medical record reminder to improve blood pressure control and provider adherence to recommended therapy	1 No effect on blood pressure control: usual care 45% controlled vs. 48% for computerized support group (adjusted OR 0.96 (95% CI 0.78–1.19)) 2 Improved provider adherence to recommended therapy: adjusted OR 1.32 (1.09–1.61)	1b
Montgomery et al [38]	Outpatient primary care practices, New Zealand	Cluster RCT (27 practices randomized, 614 hypertensive patients: 229 computerized support plus chart, 228 chart only, 157 usual care, mean age 71 years)	Electronic medical record reminder and cardiovascular risk chart vs. risk chart alone vs. usual care to reduce percentage of patients with 5-year cardiovascular risk ≥10%	Computerized support increased classification into higher cardiovascular risk group (≥10% 5-year risk): adjusted OR 2.3 (95% CI 1.1–4.8) for computerized support group vs. chart only	1b
Murray et al [39]	Outpatient primary care clinic and pharmacy, academic medical center, the United States	Cluster RCT with 2×2 factorial design (32 practices and 20 pharmacists randomized, 712 hypertensive patients: 171 usual care, 180 pharmacist intervention, 181 physician intervention, 180 both pharmacist and physician intervention, mean age 54 years)	Electronic medical record-generated care suggestions to the physician, pharmacist, or both to improve health-related quality of life measures, secondary outcomes systolic and diastolic blood pressure	1 No difference in health-related quality of life measures among groups 2 No differences in systolic or diastolic blood pressures among groups	2b

Table 2.2 *Continued*

Study Reference	Study Setting	Study Design (Number of Participants)	Intervention	Main Outcomes	Evidence Rating[a]
Roumie et al [40]	Outpatient primary care clinics, Veterans Affairs, the United States	Cluster RCT (182 providers randomized, 1341 hypertensive patients: 470 provider education plus computerized alert plus patient education, 547 provider education plus computerized alert, 324 provider education only, mean age 65 years)	E-mail-based provider education about blood pressure guidelines plus electronic medical record alert plus educational letter to patients vs. provider education plus electronic medical record alert vs. provider education alone to improve systolic blood pressure, secondary outcome diastolic blood pressure	No difference in proportion of patients with controlled systolic or diastolic blood pressure for computerized support and provider education group vs. provider education only (adjusted RR 1.00; 95% CI 0.79–1.25), but increased proportion with controlled systolic blood pressure in computerized support, provider education, and patient letter vs. provider education only (adjusted RR 1.31; 95% CI 1.06–1.62)	1b

[a]Evidence ratings according to Oxford Centre for Evidence-Based Medicine's Levels of Evidence.

many forms, from simple links and alerts to much more intricate disease management systems that integrate with EHRs, which are rich repositories of individual health information that can be processed through a CDS structure to generate clinical recommendations.

While the fundamental structure seems simple, design and application of a system becomes complex and multidimensional, confronting issues from reliability of guidelines and encoding of algorithms to interface usability and integration into clinical workflow. CDS systems have been designed to interface with the many versions of EHR and CPOE that exist in practice, and are therefore, highly variable in design. This variability makes comparison of CDS studies much more difficult than comparing studies of the same pharmaceutical agent or medical procedure. In addition to differences in the CDS per se, the implementation of a CDS system within an organization may vary markedly, so that the same CDS implemented in different sites may have different effects. The salience of the precise implementation of health information technology within the organization has given rise to study of "socio-technical integration" [45, 46]. Given the rapidly evolving na-

ture of CDS systems, EMRs, and information technology in general, reviews of evidence in the CDS field are more likely to meet the criterion for moderate quality evidence even if individual studies are high quality, namely that "further research is likely to have an important impact on our confidence in the estimate of effect and may change the estimate" [47].

Keeping in mind that CDS systems are difficult to compare to one another, the available studies examining CDS interventions to improve providers' prescribing choices in older patients suggest that the systems do have a benefit. To date, many of these CDS interventions have targeted the prescribing of psychoactive medications not recommended for use in older patients, with the goal of decreasing ADEs, including falls. Unfortunately, most studies have not examined clinical outcomes, which are more time consuming, costly, and complicated to measure. The two studies that examined clinical outcomes both suggest that these interventions may decrease falls, but these findings would need to be confirmed with larger studies.

On the other hand, the few available studies of CDS to improve hypertension management, which were primarily conducted in geriatric populations due to the high prevalence of hypertension in this population, have been disappointing in terms of improvements in blood pressure control. There is a suggestion that choice of medication may change among providers using the CDS to align more closely to national guidelines for antihypertensive therapy, which may have benefit over time since the guidelines are based on strong evidence.

These results may demonstrate the complexity of creating successful CDS for chronic disease management, as opposed to CDS that triggers simple alerts when prescribing a medication inappropriate for use in an older patient. Chronic disease management is highly multifaceted and often dependent on patient choices, requiring a much more complex ontology in the CDS structure. Integrating the CDS into the clinical workflow also becomes more challenging. Therefore, the process of creating a successful CDS for management of chronic disease is a long, iterative process, with multiple trials of the system that generate observational data and feedback [43].

A full range of issues important in geriatric care could be the subject of CDS interventions to be studied, including pharmacological and behavioral management of dementia, fall prevention, pressure ulcer prevention, urinary incontinence, osteoporosis screening and management, and mobility issues. Several CDS systems have been described in the literature that address these care areas, although the number of studies remains small and many are at the stage of describing the system features and implementation process, rather than investigating outcomes. For example, prototype CDS systems have been described for dementia care [48–51] and pressure ulcer prevention, and improved care processes in long-term care settings [52–59].

The practice of geriatrics may change significantly as the result of the transition to EHRs with integrated CDS. It has been theorized that these tools will foster the multidisciplinary management often needed in good geriatric care, linking physicians, nurses, allied health professionals, patients, and family through the EHR, and allowing the center of care for older patients to move from the hospital and clinic to the home [1]. Rapid increases in the size of the geriatric population are expected to occur simultaneously with the rapid expansion of EHRs and CDS, and these two phenomena will doubtlessly interact in some way [1].

Acknowledgment

Marina Martin was supported by Stanford Institutional National Research Service Award (5T32-HL07034).

Disclaimer

Views expressed are those of the authors and not necessarily those of the Department of Veterans Affairs.

References

1. Nebeker JR, Hurdle JF, Bair BD (2003) Future history: medical informatics in geriatrics. *J Gerontol A Biol Sci Med Sci* 58(9): M820–M825.
2. Besdine, R, et al (2005) Caring for older Americans: the future of geriatric medicine. *J Am Geriatr Soc* 53(6 Suppl): S245–S256.
3. Osheroff, JA, et al (2007) A roadmap for national action on clinical decision support. *J Am Med Inform Assoc* 14(2): 141–145.
4. Greenes RA (2007) Definition, scope, and challenges. In: RA Greenes (ed.) Clinical Decision Support: The Road Ahead. Boston, MA: Academic Press.
5. Eslami S, Abu-Hanna A, de Keizer NF (2007) Evaluation of outpatient computerized physician medication order entry systems: a systematic review. *J Am Med Inform Assoc* 14(4): 400–406.
6. Durieux P, et al (2008) Computerized advice on drug dosage to improve prescribing practice. *Cochrane Database Syst Rev* (3): CD002894.
7. Shojania KG, et al (2009) The effects of on-screen, point of care computer reminders on processes and outcomes of care. *Cochrane Database Syst Rev* (3): CD001096.
8. DesRoches CM, et al (2008) Electronic health records in ambulatory care–a national survey of physicians. *N Engl J Med* 359(1): 50–60.
9. Kawamoto K, et al (2005) Improving clinical practice using clinical decision support systems: a systematic review of trials to identify features critical to success. *BMJ* 330(7494): 765.
10. Egan BM, Zhao Y, Axon RN (2010) US trends in prevalence, awareness, treatment, and control of hypertension, 1988–2008. *JAMA* 303(20): 2043–2050.
11. Garg AX, et al (2005) Effects of computerized clinical decision support systems on practitioner performance and patient outcomes: a systematic review. *Jama* 293(10): 1223–1238.
12. Kaushal R, Shojania KG, Bates DW (2003) Effects of computerized physician order entry and clinical decision support systems on medication safety: a systematic review. *Arch Intern Med* 163(12): 1409–1416.
13. Kuperman GJ, et al (2007) Medication-related clinical decision support in computerized provider order entry systems: a review. *J Am Med Inform Assoc* 14(1): 29–40.

14. Pearson SA, et al (2009) Do computerised clinical decision support systems for prescribing change practice? A systematic review of the literature (1990–2007). *BMC Health Serv Res* 9: 154.

15. Wolfstadt JI, et al (2008) The effect of computerized physician order entry with clinical decision support on the rates of adverse drug events: a systematic review. *J Gen Intern Med* 23(4): 451–458.

16. Bates DW, et al (1995) Incidence of adverse drug events and potential adverse drug events. Implications for prevention. *ADE Prevention Study GrouJama* 274(1): 29–34.

17. Yourman L, Concato J., Agostini JV (2008) Use of computer decision support interventions to improve medication prescribing in older adults: a systematic review. *Am J Geriatr Pharmacother* 6(2): 119–129.

18. Fick DM, et al (2003) Updating the Beers criteria for potentially inappropriate medication use in older adults: results of a US consensus panel of experts. *Arch Intern Med* 163(22): 2716–2724.

19. Hanlon JT, et al (1997) Adverse drug events in high risk older outpatients. *J Am Geriatr Soc* 45(8): 945–948.

20. Beers MH (1997) Explicit criteria for determining potentially inappropriate medication use by the elderly. An update. *Arch Intern Med* 157(14): 1531–1536.

21. Beers MH, et al (1991) Explicit criteria for determining inappropriate medication use in nursing home residents. UCLA Division of Geriatric Medicine. *Arch Intern Med* 151(9): 1825–1832.

22. Agostini JV, Zhang Y, Inouye SK (2007) Use of a computer-based reminder to improve sedative-hypnotic prescribing in older hospitalized patients. *J Am Geriatr Soc* 55(1): 43–48.

23. Feldstein A, et al (2006) Electronic medical record reminder improves osteoporosis management after a fracture: a randomized, controlled trial. *J Am Geriatr Soc* 54(3): 450–457.

24. Judge J, et al (2006) Prescribers' responses to alerts during medication ordering in the long term care setting. *J Am Med Inform Assoc* 13(4): 385–390.

25. Peterson JF, et al (2005) Guided prescription of psychotropic medications for geriatric inpatients. *Arch Intern Med* 165(7): 802–807.

26. Peterson JF, et al (2007) Physicians' response to guided geriatric dosing: initial results from a randomized trial. *Stud Health Technol Inform* 129(Pt 2): 1037–1040.

27. Smith DH, et al (2006) The impact of prescribing safety alerts for elderly persons in an electronic medical record: an interrupted time series evaluation. *Arch Intern Med* 166(10): 1098–1104.

28. Tamblyn R, et al (2003) The medical office of the 21st century (MOXXI): effectiveness of computerized decision-making support in reducing inappropriate prescribing in primary care. *CMAJ* 169(6): 549–556.

29. Terrell KM, et al (2009) Computerized decision support to reduce potentially inappropriate prescribing to older emergency department patients: a randomized, controlled trial. *J Am Geriatr Soc* 57(8): 1388–1394.

30. Weber V, White A, McIlvried R (2008) An electronic medical record (EMR)-based intervention to reduce polypharmacy and falls in an ambulatory rural elderly population. *J Gen Intern Med* 23(4): 399–404.

31. Zillich AJ, et al (2008) Quality improvement toward decreasing high-risk medications for older veteran outpatients. *J Am Geriatr Soc* 56(7): 1299–1305.

32. Fick DM, et al (2008) Health outcomes associated with potentially inappropriate medication use in older adults. *Res Nurs Health* 31(1): 42–51.

33. Bejan-Angoulvant T, et al (2010) Treatment of hypertension in patients 80 years and older: the lower the better? A meta-analysis of randomized controlled trials. *J Hypertens* 28(7): 1366–1372.

34. Montgomery AA, Fahey T (1998) A systematic review of the use of computers in the management of hypertension. *J Epidemiol Community Health* 52(8): 520–525.

35. Rossi RA, Every NR (1997) A computerized intervention to decrease the use of calcium channel blockers in hypertension. *J Gen Intern Med* 12(11): 672–678.

36. Goldstein MK, et al (2005) Improving adherence to guidelines for hypertension drug prescribing: cluster-randomized controlled trial of general versus patient-specific recommendations. *Am J Manag Care* 11(11): 677–685.

37. Hicks LS, et al (2008) Impact of computerized decision support on blood pressure management and control: a randomized controlled trial. *J Gen Intern Med* 23(4): 429–441.

38. Montgomery AA, et al (2000) Evaluation of computer based clinical decision support system and risk chart for management of hypertension in primary care: randomised controlled trial. *BMJ* 320(7236): 686–690.

39. Murray MD, et al (2004) Failure of computerized treatment suggestions to improve health outcomes of outpatients with uncomplicated hypertension: results of a randomized controlled trial. *Pharmacotherapy* 24(3): 324–337.

40. Roumie CL, et al (2006) Improving blood pressure control through provider education, provider alerts, and patient education: a cluster randomized trial. *Ann Intern Med* 145(3): 165–175.

41. Persson M, et al (2000) Evaluation of a computer-based decision support system for treatment of hypertension with drugs: retrospective, nonintervention testing of cost and guideline adherence. *J Intern Med* 247(1): 87–93.

42. Dorr D, et al (2007) Informatics systems to promote improved care for chronic illness: a literature review. *J Am Med Inform Assoc* 14(2): 156–163.

43. Goldstein MK (2008) Using health information technology to improve hypertension management. *Curr Hypertens Rep* 10(3): 201–207.

44. Stead W, Lin H (eds) (2009) Computational technology for effective health care: immediate steps and strategic directions. Washington DC: The National Academies Press.

45. Berg M (2001) Implementing information systems in health care organizations: myths and challenges. *Int J Med Inform* 64(2–3): 143–156.

46. Berg M (1997) Rationalizing medical work: decision-support techniques and medical practices. In: WE Bijker, WB Carlson, T. Pinch (ed.) *Inside Technology*. Cambridge, MA: The MIT Press.

47. Guyatt GH, et al (2008) GRADE: an emerging consensus on rating quality of evidence and strength of recommendations. *BMJ* 336(7650): 924–926.

48. Lindgren H, Eklund P, Eriksson S (2002) Clinical decision support system in dementia care. *Stud Health Technol Inform* 90: 568–571.

49. Boustani M, et al (2007) A gero-informatics tool to enhance the care of hospitalized older adults with cognitive impairment. *Clin Interv Aging* 2(2): 247–253.

50. Iliffe S, et al (2002) Design and implementation of a computer decision support system for the diagnosis and management of dementia syndromes in primary care. *Methods Inf Med* 41(2): 98–104.

51. Lindgren H (2008) Decision support system supporting clinical reasoning process - an evaluation study in dementia care. *Stud Health Technol Inform* 136: 315–320.

52. Alexander GL (2008) Analysis of an integrated clinical decision support system in nursing home clinical information systems. *J Gerontol Nurs* 34(2): 15–20.

53. Alexander GL (2008) A descriptive analysis of a nursing home clinical information system with decision support. *Perspect Health Inf Manag* 5: 12.

54. Fossum M, et al (2009) Clinical decision support systems to prevent and treat pressure ulcers and under-nutrition in nursing homes. *Stud Health Technol Inform* 146: 877–878.

55. Quaglini S, et al (2000) A computerized guideline for pressure ulcer prevention. *Int J Med Inform* 58–59: 207–217.

56. Rochon PA, et al (2005) Computerized physician order entry with clinical decision support in the long-term care setting: insights from the Baycrest Centre for Geriatric Care. *J Am Geriatr Soc* 53(10): 1780–1789.

57. Subramanian S, et al (2007) Computerized physician order entry with clinical decision support in long-term care facilities: costs and benefits to stakeholders. *J Am Geriatr Soc* 55(9): 1451–1457.

58. Timm JA, et al (2008) Using expert rules to automate pressure ulcer alerts for the clinical nurse specialist. *AMIA Annu Symp Proc* 1154.

59. Zielstorff RD, et al (1997) Evaluation of a decision support system for pressure ulcer prevention and management: preliminary findings. *Proc AMIA Annu Fall Symp* 248–252.

CHAPTER 3

Simplifying the pillbox: drugs and aging

Sudeep S. Gill[1] & Dallas P. Seitz[2]

[1]*Department of Medicine, Division of Geriatric Medicine, Queen's University, Kingston, ON, Canada*
[2]*Department of Psychiatry, Division of Geriatric Psychiatry, Queen's University, Kingston, ON, Canada*

Introduction

The appropriate prescribing of medications represents a major challenge for clinicians who care for older adults, especially those with multiple medical conditions. Each of these comorbid conditions may require several drug treatments. As a result, older individuals are often prescribed many medications. Over time, the prescribing physician must remain vigilant for drug–drug and drug–disease interactions, and must balance prescribing decisions against the dynamics of physiological changes (e.g., changes in renal and hepatic functions) and changes in the patient's goals of care. An important tension also exists between avoiding inappropriate medications ("errors of commission") and avoiding the underuse of potentially beneficial drugs ("errors of omission"). As a result of these many factors, appropriate prescribing for the older patient is a highly complex and ever-shifting balancing act for clinicians.

Additional barriers to optimal prescribing for the elderly relate to potential limitations in the evidence base and its application to individual patients [1, 2]. Considerable effort is required to remain up-to-date with the best evidence about the effectiveness and safety of existing drugs and to learn about newly introduced medications. Care must be taken to avoid reliance on evidence distorted by sponsorship bias [3]. Furthermore, evidence about medications is often based on studies involving relatively young patients with limited comorbid illness. As a result, careful review is necessary to ensure findings from these studies can be generalized to frail older adults with multiple comorbidities. Elderly patients with comorbid conditions are often underrepresented in randomized controlled trials (RCTs) evaluating drug treatments [4–7]. Scott and Guyatt have pointed out that only 5% of RCTs in one review were designed specifically for older patients, and another review found 72% of trials published in major medical journals had excluded older patients [8]. Reviews have identified strategies to improve recruitment of older adults into RCTs that evaluate treatments targeted to this population (Level 2a evidence) [9, 10].

Beyond individual RCTs, problems also exist with clinical practice guidelines. Many of these guidelines are disease specific and do not consider the impact of comorbid conditions [11]. The limitations of guideline-based care are illustrated by a hypothetical 79-year-old woman with five comorbid chronic illnesses described by Boyd and colleagues [12]. If relevant disease-specific clinical practice guidelines were rigorously followed, this hypothetical patient would be prescribed a costly regimen of 12 medications requiring 19 doses per day, and would be at risk for a number of adverse drug–drug, drug–disease, and drug–diet interactions [12]. This example has several lessons. First, it reminds us that medications are a common

Evidence-Based Geriatric Medicine: A Practical Clinical Guide, First Edition. Edited by Jayna M. Holroyd-Leduc and Madhuri Reddy.
© 2012 Blackwell Publishing Ltd. Published 2012 by Blackwell Publishing Ltd.

cause of many geriatric syndromes (including cognitive impairment, injurious falls, and urinary incontinence), and that these outcomes are rarely reported in RCTs. Second, the case highlights the fact that blind adherence to current "evidence-based" clinical practice guidelines for older individuals with multiple comorbidities may have unintended adverse effects. In recognition of the tension between avoiding polypharmacy while still encouraging use of effective drug treatments, some guidelines are now addressing issues specific to the older population such as cognitive impairment, comorbid disease burden, and remaining life expectancy [13–16].

Despite the fact that polypharmacy is commonly encountered by physicians who care for elderly patients, the medical literature provides limited guidance on the clinical approach to this issue. The concept of polypharmacy as it applies to the management of older adults is of great clinical importance and continues to evolve. For example, the term "polypharmacy" has traditionally suggested suboptimal prescribing and has been linked to a heightened risk of drug interactions, adverse drug events, and reduced overall medication adherence. More recent research, however, has emphasized the underuse of beneficial medications, and this research suggests that polypharmacy may be necessary in some individuals to permit the optimal management of their multiple comorbid illnesses (Level 2c evidence) [17].

An important first step in assessing appropriate medication use in the elderly is undertaking a comprehensive and accurate medication history. Often, there are discrepancies between a physician's records of what medications the patient has been prescribed and what they are in fact taking. A common approach adopted by geriatricians is to request that the patient bring all of their medications to the clinic in one large "brown bag," including not only prescription medications but also over-the-counter medicines, vitamins, supplements, and herbal remedies. This comprehensive "brown bag" approach (also known as medication reconciliation) can highlight important discrepancies and provides the most accurate and direct assessment of the individual's current medication use. This approach encourages the physician to ask the patient about indications for each medication and to review the patient's perception of each medication's beneficial and/or harmful effects. This approach also helps

to ensure the patient is taking their medications as intended [18].

Several excellent reviews cover a variety of topics relating to how to best apply the principles of evidence-based medicine to the appropriate prescribing of medications for older individuals [8, 18–20]. This chapter reviews: definitions, epidemiology, and consequences of inappropriate prescribing and polypharmacy; the interrelated concepts of errors of commission and errors of omission; how to approach appropriate prescribing in the individual older patient; and predictors of drug adherence and strategies to maximize adherence.

Search strategy

We searched MEDLINE, Embase, and the Cochrane Library until February 2011 in order to identify existing systematic reviews and meta-analyses relevant to the topics covered in the three questions that focus on appropriate prescribing of medications for older adults: (1) what is inappropriate prescribing and how can it be prevented?; (2) what strategies can clinicians employ to optimize prescribing in individual older patients?; and (3) once we identify optimal prescribing, how can we promote long-term adherence to these medications? Our search terms included "inappropriate prescribing," "suboptimal prescribing," "polypharmacy," "multiple medications," "aged," "elderly," and "geriatric." To keep the discussion of appropriate prescribing as general as possible, we intentionally avoided a focus on a particular drug class or condition. Where reviews on interventions were not available, we described information obtained from RCTs. We also included information contained in guidelines published by medical associations and professional organizations where there were no RCTs and reviewed evidence for topics that do not relate to interventions. For this chapter, we graded relevant studies using the Oxford Centre for Evidence-Based Medicine (CEBM) Levels of Evidence.

What is inappropriate prescribing and how can it be prevented?

A comprehensive definition for inappropriate prescribing is difficult to achieve, as this concept includes several dynamic core components, such as: the use of medications that result in more harm than benefit (especially when safer alternatives are available); the misuse of medications (e.g., inappropriate dose or duration); and the potential for clinically important drug–drug or drug–disease interactions. This approach highlights the dynamic nature of inappropriate prescribing because other medications and comorbid conditions change over time, and a medication that is considered appropriate at one time may later become inappropriate. In addition, note that all these components generally involve "errors of commission" (underprescribing or "errors of omission" is discussed in greater detail later).

Several groups of investigators have published lists of inappropriate medications for the elderly, and these include the Beers Criteria [21, 22], the Inappropriate Prescribing in the Elderly Tool (IPET) [23, 24], the Medication Appropriateness Index (MAI) [25], the Screening Tool of Older Persons' Potentially Inappropriate Prescriptions (STOPP) [26], and the Screening Tool to Alert Doctors to the Right Treatment (START) [27]. Similar criteria have been developed by consensus panels in France, Australia, Japan, Norway, and Italy, and have been reviewed by Levy and colleagues [28]. The strength of evidence varies considerably for individual recommendations in these consensus lists (i.e., from Level 1a to Level 5 evidence).

The most widely used list of inappropriate prescribing in the elderly is the Beers Criteria, which was introduced in 1991 [21]. The Beers Criteria consist of two lists of medications to be avoided in older people (one list that is independent of diagnosis, and a second list that considers diagnosis). These criteria were initially developed for use in the nursing home setting, but have been revised several times and the most recent iteration published in 2003 can be used to detect inappropriate prescribing in different settings (Tables 3.1 and 3.2) [22]. These updated criteria list 48 inappropriate medications for use in older adults and categorize them as always inappropriate, potentially inappropriate, or potentially inappropriate in certain circumstances. Drugs are rated as associated with a high to low severity of adverse events. The criteria also include 20 diseases and conditions, and medications to be avoided in people with these conditions. The Beers Criteria do not address underprescribing, drug–drug interactions, or drug class duplication. In addition,

many of the drugs listed are not absolutely contraindicated.

The IPET was published in 2000 [23], and was adapted from the recommendations of a Canadian consensus panel [24]. The IPET includes 14 inappropriate prescribing errors such as adverse drug reactions and drug–disease interactions. As an example of the need to periodically revise these explicit lists to reflect current evidence, one of the IPET recommendations is to avoid beta-blockers in older adults with congestive heart failure (CHF). While this recommendation reflected consensus at the time of publication, multiple RCTs have since established the effectiveness and safety of beta-blockers in the setting of heart failure (Level 1a evidence) [29].

The MAI [25] measures prescribing appropriateness according to ten criteria, including indication, effectiveness, dose, administration, drug–drug and drug–disease interactions, and cost. The MAI does not list inappropriate medications but ranks a selected drug as indicated or not indicated based on a score generated by these ten criteria. The MAI does not address underprescribing. In contrast to the Beers Criteria and the IPET, the generic nature of the MAI makes it resistant to becoming outdated; on the other hand, clinical expertise is required to apply some MAI criteria. Because of the time required to complete the MAI and the need for clinical expertise on a wide spectrum of medications, it is not widely used in clinical practice but is instead predominantly used as a research tool.

A European consensus group developed the STOPP criteria, which list 65 potentially inappropriate prescribing practices in older adults categorized according to organ system (Table 3.3) [26]. STOPP criteria are arranged according to physiological systems, and include drug–drug and drug–disease interactions, drugs that affect older patients at risk for falls, and therapeutic duplication. The STOPP criteria are designed to be used alongside a second complementary list, the START criteria, which address underprescribing or omission of clinically indicated, evidence-based medications (Table 3.4) [27]. (Underprescribing, or errors of omission, are discussed in greater detail later.) START criteria list 22 evidence-based prescribing indications for older adults and also categorize medications according to organ system. The STOPP and START criteria have undergone consensus validation and testing for interrater reliability [26, 30]. An RCT is evaluating

Table 3.1 2002 Criteria for potentially inappropriate medication use in older adults: independent of diagnoses or conditions

Drug	Concern	Severity Rating (High or Low)
Propoxyphene (Darvon) and combination products (Darvon with ASA, Darvon-N, and Darvocet-N)	Offers few analgesic advantages over acetaminophen, yet has the adverse effects of other narcotic drugs.	Low
Indomethacin (Indocin and Indocin SR)	Of all available nonsteroidal anti-inflammatory drugs, this drug produces the most CNS adverse effects.	High
Pentazocine (Talwin)	Narcotic analgesic that causes more CNS adverse effects, including confusion and hallucinations, more commonly than other narcotic drugs. Additionally, it is a mixed agonist and antagonist.	High
Trimethobenzamide (Tigan)	One of the least effective antiemetic drugs, yet it can cause extrapyramidal adverse effects.	High
Muscle relaxants and antispasmodics; methocarbamol (Robaxin), carisoprodol (Soma), chlorzoxazone (Paraflex), metaxalone (Skelaxin), cyclobenzaprine (Flexeril), and oxybutynin (Ditropan). Do not consider the extended-release Ditropan XL.	Most muscle relaxants and antispasmodic drugs are poorly tolerated by elderly patients, since these cause anticholinergic adverse effects, sedation, and weakness. Additionally, their effectiveness at doses tolerated by elderly patients is questionable.	High
Flurazepam (Dalmane)	This benzodiazepine hypnotic has an extremely long half-life in elderly patients (often days), producing prolonged sedation and increasing the incidence of falls and fracture. Medium- or short-acting benzodiazepines are preferable.	High
Amitriptyline (Elavil), chlordiazepoxide-amitriptyline (Limbitrol), and perphenazine-amitriptyline (Triavil)	Because of its strong anticholinergic and sedation properties, amitriptyline is rarely the antidepressant of choice for elderly patients.	High
Doxepin (Sinequan)	Because of its strong anticholinergic and sedating properties, doxepin is rarely the antidepressant of choice for elderly patients.	High
Meprobamate (Miltown and Equanil)	This is a highly addictive and sedating anxiolytic. Those using meprobamate for prolonged periods may become addicted and may need to be withdrawn slowly.	High
Doses of short-acting benzodiazepines: doses greater than lorazepam (Ativan), 3 mg; oxazepam (Serax), 60 mg; alprazolam (Xanax), 2 mg; temazepam (Restoril), 15 mg; and triazolam (Halcion), 0.25 mg	Because of increased sensitivity to benzodiazepines in elderly patients, smaller doses may be effective as well as safer. Total daily doses should rarely exceed the suggested maximums.	High

Table 3.1 *Continued*

Drug	Concern	Severity Rating (High or Low)
Long-acting benzodiazepines: chlordiazepoxide (Librium), chlordiazepoxide-amitriptyline (Limbitrol), clidinium-chlordiazepoxide (Librax), diazepam (Valium), quazepam (Doral), halazepam (Paxipam), and chlorazepate (Tranxene)	These drugs have a long half-life in elderly patients (often several days), producing prolonged sedation and increasing the risk of falls and fractures. Short- and intermediate-acting benzodiazepines are preferred if a benzodiazepine is required.	High
Disopyramide (Norpace and Norpace CR)	Of all antiarrhythmic drugs, this is the most potent negative inotrope, and therefore, may induce heart failure in elderly patients. It is also strongly anticholinergic. Other antiarrhythmic drugs should be used.	High
Digoxin (Lanoxin) (should not exceed >0.125 mg/d except when treating atrial arrhythmias)	Decreased renal clearance may lead to increased risk of toxic effects.	Low
Short-acting dipyridamole (Persantine). Do not consider the long-acting dipyridamole (which has better properties than the short-acting in older adults) except with patients with artificial heart valves	May cause orthostatic hypotension.	Low
Methyldopa (Aldomet) and methyldopa-hydrochlorothiazide (Aldoril)	May cause bradycardia and exacerbate depression in elderly patients.	High
Reserpine at doses >0.25 mg	May induce depression, impotence, sedation, and orthostatic hypotension.	Low
Chlorpropamide (Diabinese)	It has a prolonged half-life in elderly patients and could cause prolonged hypoglycemia. Additionally, it is the only oral hypoglycemic agent that causes SIADH.	High
GI antispasmodic drugs: dicyclomine (Bentyl), hyoscyamine (Levsin and Levsinex), propantheline (Pro-Banthine), belladonna alkaloids (Donnatal and others), and clidinium-chlordiazepoxide (Librax)	GI antispasmodic drugs are highly anticholinergic and have uncertain effectiveness. These drugs should be avoided (especially for long-term use).	High
Anticholinergics and antihistamines: chlorpheniramine (Chlor-Trimeton), diphenhydramine (Benadryl), hydroxyzine (Vistaril and Atarax), cyproheptadine (Periactin), promethazine (Phenergan), tripelennamine, dexchlorpheniramine (Polaramine)	All nonprescription and many prescription antihistamines may have potent anticholinergic properties. Nonanticholinergic antihistamines are preferred in elderly patients when treating allergic reactions.	High
Diphenhydramine (Benadryl)	May cause confusion and sedation. Should not be used as a hypnotic, and when used to treat emergency allergic reactions, it should be used in the smallest possible dose.	High
Ergot mesyloids (Hydergine) and cyclandelate (Cyclospasmol)	Have not been shown to be effective in the doses studied.	Low

Continued

Table 3.1 *Continued*

Drug	Concern	Severity Rating (High or Low)
Ferrous sulfate >325 mg/d	Doses >325 mg/d do not dramatically increase the amount absorbed but greatly increase the incidence of constipation.	Low
All barbiturates (except Phenobarbital) except when used to control seizures	Are highly addictive and cause more adverse effects than most sedative or hypnotic drugs in elderly patients.	High
Meperidine (Demerol)	Not an effective oral analgesic in doses commonly used. May cause confusion and has many disadvantages to other narcotic drugs.	High
Ticlopidine (Ticlid)	Has been shown to be no better than aspirin in preventing clotting and may be considerably more toxic. Safer, more effective alternatives exist.	High
Ketorolac (Toradol)	Immediate and long-term use should be avoided in older persons, since a significant number have asymptomatic GI pathologic conditions.	High
Amphetamines and anorexic agents	These drugs have potential for causing dependence, hypertension, angina, and myocardial infarction.	High
Long-term use of full-dosage, longer half-life, non-COX-selective NSAIDs: naproxen (Naprosyn, Avaprox, and Aleve), oxaprozin (Daypro), and piroxicam (Feldene)	Have the potential to produce GI bleeding, renal failure, high blood pressure, and heart failure.	High
Daily fluoxetine (Prozac)	Long half-life of drug and risk of producing excessive CNS stimulation, sleep disturbances, and increasing agitation. Safer alternatives exist.	High
Long-term use of stimulant laxatives: bisacodyl (Dulcolax), cascara sagrada, and Neoloid except in the presence of opiate analgesic use	May exacerbate bowel dysfunction.	High
Amiodarone (Cordarone)	Associated with QT interval problems and risk of provoking torsades de pointes. Lack of efficacy in older adults.	High
Orphenadrine (Norflex)	Causes more sedation and anticholinergic adverse effects than safer alternatives.	High
Guanethidine (Ismelin)	May cause orthostatic hypotension. Safer alternatives exist.	High
Guanadrel (Hylorel)	May cause orthostatic hypotension.	High
Cyclandelate (Cyclospasmol)	Lack of efficacy.	Low

Table 3.1 *Continued*

Drug	Concern	Severity Rating (High or Low)
Isoxsurpine (Vasodilan)	Lack of efficacy.	Low
Nitrofurantoin (Macrodantin)	Potential for renal impairment. Safer alternatives available.	High
Doxazosin (Cardura)	Potential for hypotension, dry mouth, and urinary problems.	Low
Methyltestosterone (Android, Virilon, and Testrad)	Potential for prostatic hypertrophy and cardiac problems.	High
Thioridazine (Mellaril)	Greater potential for CNS and extrapyramidal adverse effects.	High
Mesoridazine (Serentil)	CNS and extrapyramidal adverse effects.	High
Short-acting nifedipine (Procardia and Adalat)	Potential for hypotension and constipation.	High
Clonidine (Catapres)	Potential for orthostatic hypotension and CNS adverse effects.	Low
Mineral oil	Potential for aspiration and adverse effects. Safer alternatives available.	High
Cimetidine (Tagamet)	CNS adverse effects including confusion.	Low
Ethacrynic acid (Edecrin)	Potential for hypertension and fluid imbalances. Safer alternatives available.	Low
Desiccated thyroid	Concerns about cardiac effects. Safer alternatives available.	High
Amphetamines (excluding methylphenidate hydrochloride and anorexics)	CNS stimulant with adverse effects.	High
Estrogens only (oral)	Evidence of the carcinogenic (breast and endometrial cancer) potential of these agents and lack of cardioprotective effect in older women.	Low

Source: [22].
CNS, central nervous system; COX, cyclooxygenase; GI, gastrointestinal; NSAIDs, nonsteroidal anti-inflammatory drugs; SIADH, syndrome of inappropriate antidiuretic hormone secretion.

whether clinical implementation of the STOPP and START criteria for hospitalized older patients can improve prescribing quality and prevent potentially inappropriate prescribing (ClinicalTrials.gov Identifier: NCT00915824).

There is evidence to suggest that inappropriate prescribing, defined using the measures described previously, is linked to increased health services utilization and adverse clinical outcomes (Level 2c evidence). For example, Klarin and colleagues found that inappropriate drug use (defined in part by the Beers Criteria and IPET) was common and associated with an increased risk of acute hospitalization in community-dwelling older adults. No association between

Table 3.2 2002 Criteria for potentially inappropriate medication use in older adults: considering diagnoses or conditions

Disease or Condition	Drug	Concern	Severity Rating (High or Low)
Heart failure	Disopyramide (Norpace) and high sodium content drugs (sodium and sodium salts (alginate bicarbonate, biphosphate, citrate, phosphate, salicylate, and sulfate))	Negative inotropic effect. Potential to promote fluid retention and exacerbation of heart failure.	High
Hypertension	Phenylpropanolamine hydrochloride (removed from the market in 2001), pseudoephedrine, diet pills, and amphetamines	May produce elevation of blood pressure secondary to sympathomimetic activity.	High
Gastric or duodenal ulcers	NSAIDs and aspirin (>325 mg) (coxibs excluded)	May exacerbate existing ulcers or produce new/additional ulcers.	High
Seizures or epilepsy	Clozapine (Clozaril), chlorpromazine (Thorazine), thioridazine (Mellaril), and thiothixene (Navane)	May lower seizure thresholds.	High
Blood clotting disorders or receiving anticoagulant therapy	Aspirin, NSAIDs, dipyridamole (Persantin), ticlopidine (Ticlid), and clopidogrel (Plavix)	May prolong clotting time and elevate INR values or inhibit platelet aggregation, resulting in an increased potential for bleeding.	High
Bladder outflow obstruction	Anticholinergics and antihistamines, gastrointestinal antispasmodics, muscle relaxants, oxybutynin (Ditropan), flavoxate (Urispas), anticholinergics, antidepressants, decongestants, and tolterodine (Detrol)	May decrease urinary flow, leading to urinary retention.	High
Stress incontinence	Alpha-blockers (doxazosin, prazosin, and terazosin), anticholinergics, tricyclic antidepressants (imipramine hydrochloride, doxepin hydrochloride, and amitriptyline hydrochloride), and long-acting benzodiazepines	May produce polyuria and worsening of incontinence.	High
Arrhythmias	Tricyclic antidepressants (imipramine hydrochloride, doxepin hydrochloride, and amitriptyline hydrochloride)	Concern due to proarrhythmic effects and ability to produce QT interval changes.	High
Insomnia	Decongestants, theophylline (Theodur), methylphenidate (Ritalin), MAOIs, and amphetamines	Concern due to CNS stimulant effects.	High
Parkinson disease	Metoclopramide (Reglan), conventional antipsychotics, and tacrine (Cognex)	Concern due to their antidopaminergic/cholinergic effects.	High

Table 3.2 *Continued*

Disease or Condition	Drug	Concern	Severity Rating (High or Low)
Cognitive impairment	Barbiturates, anticholinergics, antispasmodics, and muscle relaxants. CNS stimulants: dextroAmphetamine (Adderall), methylphenidate (Ritalin), methamphetamine (Desoxyn), and pemolin	Concern due to CNS-altering effects.	High
Depression	Long-term benzodiazepine use. Sympatholytic agents: methyldopa (Aldomet), reserpine, and guanethidine (Ismelin)	May produce or exacerbate depression.	High
Anorexia and malnutrition	CNS stimulants: dextroamphetamine (Adderall), methylphenidate (Ritalin), methamphetamine (Desoxyn), pemolin, and fluoxetine (Prozac)	Concern due to appetite-suppressing effects.	High
Syncope or falls	Short- to intermediate-acting benzodiazepine and tricyclic antidepressants (imipramine hydrochloride, doxepin hydrochloride, and amitriptyline hydrochloride)	May produce ataxia, impaired psychomotor function, syncope, and additional falls.	High
SIADH/hyponatremia	SSRIs: fluoxetine (Prozac), citalopram (Celexa), fluvoxamine (Luvox), paroxetine (Paxil), and sertraline (Zoloft)	May exacerbate or cause SIADH.	Low
Seizure disorder	Bupropion (Wellbutrin)	May lower seizure threshold.	High
Obesity	Olanzapine (Zyprexa)	May stimulate appetite and increase weight gain.	Low
COPD	Long-acting benzodiazepines: chlordiazepoxide (Librium), chlordiazepoxide-amitriptyline (Limbitrol), clidinium-chlordiazepoxide (Librax), diazepam (Valium), quazepam (Doral), halazepam (Paxipam), and chlorazepate (Tranxene). Beta-blockers: propranolol	CNS adverse effects. May induce respiratory depression. May exacerbate or cause respiratory depression.	High
Chronic constipation	Calcium channel blockers, anticholinergics, and tricyclic antidepressant (imipramine hydrochloride, doxepin hydrochloride, and amitriptyline hydrochloride)	May exacerbate constipation.	Low

Source: [22].

CNS, central nervous system; COPD, chronic obstructive pulmonary disease; INR, international normalized ratio; MAOIs, monoamine oxidase inhibitors; NSAIDs, nonsteroidal anti-inflammatory drugs; SIADH, syndrome of inappropriate antidiuretic hormone secretion; SSRIs, selective serotonin reuptake inhibitors.

Table 3.3 STOPP (Screening Tool of Older People's potentially inappropriate Prescriptions)

The following prescriptions are potentially inappropriate in persons aged ≥65 years of age:

A Cardiovascular System

1 Digoxin at a long-term dose >125 µg per day with impaired renal function[a] (*increased risk of toxicity*)
2 Loop diuretic for dependent ankle edema only, i.e., no clinical signs of heart failure (*no evidence of efficacy, compression hosiery usually more appropriate*)
3 Loop diuretic as first-line monotherapy for hypertension (*safer, more effective alternatives available*)
4 Thiazide diuretic with a history of gout (*may exacerbate gout*)
5 Noncardioselective beta-blocker with chronic obstructive pulmonary disease (COPD) (*risk of bronchospasm*)
6 Beta-blocker in combination with verapamil (*risk of symptomatic heart block*)
7 Use of diltiazem or verapamil with NYHA Class III or IV heart failure (*may worsen heart failure*)
8 Calcium channel blockers with chronic constipation (*may exacerbate constipation*)
9 Use of aspirin and warfarin in combination without histamine H2 receptor antagonist (except cimetidine because of interaction with warfarin) or proton pump inhibitor (PPI) (*high risk of gastrointestinal bleeding*)
10 Dipyridamole as monotherapy for cardiovascular secondary prevention (*no evidence for efficacy*)
11 Aspirin with a past history of peptic ulcer disease without histamine H2 receptor antagonist or PPI (*risk of bleeding*)
12 Aspirin at dose >150 mg per day (*increased bleeding risk, no evidence for increased efficacy*)
13 Aspirin with no history of coronary, cerebral, or peripheral arterial symptoms or occlusive arterial event (*not indicated*)
14 Aspirin to treat dizziness not clearly attributable to cerebrovascular disease (*not indicated*)
15 Warfarin for first, uncomplicated deep venous thrombosis for longer than 6-month duration (*no proven added benefit*)
16 Warfarin for first, uncomplicated pulmonary embolus for longer than 12-month duration (*no proven benefit*)
17 Aspirin, clopidogrel, dipyridamole, or warfarin with concurrent bleeding disorder (*high risk of bleeding*)

B Central Nervous System and Psychotropic Drugs

1 Tricyclic antidepressants (TCAs) with dementia (*risk of worsening cognitive impairment*)
2 TCAs with glaucoma (*likely to exacerbate glaucoma*)
3 TCAs with cardiac conductive abnormalities (*proarrhythmic effects*)
4 TCAs with constipation (*likely to worsen constipation*)
5 TCAs with an opiate or calcium channel blocker (*risk of severe constipation*)
6 TCAs with prostatism or prior history of urinary retention (*risk of urinary retention*)
7 Long-term (i.e., >1 month), long-acting benzodiazepines, e.g., chlordiazepoxide, fluazepam, nitrazepam, chlorazepate, and benzodiazepines with long-acting metabolites, e.g., diazepam (*risk of prolonged sedation, confusion, impaired balance, falls*)
8 Long-term (i.e., >1 month) neuroleptics as long-term hypnotics (*risk of confusion, hypotension, extrapyramidal side effects, falls*)
9 Long-term neuroleptics (>1 month) in those with Parkinsonism (*likely to worsen extrapyramidal symptoms*)
10 Phenothiazines in patients with epilepsy (*may lower seizure threshold*)
11 Anticholinergics to treat extrapyramidal side effects of neuroleptic medications (*risk of anticholinergic toxicity*)
12 Selective serotonin reuptake inhibitors (SSRIs) with a history of clinically significant hyponatraemia (*noniatrogenic hyponatraemia <130 mmol/L within the previous 2 months*)
13 Prolonged use (>1 week) of first-generation antihistamines, i.e., diphenydramine, chlorpheniramine, cyclizine, promethazine (*risk of sedation and anticholinergic side effects*)

C Gastrointestinal System

1 Diphenoxylate, loperamide, or codeine phosphate for treatment of diarrhea of unknown cause (*risk of delayed diagnosis, may exacerbate constipation with overflow diarrhea, may precipitate toxic megacolon in inflammatory bowel disease, may delay recovery in unrecognized gastroenteritis*)
2 Diphenoxylate, loperamide, or codeine phosphate for treatment of severe infective gastroenteritis, i.e., bloody diarrhea, high fever, or severe systemic toxicity (*risk of exacerbation or protraction of infection*)
3 Prochlorperazine (Stemetil) or metoclopramide with Parkinsonism (*risk of exacerbating Parkinsonism*).
4 PPI for peptic ulcer disease at full therapeutic dosage for >8 weeks (*earlier discontinuation or dose reduction for maintenance/prophylactic treatment of peptic ulcer disease, esophagitis, or GORD indicated*)
5 Anticholinergic antispasmodic drugs with chronic constipation (*risk of exacerbation of constipation*)

Table 3.3 *Continued*

D Respiratory System

1 Theophylline as monotherapy for COPD (*safer, more effective alternative; risk of adverse effects due to narrow therapeutic index*)
2 Systemic corticosteroids instead of inhaled corticosteroids for maintenance therapy in moderate–severe COPD (*unnecessary exposure to long-term side effects of systemic steroids*)
3 Nebulized ipratropium with glaucoma (*may exacerbate glaucoma*)

E Musculoskeletal System

1 Nonsteroidal anti-inflammatory drug (NSAID) with history of peptic ulcer disease or gastrointestinal bleeding, unless with concurrent histamine H2-receptor antagonist, PPI, or misoprostol (*risk of peptic ulcer relapse*)
2 NSAID with moderate–severe hypertension (moderate: 160/100 mmHg–179/109 mmHg; severe: ≥180/110 mmHg) (*risk of exacerbation of hypertension*)
3 NSAID with heart failure (*risk of exacerbation of heart failure*)
4 Long-term use of NSAID (>3 months) for relief of mild joint pain in osteoarthtitis (*simple analgesics preferable and usually as effective for pain relief*)
5 Warfarin and NSAID together (*risk of gastrointestinal bleeding*)
6 NSAID with chronic renal failure[b] (*risk of deterioration in renal function*)
7 Long-term corticosteroids (>3 months) as monotherapy for rheumatoid arthritis or osteoarthritis (*risk of major systemic corticosteroid side effects*)
8 Long-term NSAID or colchicine for chronic treatment of gout where there is no contraindication to allopurinol (*allopurinol first choice prophylactic drug in gout*)

F Urogenital System

1 Bladder antimuscarinic drugs with dementia (*risk of increased confusion, agitation*)
2 Bladder antimuscarinic drugs with chronic glaucoma (*risk of acute exacerbation of glaucoma*)
3 Bladder antimuscarinic drugs with chronic constipation (*risk of exacerbation of constipation*)
4 Bladder antimuscarinic drugs with chronic prostatism (*risk of urinary retention*)
5 Alpha-blockers in males with frequent incontinence, i.e., one or more episodes of incontinence daily (*risk of urinary frequency and worsening of incontinence*)
6 Alpha-blockers with long-term urinary catheter in situ, i.e., more than 2 months (*drug not indicated*)

G Endocrine System

1 Glibenclamide or chlorpropamide with type 2 diabetes mellitus (*risk of prolonged hypoglycaemia*)
2 Beta-blockers in those with diabetes mellitus and frequent hypoglycemic episodes, i.e., ≥1 episode per month (*risk of masking hypoglycemic symptoms*)
3 Estrogens with a history of breast cancer or venous thromboembolism (*increased risk of recurrence*)
4 Estrogens without progestogen in patients with intact uterus (*risk of endometrial cancer*)

H Drugs that Adversely Affect those Prone to Falls (≥1 Fall in the Past 3 Months)

1 Benzodiazepines (*sedative, may cause reduced sensorium, impair balance*)
2 Neuroleptic drugs (*may cause gait dyspraxia, Parkinsonism*)
3 First-generation antihistamines (*sedative, may impair sensorium*)
4 Vasodilator drugs known to cause hypotension in those with persistent postural hypotension, i.e., recurrent >20 mmHg drop in systolic blood pressure (*risk of syncope, falls*)
5 Long-term opiates in those with recurrent falls (*risk of drowsiness, postural hypotension, vertigo*)

I Analgesic Drugs

1 Use of long-term powerful opiates, e.g., morphine or fentanyl as first-line therapy for mild–moderate pain (*WHO analgesic ladder not observed*)

Continued

Table 3.3 *Continued*

---

2 Regular opiates for more than 2 weeks in those with chronic constipation without concurrent use of laxatives (*risk of severe constipation*)

3 Long-term opiates in those with dementia unless indicted for palliative care or management of moderate/severe chronic pain syndrome (*risk of exacerbation of cognitive impairment*)

J Duplicate Drug Classes

Any regular duplicate drug class prescription, e.g., two concurrent opiates, NSAIDs, SSRIs, loop diuretics, ACE inhibitors (*optimization of monotherapy within a single drug class should be observed prior to considering a new class of drug*). This excludes duplicate prescribing of drugs that may be required on a prn basis, e.g., inhaled beta2 agonists (long- and short acting) for asthma or COPD, and opiates for management of breakthrough pain.

---

[a]GFR <50 mL/min.
[b]Estimated GFR 20–50 mL/min.

inappropriate drug use and mortality was found in this study [31]. However, a second study conducted by Lau and colleagues used the Beers Criteria to define potentially inappropriate prescribing among nursing home residents, and found that this measure was associated with significantly increased risks of both hospitalization and death [32].

A systematic review by Kaur and colleagues identified 24 original studies of strategies to reduce inappropriate prescribing in the elderly [33]. Interventions studied included educational interventions, medication reviews, geriatrician services, multidisciplinary teams, computerized support systems, regulatory policies, and multifaceted approaches. Although the evidence base is limited, Kaur and colleagues suggest promising strategies including multidisciplinary case conferences involving a geriatrician, pharmacist-led interventions, and computerized support systems (Level 1a evidence) [33]. Another systematic review focused on pharmacist-led interventions has also suggested that pharmacist involvement in the care of hospitalized older adults can have important benefits in reducing inappropriate prescribing (Level 1a evidence) [34]. Since publication of this review, another RCT has provided further evidence to support the benefits of ward-based pharmacists. This RCT found pharmacist care was associated with significant reductions in re-hospitalizations and emergency department visits, as well as lower healthcare costs (Level 1b evidence) [35].

Polypharmacy

Although the term polypharmacy is often used, there is no consensus on its definition. The simplest definition is based on the total number of medications taken by a patient: polypharmacy is said to exist when patients take more medications than this arbitrary number. The number of medications constituting polypharmacy using this approach has been variably defined in the literature as between five and ten [36]. This definition of polypharmacy is problematic, as it is unclear which drugs should take priority and which should be discontinued when the arbitrary target number is exceeded. In addition, it is unclear whether the number of medications should include over-the-counter products, herbal drugs, or other drug preparations with systemic effects (e.g., eye drops). Thus, defining polypharmacy in terms of an arbitrary numerical threshold does not address the appropriate or inappropriate use of medications and could promote the exclusion of potentially useful drug treatments for some patients ("errors of omission"). A more practical definition of polypharmacy is, "the prescription, administration, or use of more medications than are clinically indicated" [36]. This definition emphasizes the fact that the problems of polypharmacy involve unnecessary medications, inappropriate drug combinations, and inappropriate drugs for specific patients.

Although the intentions of prescribing multidrug regimens to manage chronic diseases and their complications are usually good, unintended negative consequences become progressively more common as the number of medications prescribed to frail elderly patients increase. Such consequences include increasing costs, adverse drug reactions to a single drug, drug–drug interactions, drug–disease interactions, reduced overall medication adherence, and the

Table 3.4 START: Screening Tool to Alert doctors to Right i.e. appropriate, indicated Treatment

These medications should be considered for people ≥65 years of age with the following conditions, where no contraindication to prescription exists.

A Cardiovascular System

1 Warfarin in the presence of chronic atrial fibrillation
2 Aspirin in the presence of chronic atrial fibrillation, where warfarin is contraindicated, but not aspirin
3 Aspirin or clopidogrel with a documented history of atherosclerotic coronary, cerebral or peripheral vascular disease in patients with sinus rhythm
4 Antihypertensive therapy where systolic blood pressure consistently >160 mmHg
5 Statin therapy with a documented history of coronary, cerebral, or peripheral vascular disease, where the patient's functional status remains independent for activities of daily living and life expectancy is >5 years
6 Angiotensin converting enzyme (ACE) inhibitor with chronic heart failure
7 ACE inhibitor following acute myocardial infarction
8 Beta-blocker with chronic stable angina

B Respiratory System

1 Regular inhaled beta 2 agonist or anticholinergic agent for mild to moderate asthma or COPD
2 Regular inhaled corticosteroid for moderate–severe asthma or COPD, where predicted FEV1 <50%
3 Home continuous oxygen with documented chronic type 1 respiratory failure (pO2 <8.0 kPa, pCO2 <6.5 kPa) or type 2 respiratory failure (pO2 <8.0 kPa, pCO2 >6.5 kPa)

C Central Nervous System

1 L-DOPA in idiopathic Parkinson's disease with definite functional impairment and resultant disability
2 Antidepressant drug in the presence of moderate–severe depressive symptoms lasting at least 3 months

D Gastrointestinal System

1 Proton Pump Inhibitor (PPI) with severe gastro-esophageal acid reflux disease or peptic stricture requiring dilatation
2 Fiber supplement for chronic, symptomatic diverticular disease with constipation

E Musculoskeletal System

1 Disease-modifying antirheumatic drug (DMARD) with active moderate–severe rheumatoid disease lasting >12 weeks
2 Bisphosphonates in patients taking maintenance oral corticosteroid therapy
3 Calcium and Vitamin D supplement in patients with known osteoporosis (radiological evidence or previous fragility fracture or acquired dorsal kyphosis)

F Endocrine System

1 Metformin with type 2 diabetes +/− metabolic syndrome (in the absence of renal impairment[a])
2 ACE inhibitor or Angiotensin Receptor Blocker in diabetes with nephropathy, i.e., overt urinalysis proteinuria or microalbuminuria (>30 mg per 24 hours) +/− serum biochemical renal impairment[a]
3 Antiplatelet therapy in diabetes mellitus if one or more coexisting major cardiovascular risk factor present (hypertension, hypercholesterolemia, and smoking history)
4 Statin therapy in diabetes mellitus if one or more coexisting major cardiovascular risk factor present

[a]GFR <50 mL/min.

development of geriatric syndromes. Geriatric syndromes associated with the inappropriate use of medications include cognitive impairment, falls and consequent injuries, and urinary incontinence (Level 2c evidence) [37].

Errors of omission

With the exception of the START criteria, most published lists of inappropriate prescribing focus on "errors of commission" in drug prescribing. However, investigators have pointed out that elderly patients with multiple chronic diseases are often undertreated with potentially useful medications (i.e., "errors of omission") [17]. For example, common errors of omission include the underprescribing of osteoporosis treatments to patients who suffer hip fractures and the underprescribing of angiotensin converting enzyme (ACE) inhibitors to patients with diabetes (Level 2c evidence) [38]. Potential undertreatment is especially important for older adults who suffer from multiple chronic diseases. Concerns over polypharmacy must be balanced against the need to adequately treat associated comorbid conditions in order to reduce the risk of complications. Interestingly, one study from the Netherlands found a strong relationship between polypharmacy (defined as the concomitant use of five or more drugs) and underprescribing [39]. Another study by Steinman and colleagues found that inappropriate medication use and underuse were common in older people taking five or more medications, with both simultaneously present in more than 40% of patients studied [40]. Inappropriate medication use was most frequent in patients taking many medications, but underuse was also common and the authors felt underprescribing merits attention regardless of the total number of medications taken [40].

Clinical bottom line

Inappropriate prescribing is a complex and dynamic concept that encompasses both errors of commission and errors of omission. Various consensus groups have developed lists of common examples of errors of commission and omission in order to assist clinicians who prescribe medications for the elderly. Promising interventions to reduce inappropriate prescribing include multidisciplinary case conferences involving a geriatrician, computerized support systems, and a pharmacist in the care of hospitalized older adults [33–35].

What strategies can clinicians employ to optimize prescribing in individual older patients?

Although drugs-to-avoid criteria (such as the Beers Criteria, IPET, MAI, and STOPP) are valuable to identify medications that are generally inappropriate for most older adults, the different approaches often yield widely discordant rates of inappropriate prescribing and likely reflect different aspects of the complex, mul-

tifaceted concept of "prescribing quality" [41]. These criteria are also insufficiently accurate to act as stand-alone measures of prescribing quality, particularly in the clinical care of individual older patients [42]. Most of these criteria do not provide an integrated framework that is easy to implement in the clinic or at the bedside, and most are unable to comprehensively consider the individual patient's goals of care and treatment preferences.

What evidence-based strategies are then available to assist the clinician confronted by an elderly patient's complex and lengthy medication list? Unfortunately, evidence to support any interventions in this is limited. As described in the Introduction, geriatricians and pharmacists typically promote a strategy involving systematic review of a patient's medication list (using the "brown bag" or medication reconciliation approach). Although medication reconciliation is appealing from an intuitive perspective, a systematic review found little good quality evidence to demonstrate the effectiveness of medication reconciliation in the primary care setting (Level 1a evidence) [43]. As described previously, a systematic review of pharmacist-led interventions for hospitalized adults did find benefits from the addition of their services, but this review also recommended further study to strengthen the evidence base supporting this approach (Level 1a evidence) [34]. Of course, pharmacist expertise is not limited simply to medication reconciliation, and unfortunately many clinicians are unable to access a clinical pharmacist to assist with routine patient care. Despite the limited empirical evidence for the effectiveness of periodic medication reconciliation, the Assessing Care of Vulnerable Elders (ACOVE) project recommends medication review at least once per year as an important measure of care quality in older adults (Level 5 evidence) [44]. Functional decline or the development of geriatric syndromes such as falls are often atypical presentations of adverse drug effects in the elderly, and should also trigger careful medication review [37]. Iyer and colleagues have systematically reviewed RCTs of drug withdrawal in older adults, and these RCTs provide evidence for the short-term effectiveness and/or lack of harm associated with withdrawal of several classes of drugs (e.g., antihypertensives, benzodiazepines, and psychotropic agents) (Level 1a evidence) [45]. Garfinkel and colleagues have described the Good Palliative-Geriatric Practice algorithm for drug discontinuation, which has been used successfully in two studies to reduce medication burden in nursing home residents and community-dwelling older adults [46, 47]. One of these studies found the algorithm was associated with significant reductions in mortality, referrals to acute care, and drug costs (Level 1b evidence) [46].

Incorporating an individual's goals of care and preferences is also important, although limited empirical evidence exists to support this statement. Holmes and colleagues have proposed a practical strategy whereby life expectancy, time to realization of treatment benefit, primary goals of care (e.g., prevention, cure, or palliation), and validity of specific treatment targets (e.g., blood pressure) are integrated to decide on appropriate treatments for older individuals with the aim of minimizing unwarranted polypharmacy (Level 5 evidence) [48]. As mentioned in Introduction, caution should be exercised when applying disease-specific clinical practice guidelines to older adults with multiple chronic diseases [11, 12].

Clinical bottom line

Further research is needed to better establish effective strategies to optimize prescribing in individual older patients. Promising interventions include periodic medication reconciliation, ideally in collaboration with a pharmacist. The individual patient's goals of care and preferences should be incorporated into prescribing decisions.

Once we identify optimal prescribing, how can we promote long-term adherence to these medications?

Terminology: persistence, compliance, and adherence

Persistence generally refers to the accumulation of time during which a medication is taken, from the time it is initiated until the time it is discontinued. Compliance is the proportion of medication taken at a given time according to instructions while a patient is persistent. The term "compliance" has been viewed as having paternalistic overtones, and therefore, more recently many authors have preferred to use the term "adherence," which is thought to better reflect a therapeutic alliance between the prescribing physician and the patient [49].

Long-term adherence to effective medications is necessary to derive the full benefits of treatment. The level of adherence necessary to achieve benefit from a medication varies by drug class, but many studies use a cutoff of 80% to separate high from low adherence rates [50]. Inadequate adherence is associated with failure to reach therapeutic goals (e.g., target lipid levels or blood pressure), and worse clinical outcomes including higher mortality (Level 2c evidence) [51, 52]. In one RCT involving 7599 subjects with heart failure, good adherence (>80%) to assigned treatment—even if it was placebo—resulted in better outcomes than poor adherence to the active medication (Level 2c evidence) [50].

Factors that influence drug adherence include the patient's comprehension of the treatment regimen and its benefits, adverse effects, medication costs, and regimen complexity, as well as their comorbid conditions (especially untreated depression, cognitive impairment, and the overall burden of comorbid disease). Nonadherence rates in the elderly can run as high as 84% [8]. In general, there is a correlation between the total number of drugs prescribed and the level of nonadherence [8]. Nonadherence is underreported by patients and can be challenging to detect. Physicians should therefore remain vigilant for suboptimal adherence as an explanation for not achieving treatment goals (Level 5 evidence).

To improve long-term drug adherence, particularly for elderly patients who have complex drug regimens, effective communication between the prescribing physician and the patient is critical. It is important to set time aside to collaborate with the patient in order to reach goals of treatment tailored to the individual, and to adequately educate them about the benefits of medications, particularly those medications that are used for preventative reasons rather than immediate symptom control. Ongoing communication should also explore reasons such as adverse drug effects, low mood, cognitive impairment, and socioeconomic factors that might impact drug adherence. Simple strategies to improve adherence such as the use of pharmacy-issued weekly blister packs or dosette boxes can also provide some support for patients with complex medication regimens. More than 60 RCTs have evaluated strategies to improve adherence (Level 1a evidence) [53]. Almost all of the interventions that were effective in improving long-term adherence were complex and labor-intensive, including combinations of more convenient care, information, reminders, self-monitoring, reinforcement, counseling, family therapy, psychological therapy, crisis intervention, manual telephone follow-up, and supportive care. Although even the most effective interventions did not lead to large improvements in adherence and treatment outcomes, they can still improve important clinical outcomes and overall costs of care (Level 1a evidence) [53]. In a systematic review of eight RCTs focused on elderly individuals prescribed multiple medications, adherence was improved in relative terms by a mean of 11% through use of regularly scheduled patient follow-up visits, multicompartment dose administration aids, pharmacist-led medication reviews, and group education combined with individualized medication cards (Level 1a evidence) [54]. Another systematic review demonstrated that multidisciplinary chronic disease management programs targeted to patients with heart failure improve adherence and survival, and reduce readmissions, but such programs are resource intense (Level 1a evidence) [55].

Clinical bottom line

Clinicians should maintain a high index of suspicion for drug nonadherence in patients who fail to achieve treatment targets (e.g., blood pressure goals on antihypertensive drugs, lipid targets on lipid lowering agents). If nonadherence is suspected, physicians should look for depression and cognitive impairment as contributing factors. In addition, drug adherence may be influenced by the patient's understanding of a medication's benefits, adverse effects, and costs, as well as overall medication regimen complexity. Strategies shown to improve adherence often focus on communication and improving the patient's understanding of the indications for treatment. Although labor-intensive, effective interventions can improve clinical outcomes and long-term costs of care.

Summary

Achieving optimal medication prescribing is a constant challenge for clinicians who care for older adults with multiple comorbid conditions. It is difficult to draw general conclusions given the very broad spectrum of medications that are commonly used by older adults. Nonetheless, research detailed in this chapter has high-lighted a variety of strategies to reduce inappropriate prescribing and its consequences.

Acknowledgment

Dr. Sudeep Gill is supported by a New Investigator Award from the Canadian Institutes of Health Research (CIHR). Dr. Dallas Seitz is supported by a Postdoctoral Fellowship Award from the Alzheimer Society of Canada.

References

1. Dans AL, Dans LF, Guyatt GH, Richardson S (1998) Users' guides to the medical literature: XIV. How to decide on the applicability of clinical trial results to your patient. Evidence-Based Medicine Working Group. *JAMA* 279(7): 545–549.
2. Glasziou P, Guyatt GH, Dans AL, Dans LF, Straus S, Sackett DL (1998) Applying the results of trials and systematic reviews to individual patients. *ACP J Club* 129(3): A15–A16.
3. Sismondo S (2008) Pharmaceutical company funding and its consequences: a qualitative systematic review. *Contemp Clin Trials* 29(2): 109–113.
4. Lee PY, Alexander KP, Hammill BG, Pasquali SK, Peterson ED (2001) Representation of elderly persons and women in published randomized trials of acute coronary syndromes. *JAMA* 286(6): 708–713.
5. Evans A, Kalra L (2001) Are the results of randomized controlled trials on anticoagulation in patients with atrial fibrillation generalizable to clinical practice? *Arch Intern Med* 161(11): 1443–1447.
6. Heiat A, Gross CP, Krumholz HM (2002) Representation of the elderly, women, and minorities in heart failure clinical trials. *Arch Intern Med* 162(15): 1682–1688.
7. Gill SS, et al (2004) Representation of patients with dementia in clinical trials of donepezil. *Can J Clin Pharmacol* 11(2): e274–e285.
8. Scott IA, Guyatt GH (2010) Cautionary tales in the interpretation of clinical studies involving older persons. *Arch Intern Med* 170(7): 587–595.
9. Witham MD, McMurdo MET (2007) How to get older people included in clinical studies. *Drugs Aging* 24(3): 187–196.
10. UyBico SJ, Pavel S, Gross CP (2007) Recruiting vulnerable populations into research: a systematic review of recruitment interventions. *J Gen Intern Med* 22(6): 852–863.
11. Tinetti ME, Bogardus ST, Jr., Agostini JV (2004) Potential pitfalls of disease-specific guidelines for patients with multiple conditions. *N Engl J Med* 351(27): 2870–2874.
12. Boyd CM, Darer J, Boult C, Fried LP, Boult L, Wu AW (2005) Clinical practice guidelines and quality of care for older patients with multiple comorbid diseases: implications for pay for performance. *JAMA* 294(6): 716–724.
13. Brown AF, Mangione CM, Saliba D, Sarkisian CA (2003) Guidelines for improving the care of the older person with

diabetes mellitus. *J Am Geriatr Soc* 51(5 Suppl Guidelines): S265–S280.

14. American Heart Association Council on Clinical Cardiology, Society of Geriatric Cardiology, Alexander KP, et al (2007) Acute coronary care in the elderly, part I: non-ST-segment-elevation acute coronary syndromes: a scientific statement for healthcare professionals from the American Heart Association Council on Clinical Cardiology: in collaboration with the Society of Geriatric Cardiology. *Circulation* 115(19): 2549–2569.

15. American Heart Association Council on Clinical Cardiology, Society of Geriatric Cardiology, Alexander KP, et al (2007) Acute coronary care in the elderly, part II: ST-segment-elevation myocardial infarction: a scientific statement for healthcare professionals from the American Heart Association Council on Clinical Cardiology: in collaboration with the Society of Geriatric Cardiology. *Circulation* 115(19): 2570–2589.

16. Braithwaite RS, Concato J, Chang CC, Roberts MS, Justice AC (2007) A framework for tailoring clinical guidelines to comorbidity at the point of care. *Arch Intern Med* 167(21): 2361–2365.

17. Higashi T, et al (2004) The quality of pharmacologic care for vulnerable older patients. *Ann Intern Med* 140(9): 714–720.

18. Steinman MA, Hanlon JT (2010) Managing medications in clinically complex elders: "There's got to be a happy medium". *JAMA* 304(14): 1592–1601.

19. Spinewine A, et al (2007) Appropriate prescribing in elderly people: how well can it be measured and optimised? *Lancet* 370(9582): 173–184.

20. Mallet L, Spinewine A, Huang A (2007) The challenge of managing drug interactions in elderly people. *Lancet* 370(9582): 185–191.

21. Beers MH, Ouslander JG, Rollingher I, Reuben DB, Brooks J, Beck JC (1991) Explicit criteria for determining inappropriate medication use in nursing home residents. UCLA Division of Geriatric Medicine. *Arch Intern Med* 151(9): 1825–1832.

22. Fick DM, Cooper JW, Wade WE, Waller JL, Maclean JR, Beers MH (2003) Updating the Beers criteria for potentially inappropriate medication use in older adults: results of a US consensus panel of experts. *Arch Intern Med* 163(22): 2716–2724. *Erratum in: Arch Intern Med* 2004 164(3): 298.

23. Naugler CT, Brymer C, Stolee P, Arcese ZA (2000) Development and validation of an improving prescribing in the elderly tool. *Can J Clin Pharmacol* 7(2): 103–107.

24. McLeod PJ, Huang AR, Tamblyn RM, Gayton DC (1997) Defining inappropriate practices in prescribing for elderly people: a national consensus panel. *CMAJ* 156(3): 385–391.

25. Hanlon JT, et al (1992) A method for assessing drug therapy appropriateness. *J Clin Epidemiol* 45: 1045–51.

26. Gallagher P, Ryan C, Byrne S, Kennedy J, O'Mahony D (2008) STOPP (Screening Tool of Older Person's Prescriptions) and START (Screening Tool to Alert doctors to Right Treatment). Consensus validation. *Int J Clin Pharmacol Ther* 46(2): 72–83.

27. Barry PJ, Gallagher P, Ryan C, O'Mahony D (2007) START (Screening Tool to Alert doctors to the Right Treatment) – an evidence-based screening tool to detect prescribing omissions in elderly patients. *Age Ageing* 36: 628–631.

28. Levy HB, Marcus EL, Christen C (2010) Beyond the Beers criteria: a comparative overview of explicit criteria. *Ann Pharmacother* 44(12): 1968–1975.

29. Brophy JM, Joseph L, Rouleau JL (2001) Beta-blockers in congestive heart failure. A Bayesian meta-analysis. *Ann Intern Med* 134(7): 550–560.

30. Gallagher P, et al (2009) Inter-rater reliability of STOPP (Screening Tool of Older Persons' Prescriptions) and START (Screening Tool to Alert doctors to Right Treatment) criteria amongst physicians in six European countries. *Age Ageing* 38(5): 603–606.

31. Klarin I, Wimo A, Fastbom J (2005) The association of inappropriate drug use with hospitalisation and mortality: a population-based study of the very old. *Drugs Aging* 22(1): 69–82.

32. Lau DT, Kasper JD, Potter DE, Lyles A, Bennett RG (2005) Hospitalization and death associated with potentially inappropriate medication prescriptions among elderly nursing home residents. *Arch Intern Med* 165(1): 68–74.

33. Kaur S, Mitchell G, Vitetta L, Roberts MS (2009) Interventions that can reduce inappropriate prescribing in the elderly: a systematic review. *Drugs Aging* 26(12): 1013–1028.

34. Kaboli PJ, Hoth AB, McClimon BJ, Schnipper JL (2006) Clinical pharmacists and inpatient medical care: a systematic review. *Arch Intern Med* 166(9): 955–964.

35. Gillespie U, et al (2009) A comprehensive pharmacist intervention to reduce morbidity in patients 80 years or older: a randomized controlled trial. *Arch Intern Med* 169(9): 894–900.

36. Good CB (2002) Polypharmacy in elderly patients with diabetes. *Diabetes Spectr* 15(4): 240–248.

37. Inouye SK, Studenski S, Tinetti ME, Kuchel GA (2007) Geriatric syndromes: clinical, research, and policy implications of a core geriatric concept. *J Am Geriatr Soc* 55(5): 780–791.

38. Winkelmayer WC, Fischer MA, Schneeweiss S, Wang PS, Levin R, Avorn J (2005) Underuse of ACE inhibitors and angiotensin II receptor blockers in elderly patients with diabetes. *Am J Kidney Dis* 46(6): 1080–1087.

39. Kuijpers MA, van Marum RJ, Egberts AC, Jansen PA (2008) OLDY (OLd people Drugs & dYsregulations) Study Group. Relationship between polypharmacy and underprescribing. *Br J Clin Pharmacol* 65(1): 130–133.

40. Steinman MA, Landefeld CS, Rosenthal GE, Berthenthal D, Sen S, Kaboli PJ (2006) Polypharmacy and prescribing quality in older people. *J Am Geriatr Soc* 54(10): 1516–1523.

41. Steinman MA, Rosenthal GE, Landefeld CS, Bertenthal D, Sen S, Kaboli PJ (2007) Conflicts and concordance between measures of medication prescribing quality. *Med Care* 45(1): 95–99.

42. Steinman MA, Rosenthal GE, Landefeld CS, Bertenthal D, Kaboli PJ (2009) Agreement between drugs-to-avoid criteria and expert assessments of problematic prescribing. *Arch Intern Med* 169(14): 1326–1332.

43. Bayoumi I, Howard M, Holbrook AM, Schabort I (2009) Interventions to improve medication reconciliation in primary care. *Ann Pharmacother* 43(10): 1667–1675.

44. Shrank WH, Polinski JM, Avorn J (2007) Quality indicators for medication use in vulnerable elders. *J Am Geriatr Soc* 55(suppl 2): S373–S382.

45. Iyer S, Naganathan V, McLachlan AJ, Le Couteur DG (2008) Medication withdrawal trials in people aged 65 years and older: a systematic review. *Drugs Aging* 25(12): 1021–1031.

46. Garfinkel D, Zur-Gil S, Ben-Israel J (2007) The war against polypharmacy: a new cost-effective geriatric-palliative approach for improving drug therapy in disabled elderly people. *Isr Med Assoc J* 9(6): 430–434.

47. Garfinkel D, Mangin D (2010) Feasibility study of a systematic approach for discontinuation of multiple medications in older adults: addressing polypharmacy. *Arch Intern Med* 170(18): 1648–1654.

48. Holmes HM, Hayley DC, Alexander GC, Sachs GA (2006) Reconsidering medication appropriateness for patients late in life. *Arch Intern Med* 166(6): 605–609.

49. Badamgarav E, Fitzpatrick LA (2006) A new look at osteoporosis outcomes: the influence of treatment, compliance, persistence, and adherence. *Mayo Clin Proc* 81(8): 1009–1012.

50. Granger BB, et al (2005) Adherence to candesartan and placebo and outcomes in chronic heart failure in the CHARM programme: double-blind, randomised, controlled clinical trial. *Lancet* 366(9502): 2005–2011.

51. Simpson SH, et al (2006) A meta-analysis of the association between adherence to drug therapy and mortality. *BMJ* 333(7557): 15.

52. Sokol MC, McGuigan KA, Verbrugge RR, Epstein RS (2005) Impact of medication adherence on hospitalization risk and healthcare cost. *Med Care* 43(6): 521–530.

53. Haynes RB, Ackloo E, Sahota N, McDonald HP, Yao X (2008) Interventions for enhancing medication adherence. *Cochrane Database Syst Rev* (2): CD000011.

54. George J, Elliott RA, Stewart DC (2008) A systematic review of interventions to improve medication taking in elderly patients prescribed multiple medications. *Drugs Aging* 25(4): 307–324.

55. McAlister FA, Stewart S, Ferrua S, McMurray JJ (2004) Multidisciplinary strategies for the management of heart failure patients at high risk for admission: a systematic review of randomized trials. *J Am Coll Cardiol* 44(4): 810–819.

CHAPTER 4

Breathing easier: respiratory disease in the older adult

Salahaddin Mahmudi-Azer

Clinical Fellow, Department of Critical Care Medicine, Foothills Hospital, University of Calgary, AB Canada

Introduction

There is an accumulating body of evidence indicating that age-related cellular, structural, and physiological changes in the respiratory system contribute to alterations in organ function [1–3]. These age-related changes in the respiratory system may result in alteration of symptoms, clinical presentation, response to treatment, and can also impact the overall functioning of the older adult [4]. At a cellular level, airway receptors undergo functional changes with age and are less responsive to various medications [5–7]. Structural and physiological changes associated with aging lead to an increase in alveolar dead space, which affects arterial oxygenation without impairing carbon dioxide elimination [8]. Respiratory function and exercise capacity also change with age [9].

The prevalence of pulmonary diseases increases with age and the clinical presentation of many of these conditions may be atypical in the older patient. This difference is due in part to a decrease in respiratory reserve, blunting of hypoxic and hypercarbic drive, and decreased perception of dyspnea [10, 11]. This decreased sensation of dyspnea and diminished ventilatory response to hypoxia and hypercapnia make the older patient more vulnerable to ventilatory failure during high-demand states (i.e., heart failure, pneumonia, etc.) and possible poor outcomes [12].

In this chapter, we highlight the specific geriatric respiratory diseases in which the pathophysiology, diagnosis, and/or treatment are often different from those in younger adults. Specifically, we focus on asthma, chronic obstructive pulmonary disease (COPD), pneumonia, tuberculosis (TB), obstructive sleep apnea (OSA), and lung cancer.

Search strategy

The search was performed in MEDLINE (using OVID) in 2010. To capture pulmonary function citations, the focus MESH term for lung was exploded using "anatomy & histology," "metabolism," "physiology," "ultrastructure" as subheadings. The focused lung terms were then combined with MESH terms for "thoracic wall," "respiration" or "respiratory muscles." These sets were further combined with terms for "aging" and "aged." The search was limited to English language, humans, and specific study types such as topic reviews (Cochrane), multicenter study, and meta-analysis.

A similar strategy was used for asthma, using the exploded, focused asthma MESH terms and optimized clinical queries hedges for "therapy," "diagnosis," "prognosis," "reviews," "etiology," and "clinical prediction guides." This set was combined with terms for "aged" and "aging," and the same language and study

Evidence-Based Geriatric Medicine: A Practical Clinical Guide, First Edition. Edited by Jayna M. Holroyd-Leduc and Madhuri Reddy.
© 2012 Blackwell Publishing Ltd. Published 2012 by Blackwell Publishing Ltd.

type limitations as above were applied. The MESH term "*pulmonary disease," "chronic obstructive" with either subheadings for "diagnosis," "therapy," "drug therapy," "epidemiology," "mortality," "physiopathology," "prevention & control," or "surgery" or "clinical queries" hedges were searched as above. The MESH terms "*pneumonia," "exp *Tuberculosis," "*sleep apnea," and "exp *lung neoplasms" were all treated the same way with restrictions to aged, English language, study types. The relevant end sets were combined.

For this chapter, relevant clinical studies were graded using the Oxford Centre for Evidence-based Medicine Levels of Evidence.

How should I treat my older patient with asthma?

Asthma in the older adult is more common than was previously recognized. Symptoms of asthma in the older population may mislead physicians to consider other causes such as COPD and heart failure [13, 14]. The underrecognition and undertreatment of asthma may in part account for the rise in asthma-related deaths in individuals older than 65 years of age [15, 16]. Furthermore, older individuals with asthma tend to attribute their shortness of breath to aging and often underestimate their disease and delay seeking medical advice [17]. Patient-related factors, such as psychomotor and cognitive disabilities, may also affect the optimal management of asthma in the older adult [18–20].

A number of anatomic and physiologic changes seen in asthma have been described in the normal aging lung. The aging process and associated alterations in lung function could be a predisposing factor for asthma [21–23].

Although the evidence is limited, it appears that principles of asthma treatment (e.g., corticosteroid use for maintenance and exacerbation of asthma; inhaled β-agonists or anticholinergic as rescue medications) should not change with advancing age (Level 5 evidence) [24, 25]. In the medical management of asthma, there are a number of therapeutic concerns unique to older patients. The higher likelihood of adverse effects of asthma treatment in the setting of multiple comorbidities and problems with effective drug delivery are two important therapeutic challenges [26, 27].

Age and strength seem not to be important predictors of good inhaler technique. Cognitive function can

impact use of metered-dose inhalers (MDI) in people aged 75 and older. Assessment of cognitive function is essential in older patients in whom inhaled therapy is being contemplated [28, 29]. The choice of delivery system in cognitively impaired patients may be limited to nebulized therapy, given that nebulizers do not require patient cooperation or coordination and can facilitate the fast delivery of large doses of β2-agonist, anticholinergics, and corticosteroids to the lungs [27].

While some studies have suggested that responsiveness to β2-agonist decreases with age, β2-agonists are probably of benefit in older patients with asthma (Level 2b evidence) [30–32]. A number of side effects have been attributed to nebulized β2-agonists. Commonly documented side effects, which are caused by systemic absorption of β2-agonists, are tremors, palpitations, dysrhythmias, and hypokalemia. Patients with a history of myocardial infarction seem to be at greater risk of serious dysrhythmia following nebulized β2-agonists treatment, thus necessitating an extra level of caution in this population [33, 34]. β2-Agonists are known to cause a net influx of intravascular potassium into cells leading to hypokalemia. Given a number of other potential compounding factors in older patients including treatment with diuretics, treatment with insulin, and poor nutritional intake, they are often at greater risk of hypokalemia than other age groups [35].

Clinical bottom line

Asthma often goes unrecognized and undertreated in the older patient. Principles of asthma treatment should not change with advancing age, though caution needs to be exercised when using β2-agonists.

The choice of medication delivery may be impacted by cognitive function.

Older patients also need to be monitored more closely for medication side effects, particularly if they have comorbid diseases.

How should COPD be managed in my older patient?

COPD is one of the most common chronic diseases in the world and is the fourth leading cause of death [36]. The prevalence of COPD increases with age [37]. In addition to age, factors known to be predictors of poor survival in COPD include low FEV1, the presence of cor pulmonale, low lean body weight, and residence at higher altitudes [37–39].

COPD is considered a largely preventable condition. Cigarette smoking is the major risk factor. Other risk factors that are less common and only account for 4% of COPD include occupational exposures to mineral and grain dusts, second hand cigarette smoke, and α-1 antitrypsin deficiency [40–42]. In the center of the pathogenesis of COPD is an enhanced inflammatory response. Current research is focusing on a number of key areas including a newly discovered regulatory cytokine IL-32, antioxidant defense systems, apoptosis, and cell aging [43–46].

Smoking cessation is the most important intervention in the care of patients who have COPD. Smoking cessation is known to slow the accelerated rate of decline in lung function and in older patients improves health and reduces mortality regardless of the severity of the disease (Level 1b evidence) [47, 48]. Male smokers who quit at age 65 years stand to gain 2.0 years of life expectancy and female smokers who quit at age 65 years stand to gain 3.7 years [49]. Various interventions in smoking cessation, including physician counseling, behavioral therapy, nicotine replacement (Level 2b evidence) [50], bupropion (Level 1b evidence) [51], and varenicline (Level 1b evidence) [52, 53], are known to be effective and well tolerated in those aged 65–75 years. Despite the importance of smoking cessation, physicians are less likely to advise smoking cessation to older patients [54].

Two main categories of bronchodilators used in management of COPD are (1) β-agonists and (2) anticholinergics. Short-acting bronchodilators increase exercise tolerance, decrease hyperinflation, and decrease the sensation of dyspnea (Level 2b evidence) [55, 56]. Combination therapy with short-acting β-agonists and anticholinergics (ipratropium) seems to be superior to either of these treatments alone and may improve spirometry and reduce the need for systemic steroids (Level 1a evidence) [57–59].

Long-acting β-agonists (LABA) are effective in improving lung function, health status, and frequency of exacerbations compared with placebo (Level 1a evidence) [60, 61]. LABA have been found to be superior to short-acting ipratropium in improving lung function (Level 1b evidence) [62]. A combination therapy with LABA and ipratropium improves lung function and quality of life (QOL) more than either agent alone (Level 1a evidence) [63]. Compared with placebo and with ipratropium, the long-acting anticholinergic agent tiotropium improves lung function, dyspnea, and QOL (Level 1b evidence) [64, 65]. While no significant differences were found when tiotropium was compared with LABA in frequency of exacerbations or hospitalizations (Level 1a evidence) [66], tiotropium was found to be superior in improving lung function (Level 1b evidence) [67, 68].

The role of steroids in the management of COPD has not been definitively established. While the use of inhaled corticosteroids in COPD does not affect the progressive decline in FEV1, their use has been associated with some improvement in lung function, airway reactivity, frequency of exacerbations, and respiratory symptoms (Level 1b evidence) [69–72]. The effect of a combination of inhaled salmeterol–fluticasone on COPD progression has been compared with tiotropium in two large randomized controlled trials. The UPLIFT (Understanding Potential Long-term Impacts on Function with Tiotropium) study showed that therapy with tiotropium was associated with improvements in lung function, QOL, and exacerbations during a 4-year period but it did not significantly reduce the rate of decline in FEV1 (Level 1b evidence) [73]. The analysis from the TORCH (TOward a Revolution in COPD Health) study revealed that patients treated with salmeterol/fluticasone propionate had a slower rate of lung function decline compared with patients receiving a placebo over 3 years (Level 1b evidence) [74]. This is the first study to show that a therapeutic intervention, apart from smoking cessation, can slow the progression of COPD.

In addition to respiratory status, a number of other factors are known to impact the QOL and functional status in COPD patients. Anxiety and depression in older adults seem to influence not only respiratory symptoms but also functional status and QOL [75, 76]. In patients with COPD, new onset of depression is a risk factor for the development of cognitive decline [77, 78]. Interestingly, QOL measures seem to correlate more with depression than spirometry or exercise tolerance [79, 80]. In older patients, anxiety is associated with limitation in physical functioning and disability and is a major predictor for the frequency of hospital admission for the exacerbation of COPD [81–83]. Early detection and treatment of depression and anxiety may play an important role in improving

QOL for patients who have COPD. In a study from the United Kingdom, use of the antidepressant paroxetine for at least 3 months was associated with significant improvement in depression and exercise tolerance in those with COPD (Level 2b evidence) [84].

Palliative care, end of life, and caregiver issues are other significant aspects of COPD care in older patients. It is difficult to identify when a patient who has COPD might be entering the terminal phase. Most of the available treatments of COPD are aimed at symptom-control, so the relevance of clear distinctions between active and palliative treatment in many patients becomes only obvious in periods of severe exacerbations and respiratory instability [85–87].

Older patients need to be monitored closely for medication side effects, particularly if they have comorbid diseases.

Clinical bottom line

The prevalence of COPD increases with age.

Smoking cessation is the most important intervention in the care of patients with COPD.

Short-acting or long-acting β-agonists combined with anticholinergics seem to be superior to either treatment alone.

It is important to address concomitant depression and anxiety, as they can impact symptoms, functional status, and QOL.

How should pneumonia be treated in the older patient?

Pneumonia is associated with a high rate of morbidity and mortality in older patients. Poor prognosis of pneumonia in the older patient may be secondary to factors such as burden of other comorbidities, atypical clinical signs and symptoms, greater risk for organ failure (respiratory, renal, or cardiac), and greater functional loss [88].

Every year, approximately 5% of individuals over the age of 85 will present with a new episode of community-acquired pneumonia (CAP) [89]. The higher incidence of pneumonia among the older adult may be related to host defense factors, other comorbidities, and the frail state of the patient [90, 91].

A pathogenic etiology has been identified in 39% of patients: 15% were viruses, 20% bacteria, and 4% mixed [92–94]. The most commonly isolated bacterial pathogen seems to be *Streptococcus pneumoniae* [92, 95]. Other potential pathogens include *Mycoplasma*, *Haemophilus influenzae*, *Legionella pneumophila*, *Chlamydia pneumoniae*, and Gram-negative bacilli. The more common viral infections are influenza, human metapneumovirus (hMPV), and respiratory syncytial virus (RSV). Viral etiologies seem to be more prevalent in older patients with comorbidities such as cardiac diseases and frailty. The only symptom specifically associated with viral pneumonia is myalgia [95, 96].

The unreliability of sputum Gram's stain and culture, in addition to the impracticality of serologic testing in the acute setting, probably contribute to the low diagnostic yield in determining the etiology of pneumonia [97, 98]. Normal oropharyngeal flora is often discounted as contamination, but may in fact account for a significant number of cases of CAP. The overall incidence of anaerobic lung infection secondary to aspiration may be as high as 21%–33%. Anaerobic organisms may be second only to *S. pneumoniae* as a potential cause of pneumonia in older patients [99, 100].

Legionella pneumonia is often associated with a more severe clinical syndrome. The higher mortality rate of pneumonia in older patients may in part be accounted for by a disproportionate number of cases of *L. pneumophila* pneumonia [101, 102]. Determining the severity of pneumonia, particularly on presentation, is important in treatment and prediction of prognosis. Severity of the disease within the context of other comorbidities will help in guiding the extent of the investigations, nature of treatment (inpatient vs. outpatient), potential complications, and consideration of intensive care unit admission.

The mainstay of pneumonia treatment is the use of antibiotics and supportive care in all age groups. Pneumonia is rarely defined microbiologically at presentation, so empirical antibiotics are used for its treatment. Most of CAP can be treated successfully with a narrow-spectrum β-lactam agent and a macrolide (Level 2b evidence) [103]. Severity of the disease can be used as a guide for the type of antibiotic and method of administration (e.g., oral vs. intravenous) (Level 2a evidence) [104]. Studies have shown that treatment with intravenous and oral moxifloxacin gives similar results as ceftriaxone and levofloxacin in hospitalized patients (Level 1b evidence) [105]. Combined ceftriaxone/azithromycin treatment is as effective as ceftriaxone and clarithromycin but more comfortable for hospitalized patients (Level 1b evidence) [106]. In adult patients with moderately severe CAP, a 7-day treatment course has been found to be as well tolerated and as effective as 14 days of treatment (Level 1a evidence) [107]. Treatment with 750-mg levofloxacin for 5 days is comparable to 500-mg levofloxacin for 10 days (Level 1b evidence) [108].

Opinions are divided in regard to the use of corticosteroids as additional treatment, and currently it is not widely recommended as standard treatment (Level 2a evidence) [109]. Some authors have observed a decrease in mortality in patients with severe CAP treated with systemic antibiotics and corticosteroids (Level 2b evidence) [110–112], but they have not been recommended as adjuvant therapy for pneumonia (Level 2a evidence) [113].

Clinical bottom line

Pneumonia is associated with a high rate of morbidity and mortality in older adults.

Severity of the pneumonia within the context of other comorbidities helps to guide treatment in the older population. Most CAP can be treated successfully with a narrow-spectrum β-lactam agent and a macrolide. Antibiotic courses beyond 7 days do not appear to be required.

Is my older patient at risk for TB?

TB remains a widespread infectious disease of global significance, with more than 2 billion people estimated to be infected [114]. Over the last several decades, the proportion of older patients with TB in the economically developed world has increased significantly, a rise that is not explained by an increase in the proportion of older persons in the population. By the late 1980s, older adults comprised the single largest group of patients with active TB in the developed world and an increasing proportion of deaths attributed to TB occurred in this group [115].

While a significant percentage (80%–90%) of cases of TB in the older population occurs among patients from the community, there is a comparatively higher (two- to threefold) incidence of active TB among long-term care residents [116].

Strength of reaction to tuberculin decreases with age leading to a decrease in the sensitivity of the tuberculin skin test (PPD). PPD continues to be used for screening purposes in all age groups despite its poor sensitivity and high false-negative rate in older patients [117]. To assure that false-negative reactions in the older age group are recognized, it is recommended that all older persons who undergo a tuberculin skin test be retested within 2 weeks of a negative response [118]. Chest radiography is recommended in the setting of a positive tuberculin skin test reaction.

The majority of TB cases in the older population involve the respiratory tract, and is the result of reactivation disease. Although reactivation TB typically involves the upper lobes of the lung (apical and posterior segments), a number of studies have shown that pulmonary TB infection in many older patients manifests in either the middle or the lower lung lobes [119–121].

TB can present atypically in older patients. The classical features of TB such as cough, hemoptysis, fever, night sweats, and weight loss may be absent in older patients and it may present instead with nonspecific clinical findings such as changes in functional capacity, chronic fatigue, cognitive impairment, anorexia, or unexplained low-grade fever [122, 123]. Miliary TB, TB meningitis, and skeletal and genitourinary TB seem to be more prevalent among patients with advanced age [124, 125].

Treatment for active TB in older patients is the same as for younger adults. Most cases of active TB in older patients result from reactivation of latent infection and the vast majority of cases are caused by strains of *M. tuberculosis*, which are susceptible to regular treatments (e.g., isoniazid and rifampin). Exceptions to this includes older patients from a country or region where the prevalence of drug-resistant *M. tuberculosis* is high, patients who have had previously inadequate chemotherapy treatments, or patients who acquired the infection from a contact known to be infected with multidrug resistant TB (MDR-TB) [124]. While the presence of MDR-TB may not be as significant in the older population, the treatment of TB is complicated by a number of other factors including poor adherence with treatment, poor tolerance of therapy, and the presence of underlying or associated comorbidities [126, 127]. Therapy that is directly observed twice a week has been advocated as an extremely important measure to improve adherence with therapy and thus to limit the emergence of drug resistance [128]. The older patient also requires close monitoring for treatment side effects such as liver impairment.

The long course of TB treatment has been one of the main obstacles in its successful management. Attempts to develop therapies with shorter duration that remain effective for the treatment of MDR-TB have lead to several novel therapeutic interventions currently under different phases of clinical development [129, 130]. Preliminary animal studies replacing current chemotherapy regimes with a combination of moxifloxacin and rifapentine, or linezolid for a shorter treatment course have shown promise but require clinical trials to confirm safety and effectiveness [131–133].

Clinical bottom line

The tuberculin skin test is less sensitive in the older patient, so all older persons with negative tests should be retested in 2 weeks. If the tuberculin skin test is positive, chest radiography is the next step in diagnosis.

TB may present with nonspecific clinical findings in the older patient. Most cases of active TB in older patients result from reactivation of latent infection and are susceptible to regular treatments. Treatment for active TB in older patients is the same as for younger adults.

How do I manage my older patients with obstructive sleep apnea?

OSA is a condition characterized by repeated episodes of apnea and hypopnea during sleep. OSA occurs when there are recurrent periods of complete or partial upper airway collapse that result in inadequate airflow and oxygenation despite ongoing respiratory muscle effort [134, 135]. There is stepwise increase in the prevalence of OSA with advancing age [136, 137]. Among adults aged 30–60 years, the prevalence of OSA is 9% for women and 24% for men [138], while in adults older than 60 years the prevalence is reported in the range of 38%–62% [139, 140]. The observed higher prevalence of OSA among older adults may in part be secondary to conditions such as obesity, diabetes, renal failure, heart disease, hypothyroidism, and stroke, which are known risk factors for OSA and are common in older adults [141–144]. However, it is important to note that a number of studies have shown increased OSA prevalence with age in the absence of known comorbidities [145–147]. In addition to age, male sex, and family

Table 4.1 Potentially modifiable risk factors for obstructive sleep apnea

Alcohol consumption
Cigarette smoking
Hypertension
Obesity
Diabetes mellitus
Renal Failure
Stroke
Heart failure
Atrial fibrillation

history, there are a number of potentially modifiable risk factors for OSA (Table 4.1) [141–144, 148].

Many of the typical signs and symptoms associated with sleep apnea in the general population may be absent in the older adult (Table 4.2) [149, 150]. OSA may be underdiagnosed in older adults given they may be less likely to seek medical attention and attribute symptoms, such as sleepiness, fatigue, morning headache, and concentration difficulties, to aging or to other disorders [151].

More limited methods such as portable home studies and simple overnight oximetry may have a role in screening for OSA in certain high-risk populations,

Table 4.2 Symptoms and physical signs associated with obstructive sleep apnea

Symptoms	Physical Signs
Loud snoring[a]	Elevated BMI[a]
Witnessed apneas[a]	Truncal obesity[a]
Excessive daytime somnolence	Large neck girth[a]
Night sweats	Micrognathia
Nonrestorative sleep	Macroglossia
Headaches on awakening	Tonsillar hypertrophy

[a]Magnitude of association decreases with advancing age.

but they lack critical data obtained from overnight-attended polysomnography (the diagnostic "gold standard") and may underestimate apnea severity (Level 2a evidence) [152].

The diagnosis and treatment of OSA is critical because of its association with impaired QOL, cognitive function, and cardiovascular morbidity and mortality. Large cross-sectional studies have shown that after correcting for known confounding factors, blood pressure increases linearly with severity of OSA [153, 154]. Similarly, another observational cohort study with median follow-up time of 3.4 years has shown that OSA is significantly associated with stroke or death (adjusted hazard ratio, 1.97; 95% confidence interval (CI) 1.12–3.48) [155]. In older adults, higher severity of OSA is also associated with lower executive function, decrease in mini mental status examination scores, impaired attention, impaired memory, and sequential thinking [156, 157]. Treatment of OSA is associated with improvement in cardiac function, reduction in blood pressure, reduction in recurrent atrial fibrillation, and decrease in mortality (Level 2b evidence) [158, 159]. Much remains to be learned about the efficacy of medical management of OSA in older adults.

Weight loss, alcohol avoidance, and thyroid replacement therapy in hypothyroid patients seems to be effective in decreasing the severity and in some cases curing OSA (Level 2b evidence) [160–162]. Another management measure for OSA is the avoidance of supine positioning during sleep (Level 2b evidence) [163].

The mainstay of treatment for OSA is continuous positive airway pressure (CPAP). A systematic review of 26 studies has shown that CPAP therapy has a significant positive impact on subjective sleepiness, depression, fatigue, and general health-related QOL (Level 2a evidence) [164]. CPAP therapy may be difficult for some to tolerate. Patient education about OSA and the benefits of CPAP, as well as evaluating potential obstacles encountered during CPAP therapy, has been shown to improve compliance in older adults [165]. Patients with Alzheimer's disease and OSA tolerated CPAP treatment well, thus poor cognitive function may not be a precluding factor in a trial CPAP therapy in older adults with OSA (Level 2b evidence) [166].

Clinical bottom line

OSA may be underdiagnosed in older adults given that they may attribute symptoms to aging or to other disorders. OSA is associated with cardiovascular morbidity and mortality, as well as cognitive dysfunction.

There are several potentially modifiable risk factors for OSA (Table 4.1).

While some of the typical signs and symptoms of OSA, such as nonrestful sleep and excessive daytime somnolence may be present in older adults, others such as loud snoring, elevated BMI, and large neck circumference may be absent (Table 4.2).

Overnight-attended polysomnography should be used for the diagnosis of OSA.

Weight loss, avoiding alcohol consumption, and thyroid replacement therapy in hypothyroid patients seem to have a role in the management of OSA. However, CPAP is the main form of treatment.

How is lung cancer managed in the older patient?

Lung cancer is considered a disease of aging [166] as 80% of lung cancer deaths occur in patients over the age of 60, with approximately 20% occurring in patients over the age of 80 [167, 168]. Cigarette smoking is the major risk factor for lung cancer and is influenced by smoking intensity and duration [169, 170] and abrogated by smoking cessation over time, even in persons who have smoked into the sixth decade of life [171]. Other recognized risk factors include a family history of lung cancer, exposures to occupational carcinogens, exposure to environmental tobacco smoke, air pollution, and underlying lung disease, including chronic airflow obstruction, and fibrosing pulmonary disorders [172, 173].

Older patients with lung cancer are significantly underrepresented in all clinical trials, though data obtained from these trials are routinely extended to older patients in clinical practice [174]. This may well lead to pharmacodynamic consequences, especially with drugs that require conversion to active intermediates, given changes in total body water, and renal and hepatic functions with aging [175]. The treatment of lung cancer in the older patient is further complicated by an increased likelihood of drug–drug interactions and treatment-related toxicities, the higher prevalence of comorbid conditions, and concerns regarding increased perioperative morbidity and mortality [176, 177].

Performance status, which incorporates elements of physical activity, cognition, ability to perform work, self-care, and mobility, is widely used in the evaluation of appropriate treatment and prognosis of lung cancer treatment. Studies have shown that dementia, poor nutritional status, and the absence of social support are all associated with decreased survival [178–180].

The most common form of lung cancer is nonsmall-cell lung carcinoma (NSCLC), which is comprised of the histological categories of squamous cell, large cell, and adenocarcinomas. Until recently, treatments for all forms of NSCLC have been grouped together. However, newer treatment paradigms have focused increasingly on unique histology, tumor protein expression, and gene mutation [181, 182]. Performance status, histology, and stage are the three major determinants of optimal treatment recommendations and survival for NSCLC [183].

Surgery is considered the treatment of choice for stages I, II, and some subsets of stage IIIA NSCLC. Advances in surgical techniques have paved the way for inclusion of increasing numbers of older patients in surgical studies. Yet, the debate around age and surgical treatment of NSCLC continues. Several studies support the role of surgical interventions in the treatment of NSCLC in the older patient and do not consider age a negative prognostic factor for long-term postoperative survival (Level 2b evidence) [184, 185]. Other studies support an association between increased age and occurrence of postoperative mortality and morbidity (Level 3a-4 evidence) [186, 187].

Radiation therapy may be a potential treatment alternative for medically inoperable patients who have early stage NSCLC. Radiofrequency ablation and stereotactic body radiation are two relatively new techniques that are currently used in select patient populations with NSCLC; however, long-term survival data are not yet available [188, 189].

In advanced NSCLC, chemotherapy remains the main stay of therapy [190, 191]. An accumulating body of evidence also supports the use of adjuvant chemotherapy in patients with earlier stage disease [191]. However, a number of factors including other comorbidities, age-related decline in organ function, and pharmacological interactions make chemotherapy more challenging in the older population. Despite these challenges, retrospective and prospective trials indicate that fit older patients derive similar benefit from chemotherapy as their younger counterparts (Level 2b evidence) [190, 191].

The recent data from randomized adjuvant clinical trials and meta-analysis have changed the standard of care for patients with completely resected NSCLC. Adjuvant cisplatin-based chemotherapy is associated with a significant survival benefit, with a 5.3% absolute increase in 5-year overall survival, in favor of adjuvant chemotherapy compared with no further treatment (Level 1a evidence) [192]. A recent pooled analysis of the effect of age on outcome after adjuvant cisplatin-based chemotherapy indicated that age did not impact the benefit from cisplatin adjuvant chemotherapy and, while more older patients died from noncancer-related causes, no significant difference was observed regarding toxicity [193].

The other form of lung cancer is small-cell lung cancer (SCLC). With increasing life expectancy and the aging of our population, the number of older patients with SCLC is expected to increase [194]. About 32% of newly diagnosed SCLC cases occur in patients older than 70 years of age, whereas approximately 10% of cases are diagnosed in patients older than 80 years of age [195]. SCLC is characterized by a rapid doubling time and early dissemination, leading to its overall poor prognosis. This rapid doubling time makes SCLC highly sensitive to chemotherapy and radiotherapy, and development of drug resistance during the course of disease [196]. Staging of SCLC is based on the Veterans Administration Lung Study Group system, which classifies patients as having either limited-stage (disease that is limited to 1 hemithorax, with hilar and mediastinal nodes that can be encompassed within one tolerable radiotherapy portal) or extensive-stage disease [197]. Approximately 65%–70% of patients with SCLC have disseminated or extensive disease at presentation [198].

The standard treatment for limited disease is chemotherapy plus radiotherapy [198]. Data on overall survival and treatment toxicity in older patients with limited-stage SCLC remains divided. Some studies have shown that the overall survival rates are significantly lower and treatment toxicities significantly higher in older age groups (Level 2b evidence) [199, 200]. Other studies, including retrospective, age-specific subgroup analyses have shown that toxicity, overall response rate, progression-free survival, and overall survival did not differ significantly among patients older and younger than 70 years of age (Level 2b evidence) [201–203]. A number of studies have shown that older patients received less intensive treatment in terms of chemotherapy dose or number of cycles [199, 203]. The prognosis for extensive stage SCLC remains poor, but evidence-informed practice guidelines suggest combination chemotherapy is the treatment of choice in patients with extensive-stage SCLC; the addition of radiation does not seem to improve survival [204].

Clinical bottom line

Eighty percent of lung cancer deaths occur in patients over the age of 60.

Cigarette smoking is the major risk factor for lung cancer but the risk is abrogated by smoking cessation. Performance status is widely used in the evaluation of appropriate treatment and prognosis of lung cancer in the older patient.

Chapter summary

Age-related changes in the respiratory system may result in alteration of symptoms, clinical presentation, response to treatment, and can also impact the overall functioning of the older adult.

Asthma often goes unrecognized and undertreated in the older patient. Principles of asthma treatment should not change with advancing age, though caution needs to be exercised when using β2-agonists. The choice of medication delivery can be affected by cognitive status.

The prevalence of COPD increases with age. Smoking cessation is the most important intervention in the care of patients who have COPD. β-Agonists and anticholinergics are widely used in the management of COPD. Short-acting or long-acting β-agonists combined with anticholinergics seem to be superior to either treatment alone.

Pneumonia is associated with a high rate of morbidity and mortality in older patients. Severity of the pneumonia within the context of other comorbidities will help in guiding treatment. Most CAP can be treated successfully with a narrow-spectrum β-lactam agent and a macrolide.

The proportion of older patients with TB is on the rise, especially among long-term care residents. Since the tuberculin skin test is less sensitive in the older patient, older persons with negative tests should be retested in 2 weeks. If the tuberculin skin test is positive, chest radiography is the next step in diagnosis. TB may present with nonspecific clinical findings in the older patient. Most cases of active TB in older patients result from reactivation of latent infection and are susceptible to regular treatments. Treatment for active TB in older patients is the same as for younger adults.

OSA may be underdiagnosed in older adults, even though its prevalence increases with age. OSA is associated with cardiovascular morbidity and mortality, as well as cognitive dysfunction. There are several potentially modifiable risk factors for OSA (Table 4.1). Overnight-attended polysomnography should be used for the diagnosis of OSA. Weight loss, avoiding alcohol consumption, and thyroid replacement therapy in hypothyroid patients seem to have a role in the management of OSA. However, CPAP is the main form of treatment.

The majority of lung cancer deaths occur in patients over the age of 60. Cigarette smoking is the major risk factor for lung cancer but the risk is abrogated by smoking cessation. Performance status is widely used in the evaluation of appropriate treatment and prognosis of lung cancer in the older patient.

References

1. Sharma G, Goodwin J (2006) Effect of aging on respiratory system physiology and immunology. *Clin Interv Aging* 1(3): 253–260.
2. Tolep K, Kelsen SG. (1993) Effects of aging on respiratory skeletal muscles. *Clin Chest Med* 14: 63–378.
3. Enright PL, et al (1994) Respiratory muscle strength in the elderly. *Am J Respir Crit Care Med* 149: 30–438.
4. Britto RR, Zampa CC, de Oliveira TA, Prado LF, Parreira VF (2009) Effects of the aging process on respiratory function. *Gerontology* 55: 505–510.
5. Feldman RD, et al (1984) Alterations in leukocyte β-adrenergic affinity with aging. A potential explanation of altered β-adrenergic sensitivity in the elderly. *N Engl J Med* 310: 815–819.
6. Hopp RJ, et al (1985) The effect of age on methacholine response. *J Allergy Clin Immunol* 76: 609–613.
7. Korenblatt PE, et al (2000) Effect of age on response to zafirlucast in patients with asthma in the accolate clinical experience pharmacoepidemiology trial (ACCEPT). *Ann Allergy Asthma Immunol* 84: 217–225.
8. Knudson RJ, et al (1976) The maximal expiratory flow±volume curve: normal standards, variability, effects of age. *Am Rev Respir Dis* 113: 587–599.

9. Hollenberg M, et al (2006) Longitudinal changes in aerobic capacity: implications for concepts of aging. *J Gerontol A Biol Sci Med Sci* 61(8): 851–858.

10. Hawkins, SA, Wiswell RA (2003) "Rate and mechanism of maximal oxygen consumption decline with aging: implications for exercise training. *Sports Medicine* 33(12): 877–888.

11. Peterson DD, et al (1981) Effects of aging on ventilatory and occlusion pressure responses to hypoxia and hypercapnia. *Am Rev Respir Dis* 124: 387–391.

12. Kronenberg RS, Drage CW (1973) Attenuation of the ventilatory and heart rate responses to hypoxia and hypercapnea with aging in normal men. *J Clin Invest* 52: 1912–1919.

13. Enright PL, et al (1999) Underdiagnosis and undertreatment of asthma in the elderly. Cardiovascular health study research group. *Chest* 116: 603–613.

14. Chotirmall SH, et al (2009) Diagnosis and management of asthma in older adults. *J Am Geriatr Soc* 57: 901–909.

15. Robin ED. (1988) Risk benefit analysis in chest medicine: death from bronchial asthma. *Chest* 93: 614–618.

16. Sly RM (1984) Increases in deaths from asthma. *Ann Allergy* 53: 20–25.

17. Cuttitta G, et al (2001) Changes in FVC during methacholine induced bronchoconstriction in elderly patients with asthma. Bronchial hyperresponsiveness and aging. *Chest* 119: 1685–1690.

18. Hartert TV, et al (2000) Underutilization of controller and rescue medications among older adults with asthma requiring hospital care. *J Am Geriatr Soc* 48: 651–657.

19. Busse PJ, Kilaru K (2009) Complexities of diagnosis and treatment of allergic respiratory disease in the elderly. *Drugs Aging* 26: 1–22.

20. Barua P, O'Mahony MS (2005) Overcoming gaps in the management of asthma in older patients: new insights. *Drugs Aging* 22: 1029–1059.

21. Todo Bom A, Mota Pinto A (2009) Allergic respiratory diseases in the elderly. *Respir Med* 103: 1614–1622.

22. Braman SS, Hanania NA (2007) Asthma in older adults. *Clin Chest Med* 28: 685–702.

23. Chotirmall SH, et al (2009) Diagnosis and management of asthma in older adults. *J Am Geriatr Soc* 57: 901–909.

24. Chotirmall SH, et al (2009) Diagnosis and management of asthma in older adults. *J Am Geriatr Soc* 57(5): 901–909.

25. King MJ, Hanania NA (2010) Asthma in the elderly: current knowledge and future directions. *Curr Opin Pulm Med* 16(1): 55–59.

26. Braman SS, Hanania NA (2007) Asthma in older adults. *Clin Chest Med* 28: 685–702.

27. Barua P, O'Mahony MS (2005) Overcoming gaps in the management of asthma in older patients: new insights. *Drugs Aging* 22: 1029–1059.

28. Allen SC (1997) Competence thresholds for use of inhalers in people with dementia. *Age Ageing* 26: 83–86.

29. Hindle M, Newton DAG, Chrystyn H (1995) Dry powder inhalers are bioequivalent to metered-dose inhalers. A study using a new urinary salbutamol assay technique. *Chest* 107: 629–633.

30. Connolly MJ, et al (1994) Peripheral mononuclear leukocyte b adrenoceptors and non-specific bronchial responsiveness to metacholine in young and elderly normal subjects and asthmatic patients. *Thorax* 49: 26–32.

31. Geraghty R, et al (1993) Bronchodilator response to nebulised salbutamol in elderly patients with stable chronic airflow limitation. *Respir Med* 87: 375–378.

32. Ullah MI, Newman GB, Saunders KB (1981) Influence of ageing on response to ipratropium and salbutamol in asthma. *Thorax* 36: 523–529.

33. Brashear RE (1984) Arrhythmias in patients with chronic obstructive pulmonary disease. *Med Clin North Am* 68: 969–981.

34. Lim R, et al (1989) Cardiac arrhythmias during acute exacerbations of chronic airflow limitation: effect of fall in plasma potassium concentration induced by nebulised beta 2-agonist therapy. *Postgrad Med J* 65: 449–452.

35. Smith SR, et al (1984) Cardiovascular and biochemical responses to nebulised salbutamol in normal subjects. *Br J Clin Pharmacol* 18: 641–644.

36. Rutten-van Molken M (2009) Raising the awareness: projecting the future burden of COPD with the BOLD model, *Eur Respir J* 134: 787–789.

37. Traver GA, Cline MG, Rurrows R (1979) Predictors of mortality in chronic obstructive pulmonary disease. A 15-year follow-up study. *Am Rev Respir Dis* 119(6): 895–902.

38. Cote TR, et al (1993) Chronic obstructive pulmonary disease mortality: a role for altitude. *Chest* 103: 1194–1197.

39. Wilson DO, et al (1989) Body weight in chronic obstructive pulmonary disease: The National Institutes of Health Intermittent Positive Pressure Breathing Trial. *Am Rev Respir Dis* 139: 1435–1438.

40. Raherison C, Girodet P-O (2009) Epidemiology of COPD. *Eur Respir Rev* 18: 213–221.

41. Halbert RJ, et al (2006) Global burden of COPD: systematic review and meta-analysis. *Eur Respir J* 28: 523–532.

42. Recklake MR (1989) Occupational exposures: evidence for a causal association with chronic obstructive pulmonary disease. *Am Rev Respir Dis* 140: S85–S91.

43. Calabrese F, et al (2008) IL-32, a, novel proinflammatory cytokine in chronic obstructive pulmonary disease. *Am J Resp Care Crit Med* 178: 894–901.

44. Malhotra D, et al (2008) Decline in NRF2-regulated antioxidants in chronic obstructive pulmonary disease lungs due to loss of its positive regulator, DJ-1. *Am J Respir Crit Care Med* 78: 592–604.

45. Houben JM, et al (2009) Telomere shortening in chronic obstructive pulmonary disease. *Respir Med* 103: 230–236.

46. Morissette MC, et al (2008) Increased p53 level, Bax/Bco-XL ratio and TRAIL receptor expression in human emphysema. *Am J Respir Crit Care Med* 178: 240–247.

47. Pelkonen M, et al (2001) Smoking cessation, decline in pulmonary function and total mortality: a 30-year follow up study among the Finnish cohorts of the Seven Countries Study. *Thorax* 56(9): 703–707.

48. Vollset SE, Tverdal A, Gjessing HK (2006) Smoking and deaths between 40 and 70 years of age in women and men. *Ann Intern Med* 144(6): 381–389.

49. Taylor DH Jr, et al (2002) Benefits of smoking cessation for longevity. *Am J Public Health* 92(6): 990–996.

50. Tait RJ, et al (2007) Effectiveness of a smoking cessation intervention in older adults. *Addiction* 102(1): 148–155.

51. Hurt RD, et al (1997) A comparison of sustained-release bupropion and placebo for smoking cessation. *N Engl J Med* 337(17): 1195–1202.

52. Gonzales D, et al (2006) Varenicline, an alpha4beta2 nicotinic acetylcholine receptor partial agonist, vs sustained-release bupropion and placebo for smoking cessation: a randomized controlled trial. *JAMA* 296(1): 47–55.

53. Jorenby DE, et al (2006) Efficacy of varenicline, an alpha4beta2 nicotinic acetylcholine receptor partial agonist, vs placebo or sustained release bupropion for smoking cessation: a randomized controlled trial. *JAMA* 296(1): 56–63.

54. Maguire CP, et al (2000) Do patient age and medical condition influence medical advice to stop smoking? *Age Ageing* 29(3): 264–266.

55. Belman MJ, Botnick WC, Shin JW (1996) Inhaled bronchodilators reduce dynamic hyperinflation during exercise in patients with chronic obstructive pulmonary disease. *Am J Respir Crit Care Med* 153(3): 967–975.

56. O'Donnell DE, Lam M, Webb KA (1999) Spirometric correlates of improvement in exercise performance after anticholinergic therapy in chronic obstructive pulmonary disease. *Am J Respir Crit Care Med* 160(2): 542–549.

57. COMBIVENT Inhalation Aerosol Study Group (1994) In chronic obstructive pulmonary disease, a combination of ipratropium and albuterol is more effective than either agent alone. An 85-day multicenter trial. *Chest* 105(5): 1411–1419.

58. Appleton S, et al (2006) Ipratropium bromide versus short acting beta-2 agonists for stable chronic obstructive pulmonary disease. *Cochrane Database Syst Rev* 2: CD001387.

59. The COMBIVENT Inhalation Solution Study Group (1997) Routine nebulized ipratropium and albuterol together are better than either alone in COPD. *Chest* 112(6): 1514–1521.

60. Appleton S, et al (2006) Long-acting beta2-agonists for poorly reversible chronic obstructive pulmonary disease. *Cochrane Database Syst Rev* 3: D001104.

61. Jones PW, Bosh TK (1997) Quality of life changes in COPD patients treated with salmeterol. *Am J Respir Crit Care Med* 155(4): 1283–1289.

62. Dahl R, et al (2001) Inhaled formoterol dry powder versus ipratropium bromide in chronic obstructive pulmonary disease. *Am J Respir Crit Care Med* 164(5): 778–784.

63. Appleton S, et al (2006) Ipratropium bromide versus long-acting beta-2 agonists for stable chronic obstructive pulmonary disease. *Cochrane Database Syst Rev* 3: CD006101.

64. Casaburi R, et al (2002) A long term evaluation of once-daily inhaled tiotropium in chronic obstructive pulmonary disease. *Eur Respir J* 19(2): 217–224.

65. Vincken W, et al (2002) Improved health outcomes in patients with COPD during 1 yr's treatment with tiotropium. *Eur Respir J* 19(2): 209–216.

66. Barr RG, et al (2003) Tiotropium for stable chronic obstructive pulmonary disease: a meta-analysis. *Thorax* 61(10): 854–862.

67. Brusasco V, et al (2003) Health outcomes following treatment for six months with once daily tiotropium compared with twice daily salmeterol in patients with COPD. *Thorax* 58(5): 399–404.

68. Donohue JF, et al (2002) A 6-month, placebo-controlled study comparing lung function and health status changes in COPD patients treated with tiotropium or salmeterol. *Chest* 122(1): 47–55.

69. Wise R, et al (2000) Effect of inhaled triamcinolone on the decline in pulmonary function in chronic obstructive pulmonary disease. *N Engl J Med* 343(26): 1902–1909.

70. Burge PS, et al (2000) Randomised double blind, placebo controlled study of fluticasone propionate in patients with moderate to severe chronic obstructive pulmonary disease: the ISOLDE trial. *BMJ* 320(7245): 1297–1303.

71. Pauwels RA, et al (1999) Long-term treatment with inhaled budesonide in persons with mild chronic obstructive pulmonary disease who continue smoking. European Respiratory Society Study on chronic obstructive pulmonary disease. *N Engl J Med* 340(25): 1948–1953.

72. Vestbo J, et al (1999) Long-term effect of inhaled budesonide in mild and moderate chronic obstructive pulmonary disease: a randomized controlled trial. *Lancet* 353(9167): 1819–1823.

73. Tashkin DP, et al (2008) A 4-year trial of tiotropium in chronic obstructive pulmonary disease. *N Engl J Med* 359: 1543–1554.

74. Celli BR, et al (2008) Effect of pharmacotherapy on rate of decline of lung function in chronic obstructive pulmonary disease: results from the TORCH study. *Am J Respir Crit Care Med* 178: 332–338.

75. Cully JA, et al (2006) Quality of life in patients with chronic obstructive pulmonary disease and comorbid anxiety or depression. *Psychosomatics* 47(4): 312–319.

76. Peruzza S, et al (2003) Chronic obstructive pulmonary disease (COPD) in elderly subjects: impact on functional status and quality of life. *Respir Med* 97(6): 612–617.

77. Yohannes AM, Baldwin RC, Connolly MJ (2000) Depression and anxiety in elderly outpatients with chronic obstructive pulmonary disease: prevalence, and validation of the BASDEC screening questionnaire. *Int J Geriatr Psychiatry* 15(12): 1090–1096.

78. Incalzi RA, et al (1998) Predicting cognitive decline in patients with hypoxaemic COPD. *Respir Med* 92(3): 527–533.

79. Yohannes AM, et al (1998) Depression in elderly outpatients with disabling chronic obstructive pulmonary disease. *Age Ageing* 27(2): 155–160.

80. Engstrom CP, et al (1996) Functional status and well being in chronic obstructive pulmonary disease with regard to clinical parameters and smoking: a descriptive and comparative study. *Thorax* 51(8): 825–830.

81. Yellowlees PM, et al (1987) Psychiatric morbidity in patients with chronic airflow obstruction. *Med J Aust* 146(6): 305–307.

82. Cully JA, et al (2006) Quality of life in patients with chronic obstructive pulmonary disease and comorbid anxiety or depression. *Psychosomatics* 47(4): 312–319.

83. Bosley CM, et al (1996) Psychological factors associated with use of home nebulized therapy for COPD. *Eur Respir J* 9(11): 2346–2350.

84. Eiser N, et al (2005) Effect of treating depression on quality-of-life and exercise tolerance in severe COPD. *COPD* 2(2): 233–241.

85. Lynn J, et al (2000) Living and dying with chronic obstructive pulmonary disease. *J Am Geriatr Soc* 48(5 Suppl): S91–S100.

86. Elkington H, et al (2004) The last year of life of COPD: a qualitative study of symptoms and services. *Respir Med* 98(5): 439–445.

87. Gore JM, Brophy CJ, Greenstone MA (2000) How well do we care for patients with end stage chronic obstructive pulmonary disease (COPD)? A comparison of palliative care and quality of life in COPD and lung cancer. *Thorax* 55(12): 1000–1006.

88. Lee CC, et al (2007) Comparison of clinical manifestations and outcome of community-acquired bloodstream infections among the oldest old, elderly, and adult patients. *Medicine (Baltimore)* 86: 138–144.

89. Jackson ML, et al (2004) The burden of community acquired pneumonia in seniors: results of a population-based study. *Clin Infect Dis* 39: 1642–1650.

90. Phair JP, Kauffman CA, Rjornson A (1978) Investigation of host defense mechanisms in the aged as determinants of nosocomial colonization and pneumonia. *J Reticuloendothel Soc* 23: 397–405.

91. Miller RA (1996) The aging immune system: primer and prospectus. *Science* 273: 70–74.

92. Charles PG, et al (2008) The etiology of community-acquired pneumonia in Australia: why penicillin plus doxycycline or a macrolide is the most appropriate therapy. *Clin Infect Dis* 46: 1513–1521.

93. Johnstone J, et al (2008) Viral infection in adults hospitalized with community acquired pneumonia: prevalence, pathogens and presentation. *Chest* 134: 1141–1148.

94. Jennings LC, et al (2008) Incidence and characteristics of viral community-acquired pneumonia in adults. *Thorax* 63: 42–48.

95. Díaz A, et al (2007) Etiology of community-acquired pneumonia in hospitalized patients in Chile: the increasing prevalence of respiratory viruses among classic pathogens. *Chest* 131: 779–787.

96. Camps Serra M, et al (2008) Virological diagnosis in community-acquired pneumonia in immunocompromised patients. *Eur Respir J* 31: 618–624.

97. Miyashita N, et al (2008) Assessment of the usefulness of sputum Gram stain and culture for diagnosis of community-acquired pneumonia requiring hospitalization. *Med Sci Monit* 14(4): CR171–CR176.

98. Weatherall C, Paoloni R, Gottlieb T (2008) Point-of-care urinary pneumococcal antigen test in the emergency department for community acquired pneumonia. *Emerg Med J* 25: 144–148.

99. Hill MK, Sanders CV (1991) Anaerobic disease of the lung. *Infect Dis Clin North Am* 5: 453–456.

100. Rartlett JG (1987) Anaerobic bacterial infections in the lung. *Chest* 91: 901–909.

101. Niven DJ, Laupland KB (2009) Severe community-acquired pneumonia in adults: current antimicrobial chemotherapy. *Expert Rev Anti Infect Ther* 7(1): 69–81.

102. Janssens JP (2005) Pneumonia in the elderly (geriatric) population. *Curr Opin Pulm Med* 11(3): 226–230.

103. Charles PG, et al (2008) The etiology of community-acquired pneumonia in Australia: why penicillin plus doxycycline or a macrolide is the most appropriate therapy. *Clin Infect Dis* 46: 1513–1521.

104. Niederman MS, et al (2001) Guidelines for the management of adults with community-acquired pneumonia: diagnosis, assessment of severity, antimicrobial therapy, and prevention. *Am J RespirCrit Care Med* 163: 1730–1754.

105. Torres A, et al (2008) Moxifloxacin monotherapy is effective in hospitalized patients with community-acquired pneumonia: the MOTIV study a randomized clinical trial. *Clin Infect Dis* 46: 1499–1509.

106. Tamm M, et al (2007) Clinical and bacteriological outcomes in hospitalised patients with community-acquired pneumonia treated with azithromycin plus ceftriaxone, or ceftriaxone plus clarithromycin or erythromycin: a prospective, randomised, multicentre study. *Clin Microbiol Infect* 13: 162–171.

107. Dimopoulos G, et al (2008) Short- versus long-course antibacterial therapy for community-acquired pneumonia: a metaanalysis. *Drugs* 68: 1841–1854.

108. Shorr AF, et al (2006) Levofloxacin 750-mg for 5 days for the treatment of hospitalized fine risk class III/IV community-acquired pneumonia patients. *Respir Med* 100: 2129–2136.

109. Salluh JI, et al (2008) The role of corticosteroids in severe community-acquired pneumonia: a systematic review. *Crit Care* 12: R76.

110. Garcia-Vidal C, et al (2007) Effects of systemic steroids in patients with severe community-acquired pneumonia. *Eur Respir J* 30: 951–956.

111. Mikami K, et al (2007) Efficacy of corticosteroids in the treatment of community-acquired pneumonia requiring hospitalization. *Lung* 185: 249–255.

112. Siempos II, et al (2008) Adjunctive therapies for community-acquired pneumonia: a systematic review. *J Antimicrob Chemother* 62: 661–668.

113. Gorman SK, Slavik RS, Marin J (2007) Corticosteroid treatment of severe community-acquired pneumonia. *Ann Pharmacother* 41: 1233–1237.

114. Lonnroth K, Raviglione M (2008) Global epidemiology of tuberculosis: prospects for control. *Semin Respir Crit Care Med* 29: 481.

115. Stead WW, Lofgren JP (1983) Does the risk of tuberculosis increase in old age? *J Infect Dis* 147: 951–955.

116. Stead WW (1989) Special problems in tuberculosis: tuberculosis in the elderly and in residential homes, correctional facilities, long-term care hospitals, mental hospitals, shelters for the homeless, and jails. *Clin Chest Med* 10: 397–405.

117. Marais BJ, et al (2009) Screening and preventive therapy for tuberculosis. *Clin Chest med* 30(4): 827–846.

118. Taylor Z, Nolan CM, Blumberg HM (2005) Controlling tuberculosis in the United States. Recommendations from the American Thoracic Society, CDC, and the Infectious Diseases Society of America. *MMWR Recomm Rep* 54(RR–12): 1–81.

119. Furqan M, Butler J (2010) Miliary pattern on chest radiography: TB or not TB? *Mayo Clin Proc* 85(2): 108.

120. Yoshikawa TT (1992) Tuberculosis in aging adults. *J Am Geriatr Soc* 40: 178–187.

121. Perez-Guzman C, et al (1999) Does aging modify pulmonary tuberculosis? A meta-analytical review. *Chest* 116: 961–967.

122. Towhidi M, Azarian A, Asnaashari A (2008) Pulmonary tuberculosis in the elderly. *Tanaffos* 7(1): 52–57.

123. Yoshikawa TT (1994) The challenge and unique aspects of tuberculosis in older patients. *Infect Dis Clin Pract* 3: 62–66.

124. Yoshikawa TT (1992) Tuberculosis in aging adults. *J Am Geriatr Soc* 40: 178–187.

125. Dutt AK, Stead WW (1993) Tuberculosis in the elderly. *Med Clin North Am* 77: 1353–1368.

126. Mackoy AD, Cole RB (1984) The problems of tuberculosis in the elderly. *QJ Med* 212: 497–510.

127. Nagami PH, Yoshikawa TT (1983) Tuberculosis in the geriatric patient. *J Am Geriatr Soc* 31(6): 356–363.

128. Chaulk CP, Pope DS (1997) The Baltimore City Department Program of directly observed therapy for tuberculosis. *Clin Chest Med* 18: 149–154.

129. O'Brien RJ, Spigelman M (2005) New drugs for tuberculosis: current status and future prospects. *Clin Chest Med* 26: 327–340.

130. Spigelman MK (2007) New tuberculosis therapeutics: a growing pipeline. *J Infect Dis* 196(Suppl 1): S28–S34.

131. Rosenthal IM, et al (2007) Daily dosing of rifapentine cures tuberculosis in three months or less in the murine model. *PLoS Med* 4: e344.

132. Rosenthal IM, et al (2008) Isoniazid or moxifloxacin in rifapentine-based regimens for experimental tuberculosis? *Am J Respir Crit Care Med* 178: 989–993.

133. Alcala L, et al (2003) In vitro activities of linezolid against clinical isolates of mycobacterium tuberculosis that are susceptible or resistant to first-line antituberculous drugs. *Antimicrob Agents Chemother* 47: 416–417.

134. Horner RL, et al (1989) Pharyngeal size and shape during wakefulness and sleep in patients with obstructive sleep apnea? *Q J Med* 72(268): 719–735.

135. Tsuiki S, et al (2003) Supine-dependent changes in upper airway size in awake obstructive sleep apnea patients. *Sleep Breath* 7(1): 43–50.

136. Hoch CC, et al (1990) Comparison of sleep-disordered breathing among healthy elderly in the seventh, eighth, and ninth decades of life. *Sleep* 13: 502–511.

137. Young T, et al (2002) Predictors of sleep-disordered breathing in community dwelling adults: the Sleep Heart Health Study. *Arch Intern Med* 162(8): 893–900.

138. Young T, et al (1993) The occurrence of sleep-disordered breathing among middle-aged adults. *N Engl J Med* 328: 1230–1235.

139. Ancoli-Israel S, et al (1981) Sleep apnea and nocturnal myoclonus in a senior population. *Sleep* 4(4): 349–358.

140. Ancoli-Israel S, et al (1991) Sleep-disordered breathing in community dwelling elderly. *Sleep* 14: 486–495.

141. Ancoli-Israel S, et al (2001) Long-term follow-up of sleep disordered breathing in older adults. *Sleep Med* 2(6): 511–516.

142. Wierzbicka A, et al (2006) The incidence of sleep apnea in patients with stroke or transient ischemic attack. *J Physiol Pharmacol* 57(4): 385–390.

143. Peltier AC, et al (2007) Autonomic dysfunction in obstructive sleep apnea is associated with impaired glucose regulation. *Sleep Med* 8(2): 149–155.

144. Skjodt NM, Atkar R, Easton PA (1999) Screening for hypothyroidism in sleep apnea. *Am J Respir Crit Care Med* 160: 732–735.

145. Malhotra A, et al (2006) Aging influences on pharyngeal anatomy and physiology: the predisposition to pharyngeal collapse. *Am J Med* 119(1): 72.e9–e14.

146. Worsnop C, et al (2000) Effect of age on sleep onset-related changes in respiratory pump and upper airway muscle function. *J Appl Physiol* 88(5): 1831–1839.

147. Eikermann M, et al (2007) The influence of aging on pharyngeal collapsibility during sleep. *Chest* 131(6): 1702–1709.

148. Kaparianos A, et al (2006) Obstructive sleep apnoea syndrome and genes. *Neth J Med* 64(8): 280–289.

149. Endeshaw Y (2006) Clinical characteristics of obstructive sleep apnea in community-dwelling older adults. *J Am Geriatr Soc* 54(11): 1740–1744.

150. Cohen-Zion M, et al (2001) Changes in cognitive function associated with sleep disordered breathing in older people. *J Am Geriatr Soc* 49(12): 1622–1627.

151. Groth M (2005) Sleep apnea in the elderly. *Clin Geriatr Med* 21: 701–712.

152. Flemons WW, et al (2003) Home diagnosis of sleep apnea: a systematic review of the literature. An evidence review cosponsored by the American Academy of Sleep Medicine, the American College of Chest Physicians, and the American Thoracic Society. *Chest* 124(4): 1543–1579.

153. Young T, et al (1997) Population-based study of sleep-disordered breathing as a risk factor for hypertension. *Arch Intern Med* 157(15): 1746–1752.

154. Nieto FJ, et al (2000) Association of sleep-disordered breathing, sleep apnea, and hypertension in a large community-based study. Sleep Heart Health Study. *JAMA* 283(14): 1829–1836.

155. Yaggi HK, et al (2005) Obstructive sleep apnea as a risk factor for stroke and death. *N Engl J Med* 353(19): 2034–2041.

156. Cohen-Zion M, et al (2004) Cognitive changes and sleep disordered breathing in elderly: differences in race. *J Psychosom Res* 56(5): 549–553.

157. Aloia MS, et al (2003) Neuropsychological changes and treatment compliance in older adults with sleep apnea. *J Psychosom Res* 54(1): 71–76.

158. Shamsuzzaman AS, Gersh BJ, Somers VK (2003) Obstructive sleep apnea: implications for cardiac and vascular disease. *JAMA* 290(14): 1906–1914.

159. Doherty LS, et al (2005) Long-term effects of nasal continuous positive airway pressure therapy on cardiovascular outcomes in sleep apnea syndrome. *Chest* 127(6): 2076–2084.

160. Peppard PE, et al (2000) Longitudinal study of moderate weight change and sleep-disordered breathing. *JAMA* 284(23): 3015–3021.

161. Peppard PE, Austin D, Brown RL (2007) Association of alcohol consumption and sleep disordered breathing in men and women. *J Clin Sleep Med* 3(3): 265–270.

162. Rajagopal KR, et al (1984) Obstructive sleep apnea in hypothyroidism. *Ann Intern Med* 101(4): 491–494.

163. Berger M, et al (1997) Avoiding the supine position during sleep lowers 24 h blood pressure in obstructive sleep apnea (OSA) patients. *J Hum Hypertens* 11(10): 657–664.

164. McMahon JP, Foresman BH, Chisholm RC (2003) The influence of CPAP on the neurobehavioral performance of patients with obstructive sleep apnea hypopnea syndrome: a systematic review. *WMJ* 102(1): 36–43.

165. Aloia MS, et al (2001) Improving compliance with nasal CPAP and vigilance in older adults with OSAHS. *Sleep Breath* 5(1): 13–22.

166. Chong MS, et al (2006) Continuous positive airway pressure reduces subjective daytime sleepiness in patients with mild to moderate Alzheimer's disease with sleep disordered breathing. *J Am Geriatr Soc* 54(5): 777–781.

167. Taofeek K., et al (2007) Lung cancer in elderly patients: an analysis of the surveillance, epidemiology, and end results database. *Journal of Clinical Oncology* 25(35): 5570–5577.

168. Jemal A, et al (2007) Cancer statistics, 2007. *CA Cancer J Clin* 57(1): 43–66.

169. Bach PB, et al (2003) Variations in lung cancer risk among smokers. *J Natl Cancer Inst* 95(6): 470–478.

170. Woloshin S, Schwartz LM, Welch HG (2002) Risk charts: putting cancer in context. *J Natl Cancer Inst* 94(11): 799–804.

171. Peto R, et al (2000) Smoking, smoking cessation and lung cancer in the UK since 1950: combination of national statistics with two case control studies. *BMJ* 321(7257): 323–329.

172. Alberg AJ, Samet JM (2003) Epidemiology of lung cancer. *Chest* 123(1 Suppl): 21S–49S.

173. Calabrò E, et al (2010) Lung function predicts lung cancer risk in smokers: a tool for targeting screening programmes. *Eur Respir J* 35: 146–151.

174. Jatoi A, et al (2005) Should elderly non–small-cell lung cancer patients be offered elderly-specific trials? Results of a pooled analysis from the North Central Cancer Treatment Group. *J Clin Oncol* 23: 9113–9119.

175. McLean AJ, Le Couteur DG (2004) Aging biology and geriatric clinical pharmacology. *Pharmacol Rev* 56: 163–184.

176. Rostad H, et al Lung cancer surgery (2006) The first 60 days—A population-based study. *Eur J Cardiothorac Surg* 29: 824–828.

177. Matsuoka H, et al (2005) Complications and outcomes after pulmonary resection for cancer in patients 80 to 89 years of age. *Eur J Cardiothorac Surg* 28: 380–383.

178. Hurria A, Kris MG (2003) Management of lung cancer in older adults. *CA Cancer J Clin* 53(6): 325–341.

179. Landi F, et al (1999) Body mass index and mortality among older people living in the community. *J Am Geriatr Soc* 47(9): 1072–1076.

180. Fukuse T, et al (2005) Importance of a comprehensive geriatric assessment in prediction of complications following thoracic surgery in elderly patients. *Chest* 127(3): 886–891.

181. Kris MG, et al (2006) Systemic therapy of bronchioloalveolar carcinoma: results of the first IASLC/ASCO consensus conference on bronchioloalveolar carcinoma. *J Thorac Oncol* 1(9 Suppl): S32–S36.

182. Lynch TJ, et al (2006) Summary statement: novel agents in the treatment of lung cancer: advances in epidermal growth factor receptor-targeted agents. *Clin Cancer Res* 12(14 Pt 2): 4365s–4471s.

183. Mountain CF (1997) Revisions in the international system for staging lung cancer. *Chest* 111(6): 1710–1717.

184. Janssen-Heijnen ML, et al (2004) Effect of comorbidity on the treatment and prognosis of elderly patients with non-small cell lung cancer. *Thorax* 59: 602–607.

185. O'Connell JB, Maggard MA, Ko CY (2004) Cancer-directed surgery for localized disease: decreased use in the elderly. *Ann Surg Oncol* 11: 962–969.

186. Cerfolio RJ, Bryant AS (2006) Survival and outcomes of pulmonary resection for nonsmall cell lung cancer in the elderly: a nested case-control study. *Ann Thorac Surg* 82: 424–429.

187. Sirbu H, et al Surgery for non-small cell carcinoma in geriatric patients: 15-year experience. *Asian Cardiovasc Thorac Ann* 13: 330–336.

188. Powell J, et al Treatment advances for medically inoperable non-small-cell lung cancer: emphasis on prospective trials. *The Lancet Oncology* 10(9): 885–894.

189. Zimmermann F, et al (2010) Stereotactic body radiation therapy for early non-small cell lung cancer. *Front Radiat Ther Oncol* 42: 94–114.

190. Chrischilles EA, et al (2010) Adverse events among the elderly receiving chemotherapy for advanced non-small-cell lung cancer. *J Clin Oncol* 28(4): 620–627.

191. Pallis AG, et al (2010) EORTC Elderly Task Force and Lung Cancer Group and International Society for Geriatric Oncology (SIOG) experts' opinion for the treatment of

non-small-cell lung cancer in an elderly population. *Ann Oncol* 21(4): 692–706.

192. Pignon JP, et al (2008) Lung adjuvant cisplatin evaluation: a pooled analysis by the LACE collaborative group. *J Clin Oncol* 26: 3552–3559.

193. Fruh M, et al (2008) Pooled analysis of the effect of age on adjuvant cisplatin-based chemotherapy for completely resected non-small-cell lung cancer. *J Clin Oncol* 26: 3573–3581.

194. Sekine I, et al (2004) Treatment of small cell lung cancer in the elderly based on a criteria literature review of clinical trials. *Cancer Treat Rev* 30: 359–368.

195. Owonikoko TK, et al (2007) Lung cancer in elderly patients: an analysis of the surveillance, epidemiology, and end results database. *J Clin Oncol* 25: 5570–5577.

196. Gridelli C, De Vivo R, Monfardim S (2002) Management of small cell lung cancer in the elderly. *Crit Rev Oncol Hematol* 41: 79–88.

197. Jackman DM, Johnson BE (2005) Small-cell lung cancer. *Lancet* 366: 1385–1396.

198. Puglisi M, et al (2010) Treatment options for small cell lung cancer – do we have more choice? *Br J Cancer* 102(4): 629–638.

199. Ludbrook JJ, et al (2003) Do age and comorbidity impact treatment allocation and outcomes in limited stage small-cell lung cancer? A community-based population analysis. *Int J Radiat Oncol Biol Phys* 55: 1321–1330.

200. Nou E (1996) Full chemotherapy in elderly patients with small cell bronchial carcinoma. *Acta Oncol* 35: 399–406.

201. Jara C, et al (1999) Small-cell lung cancer in the elderly – is age of patient a relevant factor? *Acta Oncol* 38: 781–786.

202. Siu LL, et al (1996) Influence of age on the treatment of limited-stage small-cell lung cancer. *J Clin Oncol* 14: 821–828.

203. Dajczman E, et al (1996) Treatment of small cell lung carcinoma in the elderly. *Cancer* 77: 2032–2038.

204. Simon GR, Turrisi A (2007) Management of small cell lung cancer: ACCP evidence-based clinical practice guidelines (2nd edition). *Chest* 132(3 suppl): 324S–339S.

CHAPTER 5

Breathing easier: an approach to heart failure in a patient with an aging heart

Jayna M. Holroyd-Leduc[1], Madhuri Reddy[2,3], & Anita Asgar[4]

[1]*Departments of Medicine and Community Health Sciences, Division of Geriatrics, University of Calgary, Calgary, AB, Canada*
[2]*Hebrew Senior Life, Boston, MA, USA*
[3]*Hebrew Senior Life, Boston, MA, USA*
[4]*Transcatheter Valve Therapy Clinic, Universite de Montreal, Institut de Cardiologie de Montreal, Montreal, QC, Canada*

Introduction

The incidence and prevalence of heart failure increases with advancing age, making heart failure one of the commonest causes for hospitalization among older adults [1, 2]. The age-associated increase in heart failure can be attributed to the combination of two factors: (1) normal age-related changes to the cardiovascular system; and (2) the high prevalence of hypertension, cardiovascular disease, and valvular heart disease at older ages [1].

Adult cardiomyocytes are terminally differentiated cells that lack the ability to regenerate [3]. In older adults, the myocardium loses myocytes, while the remaining viable myocytes hypertrophy. As a result, ventricular mass is usually preserved or increased with aging. As myocytes are lost, fibroblasts continue to divide and produce collagen. This results in a ventricle that becomes stiffer and less compliant with age.

Older hearts experience prolonged contraction duration and myocardial relaxation phase due to prolonged calcium entry during an extended sarcolemmal depolarization, along with decreased velocity of calcium uptake from the sarcoplasmic reticulum after depolarization [3]. This results in prolonged duration of ventricular relaxation.

The combination of prolonged relaxation and increased stiffness of the ventricle results in elevated left ventricular end-diastolic pressure [3]. In older adults there is decreased early diastolic filling and relatively more filling in late diastole. The atrial kick is needed to enhance total diastolic filling and preserve cardiac output. Although diastolic dysfunction is common in older adults, only a minority of older adults develop clinically significant diastolic heart failure despite these age-related changes [3, 4].

Other age-related cardiac changes include: (1) increased stiffness in the arterial walls, particularly in large arteries; (2) impaired responsiveness to beta-adrenergic stimulation; and (3) decline in sinus node function [4]. The net effect of all these age-related changes is a reduction in cardiovascular reserve and a decreased ability to compensate during stressful situations, such as in times of ischemia or infection. Age-related changes within other organs, including the kidneys and lungs, can further contribute to the increased risk of developing heart failure.

In this chapter, we review the nonpharmacological, pharmacological, and surgical evidence around the management of heart failure. We look at the literature overall, with a particular focus on older adults where the data are available.

Search strategy

MEDLINE, EMBASE, and the Cochrane Database of Systematic Reviews were searched for potentially relevant articles from 2009 to July 2011. The keywords used for all databases were "heart failure" or "congested heart failure." The search was limited to systematic reviews, Cochrane reviews, and meta-analyses. The search yielded 100 unique citations.

All the citations were screened to meet the following inclusion criteria: (1) systematic review or meta-analyses published between 2009 and July 2011, or the latest updated version of any relevant Cochrane reviews from 2008 to 2011; (2) involves management of congestive heart failure; and (3) English language. We did not limit our inclusion only to articles involving those aged 65 years or older, but focused on older adults when the data were provided. Twenty-eight systematic reviews met these inclusion criteria.

For this chapter, we graded relevant clinical studies using the Oxford Centre for Evidence-based Medicine Levels of Evidence.

What role does exercise play in the management of heart failure?

Two systematic reviews examined the role of exercise training in heart failure management (Level 1a evidence) [5, 6]. Patients with heart failure experience marked reductions in their exercise capacity, which can negatively impact activities of daily living and quality of life, and increases hospitalization and mortality rates.

Exercise programs that incorporate aerobic training, with or without resistance training, have not been found to decrease pooled all-cause mortality compared to usual medical care (relative risk (RR) 1.02; 95% confidence interval (CI) 0.70–1.51). However, they appear to reduce heart failure hospital admission rates (RR 0.72; 95% CI 0.52–0.99) [5]. There also appears to be positive impacts on health-related quality of life (standard mean difference (SMD) −0.57; 95% CI −0.83 to −0.31).

Home-based exercise programs, with or without first attending a center-based program, may be an option for some individuals with heart failure (Level 1a evidence) [6]. Compared to usual medical care, exercise duration has been shown to increase by approximately 2 minutes (95% CI 0.9–3.0) and the 6-minute walk by 30.4 m (95% CI 6.1–54.7). However, the long-term effects of home exercise are unclear.

Given their health status, not all older adults with heart failure can participate in exercise programs. Therefore, functional electrical stimulation of muscles

Table 5.1 Evidence-based treatment options for heart failure

Nonpharmacological
 Exercise training
 Functional electrical stimulation

Pharmacological
 Angiotensin converting enzymes inhibitors
 Angiotensin receptor antagonists
 Aldosterone blockers
 Beta-blockers
 Diuretics
 Digoxin
 Statins

Surgical
 Cardiac resynchronization
 Implantable cardioverter defibrillators

has been explored as an alternative. Based on a systematic review of seven randomized trials, functional electrical stimulation has been found to have similar effects on muscle strength and in the distance achieved during the 6-minute walk test (2.7 m; 95% CI −15.4 to 20.9) when compared to conventional aerobic exercise (Level 1a evidence) [7].

Clinical bottom line

Exercise training appears to have positive effects on quality of life and decreases heart failure-related hospitalizations (Table 5.1). For those with heart failure, who are unable to participate in exercise programs, there may be a role for functional electrical stimulation.

Which pharmacological agents should be used in the management of heart failure?

Although there are numerous randomized controlled trials exploring the role of pharmacological treatments among those with heart failure and guidelines often support the concomitant use of multiple agents, the effects of these agents on the frail older adult is less clear. There are a number of limitations to the currently available literature: (1) many trials exclude adults over 75 years of age; (2) those trials that include older adults often enroll small numbers of older adults, most of whom are relatively healthy with few comorbidities; and (3) few studies focus on diastolic heart failure, which accounts for a large number of heart failure cases in adults over age 75 [4].

Angiotensin converting enzyme inhibitors and angiotensin receptor antagonists

One systematic review explored whether drugs that inhibit the renin–angiotensin system prevent congestive heart failure through mechanisms beyond just reduction in blood pressure (Level 1a evidence) [8]. Thirty-one trials were identified, which compared newer antihypertensive drugs (angiotensin converting enzymes (ACE) inhibitors, angiotensin receptor antagonists (ARBs), calcium channel blockers) to older antihypertensive agents (diuretics, beta-blockers) or placebo. ACE inhibitors were associated with a significantly lower risk of heart failure compared to placebo (all $P < 0.001$). Calcium channel blockers were associated with a higher risk of heart failure compared to diuretics/beta-blockers (all $P < 0.05$). For each 5-mmHg reduction in systolic blood pressure, there was a 24% reduction in risk of heart failure ($P < 0.001$). Over and beyond the blood pressure difference, the risk of heart failure was 19% lower with ACE inhibitors/ARBs than with calcium channel blockers ($P < 0.001$). Therefore, the protective effects of ACE inhibitors and ARBs appear to be over and above just the reduction achieved in blood pressure.

A systematic review of particular relevance to the treatment older heart failure patients examined the effect of renin–angiotensin system inhibitors in persons with heart failure and preserved left ventricular ejection fraction (Level 1a evidence) [9]. Three randomized clinical trials were identified. The first compared perindopril with placebo in subjects older than 70 years with diastolic dysfunction (predominantly nonischemic, hypertensive). There was no benefit in death or heart failure hospitalization rates at 3 years. The second trial, which enrolled adults older than 18 (mean age 67), with symptomatic heart failure and a left ventricular ejection fraction >0.40, also found no benefit with respect to death or heart failure hospitalization with candesartan. The last trial enrolled patients older than 60 with symptomatic heart failure and left ventricular ejection fraction >0.45. At a mean follow-up of 50 months, there was no difference between irbesartan and placebo in the combined outcome of all-cause mortality or cardiovascular hospitalization. There was also no reduction in heart failure-related hospitalizations. A pooled analysis of the three trials found no benefit with regard to all-cause mortality (odds ratio (OR) 1.03; 95% CI 0.92–1.15) or heart failure

hospitalization (OR 0.90; 95% CI 0.80–1.02). Therefore, the role for ACE inhibitors and ARBs in older adults with diastolic dysfunction is as yet unproven.

In order to determine if there is benefit to combining ACE inhibitors with ARBs for the treatment of heart failure, a meta-analysis was recently completed (Level 1a evidence) [10]. Within the eight included trials, the mean age ranged from 54 to 69 years and the vast majority had NYHA (New York Heart Association) class II–III symptoms with impaired left ventricular ejection fraction. There was no difference in overall mortality between combination therapy and ACE inhibitors alone (RR 0.97; 95% CI 0.92–1.03). However, there were fewer heart failure-related hospital admissions with combination therapy (RR 0.81; 95% CI 0.72–0.91). Combination therapy was associated with a higher risk of worsening renal function (RR 1.91; 95% CI 1.40–2.60), symptomatic hypotension (RR 1.57; 95% CI 1.44–1.71), and hyperkalemia (RR 1.95; 95% CI 0.85–4.48). Combination therapy was more commonly discontinued (RR 1.21; 95% CI 1.07–1.37). Given the side effect profile, combination therapy should probably be avoided in the frail older adult.

ACE inhibitors (OR 0.71; 95% credibility interval (CrI) 0.59–0.85) and ARBs (OR 0.76; 95% CrI 0.62–0.90) were among the most efficient drug classes to reduce heart failure onset compared to placebo, in a Bayesian network meta-analysis [11].

Aldosterone blockade

One systematic review examined the role of aldosterone blockers in adults with left ventricular dysfunction (Level 1a evidence) [12]. Nineteen trials were included, among which 14 used spironolactone and 15 were conducted in patients with heart failure. All but three trials used placebo controls; of the three remaining trials, two used usual care as the comparator and one used metoprolol as an active comparator. Data from 14 heart failure trials revealed a 25% reduction in all-cause mortality (RR 0.75; 95% CI 0.67–0.84). All-cause hospitalizations were reduced by 27% in seven heart failure trials (RR 0.73; 95% CI 0.63–0.84). More people on aldosterone blockers developed hyperkalemia (6% vs. 3% of controls) and renal failure (9% vs. 2%). Older adults with heart failure treated with both aldosterone blockade and ACE inhibitors are at particularly high risk for hyperkalemia-related hospitalization and death [13]. Frequent laboratory monitoring is recommended.

Beta-blockers

A meta-analysis explored whether survival benefits seen with beta-blockade in heart failure is associated with the magnitude of heart rate reduction or the beta-blocker dose (Level 1a evidence) [14]. The majority of those studied had systolic dysfunction and NYHA class III or IV symptoms. Overall the risk of death was reduced (RR 0.76; 95% CI 0.68–0.84), though there was moderate heterogeneity among trials related to the magnitude of heart rate reduction. Every 5 beats/minute reduction in heart rate was associated with an 18% reduction in the risk of death (95% CI 6%–29%). There was no relationship seen between all-cause mortality and drug dose. Age did not appear to influence the mortality benefit seen from reducing heart rate. Therefore, beta-blockers should be titrated to heart rate, though the optimal or target heart rate is unknown because no trial randomly assigned participants to different target heart rates.

Diuretics

Based on a Cochrane review that included 14 randomized controlled trials (Level 1a evidence), mortality was lower among those treated with diuretics compared to placebo (OR 0.24; 95% CI 0.07–0.83) [15]. Diuretics also appear to decrease hospital admissions for worsening heart failure (OR 0.07; 95% CI 0.01–0.52). Compared to other agents, diuretics appear to improve exercise capacity in individuals with heart failure (weighted mean difference (WMD) 0.72; 95% CI 0.40–1.04). Diuretics need to be used judiciously among frail older adults, as they are more susceptible to hyponatremia and to excessive diuresis that can decrease preload and reduce cardiac output [3].

Among adults with NYHA class III–IV symptoms, loop diuretics given as continuous infusions appear to provide greater diuresis and a better safety profile compared to intravenous bolus dosing (Level 1a evidence) [16]. Urine output is greater in those given continuous infusions (WMD 271 cc/24 hours; 95% CI 93–449). Although electrolyte disturbances do not appear to differ, continuous infusion appears to be associated with fewer other adverse effects (e.g., tinnitus and hearing loss) (RR 0.6; 95% CI 0.01–0.44). There is also some evidence to suggest shorter hospital stays

and decreased all-cause mortality among those treated with continuous infusions.

A recent Bayesian network meta-analysis showed diuretics to be one of the most efficient drug classes to reduce heart failure onset compared with placebo (OR 0.59; 95% CrI 0.47–0.73) [11]. Diuretics were even more efficient than ACE inhibitors (OR 0.83; 95% CrI 0.69–0.99) and ARBs (OR 0.78; 95% CrI 0.63–0.97).

Digitalis

Digitalis glycosides have been used to treat heart failure for over 200 years. However, a recent systematic review examining the effectiveness of digitalis in treating heart failure among adults in sinus rhythm found no difference in mortality between digitalis and placebo (Level 1a evidence) [17]. Digitalis does appear to be associated with lower rates of hospitalization and clinical deterioration. Of note, the frail older adult is more susceptible to the toxic effects of digitalis, often even at therapeutic drug levels.

Antiplatelets and anticoagulation

Although the role for anticoagulation and antiplatelets among those with atrial fibrillation and heart failure appears to be clear, the role for these agents in individuals in sinus rhythm with heart failure remains uncertain. A recent Cochrane review found no evidence from randomized control trials to recommend the use of aspirin to prevent thromboembolism among those with heart failure and sinus rhythm, and evidence from cohort studies is conflicting (Level 2a evidence) [18]. A separate Cochrane review found only one pilot randomized controlled trial comparing warfarin, aspirin, and no antithrombotics therapy, with a second large trial comparing warfarin and antiplatelet therapy pending evaluation [19]. Although early evidence from these trials, along with evidence from observational studies, suggests a possible benefit from anticoagulation, there is currently insufficient evidence to recommend the routine use of anticoagulants among heart failure patients in sinus rhythm (Level 2a evidence).

Statins

Statin therapy appears to have no effect on the risk of all-cause mortality (OR 0.89; 95% CI 0.72–1.10), cardiovascular mortality (OR 0.89; 95% CI 0.71–1.1.3), or sudden cardiac death (OR 0.94; 95% CI 0.68–1.29), based on a systematic review combining ten trials comparing statins to placebo in adults with heart failure (weighted mean age 69 years) (Level 1a evidence) [20]. Statins do appear to help decrease hospitalizations for worsening heart failure (OR 0.67; 95% CI 0.50–0.90). One hospital admission for worsening heart failure will be prevented for every 52 treated with a statin for a weighted mean of 38 months.

Focusing on therapy for heart failure with preserved ejection fraction

As already outlined, older adults more frequently have diastolic heart failure instead of systolic failure. A recent systematic review attempted to determine the benefits of pharmacological agents for adults experiencing heart failure with preserved ejection fraction [21]. Combined therapy, from data within randomized control trials, did not improve mortality (RR 0.99; 95% CI 0.92–1.06) or diastolic function (WMD −0.01; 95% CI −0.03 to 0.02) (Level 1a evidence). There was also no significant improvement in these outcomes with individual therapies. Exercise capacity did improve with combined therapy (WMD 51.5; 95% CI 27.3–75.7) (Level 1a evidence). The two individual drug classes that improved exercise capacity were (1) vasodilator therapy and (2) chronotropic agents (including digoxin, verapamil, and beta-blockers).

Clinical bottom line

Both ACE inhibitors and ARBs are effective in the treatment of heart failure, though their role in diastolic heart failure is less clear. Although the combination of these two agents reduces heart failure-related hospitalizations, they do not decrease mortality and are associated with increased adverse effects.

Aldosterone blockade appears to be an effective treatment option. However, older adults are at risk for adverse effects, particularly when these agents are used in combination with ACE inhibitors.

Beta-blockers are an effective treatment option and should be titrated to heart rate.

Diuretics are an important treatment option in the management of heart failure.

Although digoxin does not decrease mortality, it does appear to be associated with decreased hospitalizations and reduced clinical deterioration.

The role for anticoagulants and antiplatelets among those with heart failure in sinus rhythm is unclear.

Statins have been shown to decrease heart failure-related hospital admissions.

The overall role for many of these agents in the treatment of diastolic heart failure, which is common among older adults, is unclear. Frail older adults need to be monitored for side effects when on any of these agents, particularly when they are used in combination and when the person becomes acutely ill.

What is the role for cardiac resynchronization and implantable cardioverter defibrillators?

The clinical symptoms of congestion are often related to electromechanical dyssynchrony that contributes to inefficient ventricular contraction, mitral regurgitation, and worsening ventricular dilation [22]. Practice guidelines recommend cardiac resynchronization therapy (CRT), using a left ventricular lead implanted via the coronary sinus, for individuals with left ventricular ejection fractions ≤35%, QRS duration ≥120 minutes, sinus rhythm, and advanced heart failure symptoms despite optimal medical therapy [23, 24]. More recent systematic reviews have suggested that there may also be benefit among individuals with milder heart failure (NYHA class I–II) (Level 1a to 2a evidence) [25, 26].

Implantable cardioverter defibrillators (ICD) are used for the prevention of sudden cardiac death in selected patients with heart failure. Compared to conventional or antiarrhythmic drug therapy, ICD therapy reduced or showed a trend towards reduced mortality in six randomized controlled trials [27]. Subgroup analysis did not reveal attenuation of benefit with higher NYHA class or lower left ventricular ejection fraction. Although there appears to be a decrease in mortality rates in men with heart failure and reduced left ventricular ejection fraction who received ICD for primary prevention of sudden cardiac death (HR 0.78; 95% CI 0.70–0.87), the benefit is less clear in women (HR 1.01; 95% CI 0.76–1.33) [28].

CRT and ICD are often used together. A recent systematic review found that the combination of CRT and ICD for the treatment of heart failure, compared to no CRT or ICD, reduced all-cause mortality (OR 0.55; 95% CI 0.40–0.76) (Level 1a evidence) [29].

Clinical bottom line

Select patients with heart failure may benefit from CRT and ICD therapies.

How should heart failure patients be monitored?

B-type natriuretic peptide (BNP), a neurohormone secreted predominately from the ventricle in response to intracardiac volume loading, can be used to diagnose acute decompensated heart failure and as a prognostic indicator of mortality and clinical outcomes. More recent systematic reviews have shown that BNP-guided drug therapy in those with chronic heart failure can reduce mortality (Level 1a evidence) [30, 31]. However, in those over 75 years of age, the mortality benefit is not as clear (RR 0.94; 95% CI 0.71–1.25) [31]. Although the percentage of patients achieving target doses of ACE inhibitors and beta-blockers increases, there does not appear to be an impact on all-cause hospitalizations (RR 0.82; 95% CI 0.64–1.05) [31].

A Cochrane review identified 16 trials evaluating the effectiveness of disease management interventions, including multidisciplinary interventions, case management interventions, and clinic interventions, but found insufficient data to form treatment recommendations [32]. More recently published reviews of telemonitoring and structured telephone support have shown promising results [33–35]. Telemonitoring involves home monitoring of patients using special telecare devices in conjunction with a telecommunication system. Telemonitoring reduces all-cause mortality (RR 0.66; 95% CI 0.54–0.81) and heart failure-related hospitalizations (RR 0.79; 95% CI 0.67–0.94) (Level 1a evidence) [33]. There may also be benefits in terms of quality of life and patient satisfaction [33, 34]. Structured telephone support has not been shown to reduce all-cause mortality (RR 0.88; 95% CI 0.76–1.01), but does appear to reduce heart failure-related hospitalizations (RR 0.77; 95% CI 0.68–0.87) (Level 1a evidence) [33]. A recent review of self-management interventions for patients with chronic heart failure indicated a positive effect, although not always significant, on hospital readmissions, heart failure-related hospitalizations, mortality rates, and quality of life (Level 1a evidence) [36].

Clinical bottom line

BNP-guided drug therapy is effective in those with chronic heart failure. However, the benefit in those over 75 years of age is less clear. Both telemonitoring and structured telephone support appear to have a role in the monitoring of heart failure, as do self-management interventions.

Summary

Heart failure is one of the commonest cardiac diagnoses in the older adult. In particular, the prevalence of diastolic dysfunction increases with age. There is evidence to support exercise training and use of several different pharmacologic agents in the management of heart failure. In select patients, CRT and ICD therapies may be indicated. Older adults with heart failure require frequent monitoring of both cardiac symptoms and drug-related adverse effects. Effective monitoring might include telemonitoring, structured telephone support, and self-management interventions.

References

1. Rich MW (2001) Heart failure in the 21st century: a cardiogeriatric syndrome. *J Gerontol Med Sci* 56A: M88–M96.
2. Popovic JR (1999) National Hospital Discharge Survey: Annual Summary with Detailed Diagnosis and Procedure Data. Hyattsville, MD: National Center for Health Statistics; 2001. *Vital Health Stat* 13(151).
3. Pugh KG, Wei JY (2001) Clinical implications of physiological changes in the aging heart. *Drugs Aging* 18(4): 263–276.
4. Rich MW (2003) Heart failure in the elderly: strategies to optimize outpatient control and reduce hospitalizations. *AJGC* 12: 19–27.
5. Davies EJ, et al (2010) Exercise training for systolic heart failure: Cochrane systematic review and meta-analysis. *Eur J Heart Fail* 12: 706–715.
6. Hwang RA, Thomas AB (2009) Efficacy of home-based exercise programmes for people with chronic heart failure: a meta-analysis. *Eur J Cardiovasc Prev Rehabil* 16: 527–535.
7. Sbruzzi GA, et al (2010) Functional electrical stimulation in the treatment of patients with chronic heart failure: a meta-analysis of randomized controlled trials. *Eur J Cardiovasc Prev Rehabil* 17: 254–260.
8. Verecchia P, et al (2009) Blood pressure reduction and rennin-angiotensin system inhibition for prevention of congestive heart failure: a meta-analysis. *Eur Heart J* 30: 679–688.
9. Shah RV, Desal AS, Givertz MM (2010) The effect of renin-angiotensin system inhibitors on mortality and heart failure hospitalization in patients with heart failure and preserved ejection fraction: a systematic review and meta-analysis. *J Cardiac Fail* 16: 260–267.
10. Kuenzli A, et al (2010) Meta-analysis of combined therapy with angiotensin receptor antagonists versus ACE inhibitors alone in patients with heart failure. *PLoS ONE* 5(4): e9946.

11. Sciarretta S, et al (2011) Antihypertensive treatment and development of heart failure in hypertension. *Arch Intern Med* 171: 384–394.

12. Ezekowitz JA, McAlister FA (2009) Aldosterone blockade and left ventricular dysfunction: a systematic review of randomized clinical trials. *Eur Heart J* 30: 469–477.

13. Juurlink DN, et al (2004) Rates of hyperkalemia after publication of the Randomized Aldactone Evaluation Study. *N Engl J Med* 351: 543–551.

14. McAlister FA, et al (2009) Meta-analysis: beta-blocker dose, heart rate reduction, and death in patients with heart failure. *Ann Intern Med* 150: 784–794.

15. Faris RF, et al (2008) Diuretics for heart failure. *Cochrane Database Syst Rev* CD003838.

16. Salvador DRK, Punzalan FE, Ramos GC (2008) Continuous infusion versus bolus injection of loop diuretics in congestive heart failure. *Cochrane Database Syst Rev* CD003178.

17. Hood WB, et al (2009) Digitalis for treatment of congestive heart failure in patients in sinus rhythm. *Cochrane Database Syst Rev* CD002901.

18. Lip YHG, Chung I (2011) Antiplatelet agents versus control or anticoagulation for heart failure in sinus rhythm. *Cochrane Database Syst Rev* CD003333.

19. Lip YHG, Chung I (2011) Anticoagulation for heart failure in sinus rhythm. *Cochrane Database Syst Rev* CD003336.

20. Lipinski MJ, et al (2009) Meta-analysis of randomized controlled trials of statins versus placebo in patients with heart failure. *Am J Cardiol* 104: 1708–1716.

21. Holland DJ, Kumbhani DJ, Ahmed SH, Marwick TH (2011) Effects of treatment on exercise tolerance, cardiac function, and mortality in heart failure with preserved ejection fraction. *J AM Coll Cardiol* 57: 1676–1686.

22. Bilchick KC, Helm RH, Kass DA (2007) Physiology of biventricular pacing. *Curr Cardiol Rep* 9: 358–365.

23. Hunt SA, et al (2009) Focused update incorporated into the ACC/AHA 2005 guidelines for the diagnosis and management of heart failure in adults. *J Am Coll Cardiol* 53: e1–e90.

24. Dickstein K, et al (2008) ESC guidelines for the diagnosis and treatment of acute and chronic heart failure. *Eur J Heart Fail* 10: 933–989.

25. Lubitz S, et al (2010) Effectiveness of cardiac resynchronization therapy in mild congestive heart failure: a systematic review and meta-analysis of randomized trials. *Eur J Heart Fail* 12: 360–366.

26. Wein S, et al (2010) Extending the boundaries of cardiac resynchronization therapy: efficacy in atrial fibrillation, New York Heart Association class II, and narrow QRS heart failure patients. *J Cardiac Fail* 16: 432–438.

27. Salukhe TV, et al (2010) Is there benefit in implanting defibrillators in patients with severe heart failure? *Heart* 96: 599–603.

28. Ghanbari H, et al (2009) Effectiveness of implantable cardioverter-defibrillators for primary prevention of sudden cardiac death in women with advanced heart failure. *Arch Intern Med* 169: 1500–1506.

29. Huang Y, Wu W, Cao Y, Qu N (2010) All cause mortality of cardiac resynchronization therapy with implantable cardioverter defibrillator: a meta-analysis of randomized controlled trials. *Int J Cardoil* 145: 413–417.

30. Felker GM, Hasselblad V, Hernandez AF, O'Connor CM (2009) Biomarker-guided therapy in chronic heart failure: a meta-analysis of randomized controlled trials. *Am Heart J* 158: 422–430.

31. Porapakkham P, et al (2010) B-type natriuretic peptide-guided heart failure therapy. *Arch Intern Med* 170: 507–514.

32. Taylor JCS, et al Clinical services organization for heart failure. *Cochrane Database Syst Rev* CD002752.

33. Inglis SC, et al Structured telephone support and telemonitoring programmes for patients with chronic heart failure. *Cochrane Database Syst Rev* CD007228.

34. Polisena J, et al (2010) Home telemonitoring for congestive heart failure: a systematic review and meta-analysis. *J Telemed Telecare* 16: 68–76.

35. Klersy C, et al (2009) A meta-analysis of remote monitoring of heart failure patients. *J Am Coll Cardiol* 54: 1683–1694.

36. Ditewig JB, Blok H, Havers J, van Veenendall H (2010) Effectiveness of self-management interventions on mortality, hospital readmissions, chronic heart failure hospitalization rates and quality of life in patients with chronic heart failure: a systematic review. *Patient Educ Couns* 78: 297–315.

CHAPTER 6

Clarifying confusion: preventing and managing delirium

Ranjani Aiyar[1] & Jayna M. Holroyd-Leduc[2]
[1]*Division of General Internal Medicine, Department of Medicine, University of Calgary and Alberta Health Services, Calgary, AB, Canada*
[2]*Departments of Medicine and Community Health Sciences, Division of Geriatrics, University of Calgary, Calgary, AB, Canada*

Introduction

Delirium is defined as an acute disturbance of consciousness, change in cognition, and a reduced ability to focus, sustain, or shift attention [1]. The disturbance develops over a short period of time, tends to fluctuate over the course of the day, and is the consequence of a general medical condition, an intoxicating substance, and/or medication use [1]. It can be challenging to distinguish delirium from dementia. Some of the key features to consider when diagnosing delirium include the sudden onset of symptoms and the associated impairment in attention (Table 6.1).

Delirium occurs in 25%–65% of hospitalized older patients but often goes unrecognized [2, 3]. It requires appropriate focus on prevention and management by healthcare workers because it is associated with increased mortality, longer length of hospital stay, increased hospital-acquired complications, persistent cognitive deficits, and increased discharge to long-term care [4–7].

Among medical patients presenting to hospital, delirium is more likely to occur in persons with sensory impairment, severe illness, cognitive impairment, and/or a high urea/creatinine ratio suggestive of dehydration [8]. Other factors that can contribute to the development of delirium include medications (e.g., sedatives, narcotics, anticholinergics, psychotropic drugs), any acute illness such as infection or organ impairment, biochemical disturbances such as abnormal electrolytes or glucose, the presence of comorbid diseases, functional impairment, depression, and alcohol or drug withdrawal. Hospital-related factors associated with an increased delirium risk include the use of physical restraints, malnutrition, the addition of more than three medications, use of bladder catheter, and any iatrogenic event [9].

Delirium occurs as a common perioperative complication in older adults and results in increased morbidity [10, 11]. It is predictive of poor postoperative function and mobility [5]. Risk factors for postoperative delirium include advanced age, history of alcohol abuse, psychotropic drug use, functional and cognitive impairment, history of depression, presence of comorbid diseases, sensory impairment, current living arrangement, abnormal preoperative blood work, and the type of surgery being considered [10, 11]. Preoperative delirium risk assessment is important to guide informed decision-making and possible preventative options (Table 6.2) [10, 12].

In this chapter, we review the screening, prevention, and management of delirium among the older hospitalized patient.

Search strategy

MEDLINE (using Ovid), EMBASE, and the Cochrane Database of Systematic Reviews were searched for

Evidence-Based Geriatric Medicine: A Practical Clinical Guide, First Edition. Edited by Jayna M. Holroyd-Leduc and Madhuri Reddy.
© 2012 Blackwell Publishing Ltd. Published 2012 by Blackwell Publishing Ltd.

Table 6.1 Distinguishing delirium from dementia

	Onset	Duration/ Course	Attention Span	Psychomotor Activity	Mood	Psychotic Features
Delirium	Sudden (hours to days)	Usually short though variable	Decreased	Increased or decreased	Normal to anxious	Visual and tactile hallucinations; frequent misinterpretation of visual stimuli
Dementia	Insidious (over months to years)	Usually slowly progressive	Normal	Usually normal to decreased	Usually normal but apathy is common	Paranoid delusions; occasional visual hallucinations

Table 6.2 Multivariate predictors of postoperative delirium (a) Validated Clinical Prediction Rule developed among patients over 50 years of age scheduled for elective noncardiac surgery

Risk Factor	Points
Age ($\geq$70 years)	1
Current alcohol abuse (self-report)	1
Poor baseline cognitive status (TICS score <30)	1
Poor baseline functional status (SAS class IV)	1
Abnormal preoperative blood work	
(Na <130 or >150 mmol/L; K <3.0 or >6.0 mmol/L; glucose <3.3 or >16.7 mmol/L)	1
Noncardiac thoracic surgery	1
Aortic aneurysm surgery	2

TICS, Telephone Interview for Cognitive Status; SAS, Specific Activity Scale.

Total Points	Risk of Postoperative Delirium (%)
0	2
1	8
2	13
$\geq$3	50

Source: Reproduced with permission from [10].

Table 6.2 *Continued*

(b) Validated Clinical Prediction Rule developed among patients over 60 years of age undergoing nonemergent cardiac surgery (coronary artery bypass or valve surgery)

Risk Factor	Points
Preoperative MMSE score $\leq 23^a$	2
Between 24 and –27	1
History of TIA[a]/stroke	1
Depressive symptoms preoperatively (GDS>4^a)	1
Abnormal preoperative albumin (≤ 3.5 or ≥ 4.5 g/dL)	1

Source: [12].
MMSE, Mini Mental State Exam; TIA, transient ischemic attack; GDS, Geriatric Depression Scale.

Total Points	Risk of Postoperative Delirium (%)
0	18
1	43
2	60
≥ 3	87

potentially relevant articles from 2005 to 2010. The keywords used for all databases were "delirium" or "confusion," "elderly" or "old" or "aged" or "senior" or "geriatric." The search was limited to evidence-based medicine reviews, Cochrane reviews, meta-analyses, evidence-based practice guidelines, and clinical prediction rules. The search yielded 288 unique citations. We also obtained additional references by consulting an expert in the field.

To answer the three clinical questions as outlined in this chapter ((1) How can I screen for delirium?; (2) How can I prevent this older hospitalized patient from becoming delirious?; (3) How can I best manage this older hospitalized patient with delirium?), all the citations were screened to meet the following four inclusion criteria: (1) systematic review or meta-analyses published/available between November 2008 and March 2010; (2) involves delirium; (3) focuses primarily on studies involving patients over 65 years of age; and (4) English language. Seven systematic reviews met these inclusion criteria.

For this chapter, we graded relevant clinical studies using the Oxford Centre for Evidence-based Medicine Levels of Evidence.

How can I screen for delirium?

We identified three systematic reviews relevant to the topic of screening [13–15]. Two focused on screening tools and met Level 1a evidence [13, 14], and one focused on nurses' recognition of delirium and met Level 2a evidence [15].

The diagnosis of delirium is mostly clinical and requires careful observation of key features.

Delirium often goes undetected, particularly in the presence of hypoactive delirium, age 80 years or older, vision impairment, and dementia [15]. Although nurses are potentially the best resource for initial detection of delirium, the recognition of delirium by this group ranges widely (from 26% to 83%) [15]. Poor communication between nurses and physicians may also act as a barrier to recognizing delirium [15].

Tools for delirium screening

The DSM criteria for delirium is the usual gold standard for diagnosis, but this requires an in-depth interview and a series of cognitive tests performed by a specialist physician (e.g., geriatrician, neurologist, or psychiatrist) [13]. Bedside delirium-screening tools should be simple and feasible for use by a broad array of healthcare providers.

Eleven screening tools of sufficient quality were identified in a recent systematic review [14]. Of these, the tests that best detect the presence of delirium (positive likelihood ratio (LR) >5.0) include the Confusion Assessment Method (CAM), the Global Attentiveness Rating Scale (GAR), the Memorial Delirium Assessment Scale (MDAS), the Delirium Rating Scale-Revised-98 (DRS-R-98), the Clinical Assessment of Confusion (CAC), and the Delirium Observation Screening Scale (DOSS). The best tests at helping to exclude a diagnosis of delirium (negative LR <0.2) include the CAM, the GAR, the MDAS, the Delirium Rating Scale (DRS), the DRS-R-98, the DOSS, the Nursing Delirium Screening Scale (Nu-DESC), and the Mini-Mental State Examination (MMSE).

As a bedside instrument, the CAM appears to have the best test characteristics including ease of use and test performance (Level 1a evidence) [14]. The CAM has a diagnostically helpful summary positive LR of 9.6 (95% confidence interval (CI) 5.8–16) and a diagnostically helpful summary negative LR of 0.16 (95% CI 0.09–0.29) [13, 14]. Additionally, its good interrater reliability means the results are comparable between assessors. The CAM instrument is based on the DSM criteria for delirium that includes assessing the presence, severity, and fluctuation of nine delirium features: (1) acute onset, (2) inattention, (3) disorganized thinking, (4) altered level of consciousness, (5) disorientation, (6) memory impairment, (7) perceptual disturbances, (8) psychomotor agitation or retardation, and (9) altered sleep–wake cycle. The CAM diagnostic algorithm is based on four cardinal features of delirium: (1) acute onset and fluctuating course, (2) inattention, (3) disorganized thinking, and (4) altered level of consciousness (Table 6.3) [16]. The CAM has been translated into ten languages and adapted for use in numerous clinical settings such as the intensive care unit, the emergency department, and long-term care settings [13]. The CAM can be completed at the bedside within a few minutes.

Clinical bottom line

Among the many delirium-screening tools, the CAM appears to be the best tool to use at the bedside. It gives similar results when administered by different healthcare providers (good interrater reliability) and is easy to use in a number of different clinical settings.

Table 6.3 The Confusion Assessment Method (CAM)

1 Acute Onset and Fluctuating Course
Is there an acute change from the patient's baseline cognition as reported by family/caregiver/healthcare provider? Does this change fluctuate over time?

2 Inattention
Does the patient have difficulty focusing on topic or is easily distracted? Can the patient not count back from 10, recite months of year backward, or spell WORLD backward?

3 Disorganized Thinking
Does the patient have rambling or incoherent speech? Do they unpredictably switch from topic to topic?

4 Altered level of consciousness
Is the patient's level of consciousness hyperalert (agitated), drowsy, stuporous or comatose?

A diagnosis of delirium requires the presence of features 1, 2, and either 3 or 4.

Source: Reproduced with permission from [16].

The CAM can help both to rule in a diagnosis of delirium ($+$LR $= 9.6$) or to exclude it ($-$LR $= 0.16$).

How can I prevent this older hospitalized patient from becoming delirious?

We identified two systematic reviews relevant to the topic of delirium prevention [17, 18]. Preventative strategies are more effective than management strategies for delirium. Since delirium generally occurs in the presence of several precipitating factors, multicomponent strategies aimed at reducing potential risk factors are most successful [17]. These strategies include avoiding factors which are known to cause delirium, identifying and treating underlying acute medical issues, and providing supportive care in order to prevent further physical and cognitive decline (Table 6.4).

Three randomized control trials ($N = 646$) have demonstrated that multicomponent delirium prevention strategies are effective among patients admitted to hospital with a hip fracture (summary RR (relative risk) 0.75; 95% CI 0.64–0.88) (Level 1a evidence) [17]. Only seven patients need to be treated with such a strategy to prevent one case of delirium.

A similar study, which used matching instead of randomization, evaluated the effectiveness of a multicomponent preventative intervention among hospitalized medical patients aged 70 or older ($N = 852$) [2]. Compared with usual care, the intervention resulted in a significant reduction in delirium rates (odds ratio (OR) 0.6; 95% CI 0.4–0.9) (Level 2b evidence). Other hospitals have also been able to successfully implement this intervention when there was a commitment of resources by hospital leadership and appropriate adaptation of protocols to local needs [19]. One successful adaptation to the original intervention has been the use of hospital volunteers to help implement the preventative protocols.

There is insufficient evidence to support pharmacological strategies in the prevention of delirium [17]. Cholinesterase inhibitors have been proposed as prophylaxis to prevent delirium [18]. However, one small clinical trial identified in systematic reviews did not support their use in the prevention of delirium (Level 1b evidence) [17, 18]. The prophylactic use of antipsychotic agents has also been studied but the evidence does not currently support their general use (Level 1b evidence) [17].

Clinical bottom line
Multicomponent preventive strategies that target delirium risk factors are effective (Table 6.4). Only seven patients need to be treated with such a strategy to prevent one case of delirium. It is important to stress the need for implementing and adhering to these strategies in everyday clinical practice.

There is insufficient evidence to support the use of pharmacological agents in the prevention of delirium.

How can I best manage this older hospitalized patient with delirium?

Management of delirium should involve removal of the cause(s) when possible, symptom management, prevention of complications, and education of patient and their family/caregivers [20]. We identified three systematic reviews relevant to the topic of delirium management [17, 21, 22].

A recent systematic review identified three randomized controlled trials ($N = 489$) that evaluated the role of comprehensive geriatric assessment and multicomponent interventions targeted at precipitants of delirium among medical inpatients [17]. Interventions focused on optimizing sensory input, orientation protocols, provision of familiar items and family presence, avoidance of restraints, optimizing mobility and encouragement of self-care, use of atypical antipsychotics where indicated, nutritional supplements where indicated, screening for treatable causes, and discharge planning. These multicomponent interventions did not decrease mortality and had no significant effect on length of hospital stay, functional status at discharge, or long-term care placement (Level 1a evidence). There were no randomized controlled trials of pharmacologic management options identified in this review. Despite the limited evidence, a recent clinical practice guideline on the management of delirium recommends a multifaceted approach to management (Table 6.5) [20].

Behavioral symptoms associated with delirium, such as agitation, aggression, calling out, and wandering, are often challenging to manage. Nonpharmacological management strategies can be attempted that include approaching the patient calmly, reassuring the patient

Table 6.4 Examples of preventative strategies that target delirium risk factors

Targeted Risk Factors and Associated Preventive Strategies

Cognitive Impairment
- Orient patient to date and place daily, and as needed
- Provide clocks and calendars

Functional Impairment
- Mobilize early and regularly
- Consult physiotherapy and occupational therapy as needed

Fluid and Electrolyte Imbalances
- Restore electrolyte and glucose levels to normal limits
- Detect and treat dehydration or fluid overload

High-Risk Medications
- Discontinue or minimize use of benzodiazepines, anticholinergics, antihistamines, and meperidine
- Modify dosages or discontinue drugs in order to minimize drug interactions and adverse effects

Pain
- Use standing orders for acetaminophen rather than as needed
- Treat breakthrough pain starting with low dose narcotics and titrating up slowly; avoid meperidine

Impaired Vision and Hearing
- Ensure appropriate use of glasses, hearing aids, and adaptive equipment
- Optimize communication strategies: avoid speaking in a high pitched voice, ensure patient can see your mouth to aid in lip reading, optimize lighting and decrease environmental noise, ask patient to repeat what they heard you say to ensure understanding

Malnutrition
- Ensure proper use of dentures, proper positioning, assistance with eating if required, and use of supplements if required

Iatrogenic Complications
- Avoid urinary catheters when possible
- If urinary catheters are used, remove them as soon as possible
- Screen for urinary retention and incontinence
- Screen for and treat symptomatic urinary tract infections
- Implement a skin care program
- Implement a bowel regimen to ensure regular bowel movements
- Provide chest physiotherapy and supplemental oxygen if indicated
- Use appropriate deep vein thrombosis prevention therapy
- Avoid restraints

Sleep Deprivation
- Implement unitwide strategies to reduce noise at night: lowered voices, pagers turned on vibrate mode, minimize overhead announcements
- Schedule medications and procedures to allow for proper sleep at night
- Use nonpharmacologic measures to promote sleep: warm milk, back rubs, hand massages, relaxing music

Source: Reproduced with permission from [17].

you are there to help, considering unmet needs (toileting, hunger/thirst, and pain), optimizing vision and hearing, enabling a safe area to move around, placing identifying signs/pictures outside the patient's room and on bathroom doors, placing large paper stop signs on exit doors, and optimizing sleep at night.

A recent systematic review, which included case reports and low quality clinical trials, examined the role

Table 6.5 Delirium management strategy

General Management
- Investigate the underlying cause(s)/precipitant(s) of delirium
- Treat the potential precipitating factor(s)
- Nonpharmacological strategies should be utilized first in the management of delirium symptoms
- Delirium management should involve a multidisciplinary team
- Provide appropriate education to healthcare providers, patients, and family members

Management of Severe Behavioral and/or Emotional Symptoms
- Attempt nonpharmacological strategies first
- Use one-on-one nursing or a trained support person
- Encourage family members/caregivers to sit with the patient
- Use consistent staff members in the care of the person
- Provide nonpharmacological strategies to assist with sleep
- Consider specialized delirium rooms
- Consider geriatric medicine or geriatric psychiatry consultation
- Antipsychotic medications should be prescribed with caution (i.e., to manage severe agitation or aggression not successfully managed by nonpharmacological approaches) starting at a low dose and then carefully titrating up for effect, while monitoring closely for adverse effects
- Olanzapine 2.5 mg orally
- Risperidone 0.25 mg orally
- Quetiapine 12.5 mg orally
- Haloperidol 0.25–0.50 mg

Source: [20].

of atypical antipsychotics for the treatment of delirium in older adults [22]. Risperidone, at a dosage of 0.5–4 mg daily, was found to be effective in treating the behavioral disturbances of delirium (Level 2a evidence). Olanzapine, at doses of 2.5–11.6 mg daily was also effective (Level 2a evidence). Additionally, quetiapine between 50 and 200 mg appears to be an option (Level 2a evidence). Atypical antipsychotics may be an effective alternative to high-potency antipsychotics. In comparison to haloperidol, the frequency of adverse reactions and side effects, in particular extrapyramidal effects, appears to be lower with atypical antipsychotic medications. However, similar to haloperidol, atypical antipsychotics have been associated with increased risk of death (1% absolute increase) [23] and stroke (1%–2% absolute increase) [24] among the frail older adult. Therefore, these medications should be used judiciously for the management of agitated or aggressive

behaviors that place the patient or others at risk of harm and that are not responsive to nonpharmacological strategies. Other behaviors, such as wandering and calling out, should be managed by nonpharmacological strategies.

A systematic review of benzodiazepine treatment of nonalcohol-related delirium found no evidence to support the use of benzodiazepines in the treatment of nonalcohol-related delirium among hospitalized patients (Level 2a evidence) [21]. Benzodiazepines may actually worsen delirium, given their sedative properties.

Clinical bottom line

Based on the current evidence, efforts appear best targeted at prevention of delirium in high-risk patients, rather than management of delirium.

Although the evidence is inconclusive, delirium management should involve a multifaceted approach that addresses potential precipitants, manages associated symptoms, and educates patients/family members/caregivers. Multicomponent interventions aimed at managing delirium have not been found to decrease mortality or length of hospital stay.

The role for atypical antipsychotics is unclear and they should be used with caution.

Benzodiazepine use is not recommended for nonalcohol-related delirium.

Summary

Delirium is a common condition, occurring in 25%–65% of hospitalized older patients. It is associated with increased mortality, increased length of hospital stay, increased hospital-acquired complications, persistent cognitive deficits, and increased rate of discharge to long-term care. Delirium often goes undiagnosed. The CAM appears to be the best delirium-screening tool to use at the bedside and can help both to rule in (+LR = 9.6) or exclude (−LR = 0.16) a diagnosis of delirium.

Multicomponent preventive strategies that target delirium risk factors are effective. Only seven patients need to be treated with such a strategy to prevent one case of delirium. Delirium management should also involve a multifaceted approach that addresses potential precipitants, manages associated symptoms, and educates patients/family members/caregivers. There is no clear evidence to support the role for medications in either the prevention or management of delirium.

References

1. Association AP (2000) *Diagnostic and Statistical Manual of Mental Disorders (DSM-IV-TR*, Fourth Edition. Washington: American Psychiatric Association.

2. Inouye SK, et al (1999) A multicomponent intervention to prevent delirium in hospitalized older patients. *N Engl J Med* 340(9): 669–676.

3. Williams-Russo P, Urquhart BL, Sharrock NE, Charlson ME (1992) Post-operative delirium: predictors and prognosis in elderly orthopedic patients. *J Am Geriatr Soc* 40(8): 759–767.

4. Francis J, Kapoor WN (1992) Prognosis after hospital discharge of older medical patients with delirium. *J Am Geriatr Soc* 40(6): 601–606.

5. Gustafson Y, et al (1988) Acute confusional states in elderly patients treated for femoral neck fracture. *J Am Geriatr Soc* 36(6): 525–530.

6. Inouye SK, Rushing JT, Foreman MD, Palmer RM, Pompei P (1998) Does delirium contribute to poor hospital outcomes? A three-site epidemiologic study. *J Gen Intern Med* 13(4): 234–242.

7. O'Keeffe S, Lavan J (1997) The prognostic significance of delirium in older hospital patients. *J Am Geriatr Soc* 45(2): 174–178.

8. Inouye SK, Viscoli CM, Horwitz RI, Hurst LD, Tinetti ME (1993) A predictive model for delirium in hospitalized elderly medical patients based on admission characteristics. *Ann Intern Med* 119(6): 474–481.

9. Inouye SK, Charpentier PA (1996) Precipitating factors for delirium in hospitalized elderly persons. Predictive model and interrelationship with baseline vulnerability. *JAMA* 275(11): 852–857.

10. Marcantonio ER, et al (1994) A clinical prediction rule for delirium after elective noncardiac surgery. *JAMA* 271(2): 134–139.

11. Dasgupta M, Dumbrell AC (2006) Preoperative risk assessment for delirium after noncardiac surgery: a systematic review. *J Am Geriatr Soc* 54(10): 1578–1589.

12. Rudolph JL, et al (2009) Derivation and validation of a preoperative prediction rule for delirium after cardiac surgery. *Circulation* 119(2): 229–236.

13. Wei LA, Fearing MA, Sternberg EJ, Inouye SK (2008) The Confusion Assessment Method: a systematic review of current usage. *J Am Geriatr Soc* 56(5): 823–830.

14. Wong CL, Holroyd-Leduc J, Simel DL, Straus SE (2010) Does this patient have delirium? Value of bedside instruments. *JAMA* 304(7): 779–786.

15. Steis MR, Fick DM (2008) Are nurses recognizing delirium? A systematic review. *J Gerontol Nurs* 34(9): 40–48.

16. Inouye SK, van Dyck CH, Alessi CA, Balkin S, Siegal AP, Horwitz RI (1990) Clarifying confusion: the confusion assessment method. A new method for detection of delirium. *Ann Intern Med* 113(12): 941–948.

17. Holroyd-Leduc JM, Khandwala F, Sink KM (2010) How can delirium best be prevented and managed in older patients in hospital?. *CMAJ* 182(5): 465–470.

18. Overshott R, Karim S, Burns A (2008) Cholinesterase inhibitors for delirium. *Cochrane Database Syst Rev* (1): CD005317.

19. Inouye SK, Baker DI, Fugal P, Bradley EH (2006) Dissemination of the hospital elder life program: implementation, adaptation, and successes. *J Am Geriatr Soc* 54(10): 1492–1499.

20. Tropea J, Slee JA, Brand CA, Gray L, Snell T (2008) Clinical practice guidelines for the management of delirium in older people in Australia. *Australas J Ageing* 27(3): 150–156.

21. Lonergan E, Luxenberg J, Areosa Sastre A (2009) Benzodiazepines for delirium. *Cochrane Database Syst Rev* (4): CD006379.

22. Ozbolt LB, Paniagua MA, Kaiser RM (2008) Atypical antipsychotics for the treatment of delirious elders. *J Am Med Dir Assoc* (1): 18–28.

23. Schneider LS, Dagerman KS, Insel P (2005) Risk of death with atypical antipsychotic drug treatment for dementia: meta-analysis of randomized placebo-controlled trials. *JAMA* 294(15): 1934–1943.

24. Sink KM, Holden KF, Yaffe K (2005) Pharmacological treatment of neuropsychiatric symptoms of dementia: a review of the evidence. *JAMA* 293(5): 596–608.

CHAPTER 7

Preserving memories: managing dementia

Dallas P. Seitz[1,2], Philip E. Lee[3], Sudeep S. Gill[4], & Paula A. Rochon[2,5,6]

[1]*Department of Psychiatry, Division of Geriatric Psychiatry, Queen's University, Kingston, ON, Canada*
[2]*Women's College Research Institute, Toronto, ON, Canada*
[3]*Division of Geriatric Medicine, University of British Columbia, Vancouver, BC, Canada*
[4]*Department of Medicine, Division of Geriatric Medicine, Queen's University, Kingston, ON, Canada*
[5]*Institute for Clinical Evaluative Sciences, Toronto, ON, Canada*
[6]*Department of Medicine, University of Toronto, Toronto, ON, Canada*

Introduction

Dementia is one of the most prevalent medical conditions in older adults [1, 2] affecting between 5% and 8% of individuals aged 65 and older, increasing to 30% of individuals over age 85 years. The number of older adults with dementia is also increasing [3]. Estimated 24 million individuals have dementia and over 4 million individuals will develop dementia each year [4], the majority of whom have Alzheimer's disease (AD) [1, 3]. Given the numbers of older adults with dementia, the management of most individuals with dementia will continue to rest with primary care physicians with support from community agencies and specialized dementia or geriatric services where these are available.

Management of dementia is complex and multifaceted and includes: identifying and reducing risk factors for dementia; screening and early diagnosis; initiating treatments for cognitive symptoms; and interventions for the challenging behavioral symptoms that frequently accompany dementia. Supporting patients with dementia involves complex ethical and medicolegal issues around capacity for decision-making and safety that are important to assess and monitor. Individuals with dementia also live with and frequently depend on family members for support and assisting family members is an important aspect of dementia care.

This chapter is written for primary care physicians who are not specialists in dementia care and focuses on the office-based management of community-dwelling older adults with AD and related forms of dementia. This chapter reviews dementia risk factors and evidence-based screening tools. We also review important issues related to capacity, driving safety, and caregiver supports. Finally, we review interventions for the cognitive symptoms of dementia as well as pharmacological and nonpharmacological treatments for behavioral symptoms associated with dementia. The chapter sections are organized in a sequence that follows a typical time course of when certain inventions or strategies are typically implemented during the course of illness as outlined in Figure 7.1. A detailed discussion of interventions for cognitive and behavioral symptom of dementia and the corresponding chapter sections are outlined in Figure 7.2.

Search strategy

We searched MEDLINE, EMBASE, and the Cochrane Library first for existing systematic reviews and meta-analyses of the topics. Where systematic reviews on topics were not available, we described information obtained from randomized controlled trials identified from searching MEDLINE, EMBASE, the Cochrane Library, and Google Scholar in July 2010 to identify relevant articles. We used the following search terms

Evidence-Based Geriatric Medicine: A Practical Clinical Guide, First Edition. Edited by Jayna M. Holroyd-Leduc and Madhuri Reddy.
© 2012 Blackwell Publishing Ltd. Published 2012 by Blackwell Publishing Ltd.

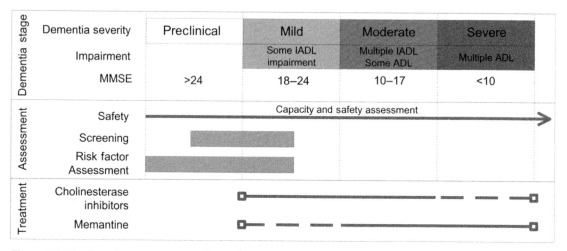

Figure 7.1 Timeline of symptom presentation and interventions for dementia. Solid line indicates strong evidence in support of a therapy, and dashed line indicates a potentially beneficial therapy.

to identify relevant citations: "dementia" "Alzheimer's disease", "cognitive impairment", "cognitive decline", "risk factors", "prevention", "screening tests", "cognitive test", "diagnosis", "cholinesterase inhibitor", "cognitive enhancer", "memantine", "behavioral symptoms", "psychosis", "agitation", "depression", "antipsychotic", "antidepressant", "behavioral", "nonpharmacological", and "psychosocial". We also included information contained in guidelines published by medical associations and professional organizations where there were no randomized controlled trials or systematic reviews for evidence on topics that did not involve interventions.

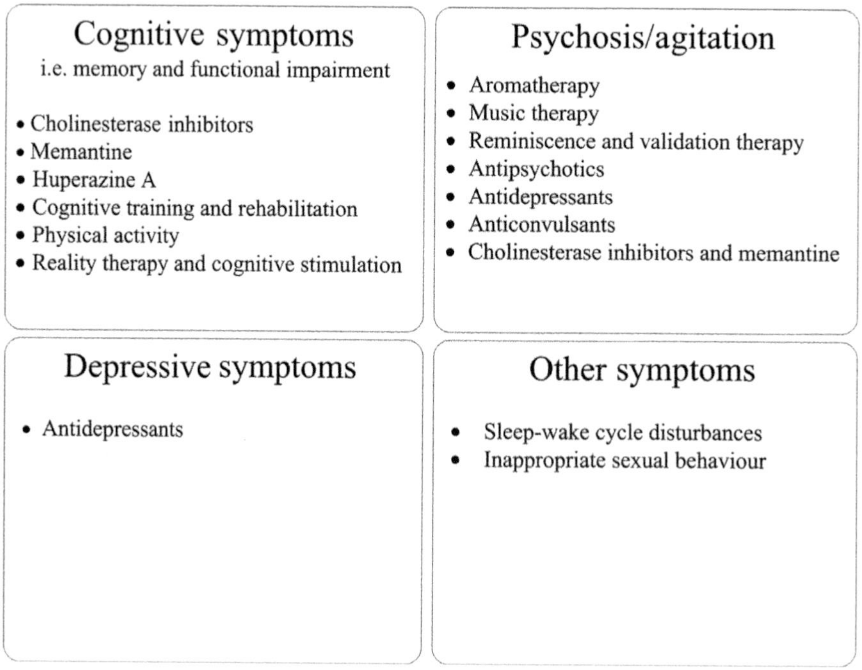

Cognitive symptoms
i.e. memory and functional impairment

- Cholinesterase inhibitors
- Memantine
- Huperazine A
- Cognitive training and rehabilitation
- Physical activity
- Reality therapy and cognitive stimulation

Psychosis/agitation

- Aromatherapy
- Music therapy
- Reminiscence and validation therapy
- Antipsychotics
- Antidepressants
- Anticonvulsants
- Cholinesterase inhibitors and memantine

Depressive symptoms

- Antidepressants

Other symptoms

- Sleep-wake cycle disturbances
- Inappropriate sexual behaviour

Figure 7.2 Interventions for cognitive and behavioral symptoms of dementia. ● indicates relevant chapter sections.

A total of 194 articles were included in this chapter including 68 systematic reviews, 24 randomized controlled trials, 6 guidelines, and 97 observational studies or other studies.

For this chapter, we graded relevant clinical studies using the Oxford Centre for Evidence-based Medicine Levels of Evidence.

What are the risk factors for Alzheimer's dementia?

Increased recognition of the importance of preventing or delaying AD is one of the principal recommendations as part of reducing the impact of dementia on society [3, 5]. Information about modifiable risk factors offers potential opportunity to intervene, while knowledge about nonmodifiable risk factors may still be valuable in estimating potential risk for the development of AD. In this section, we summarize the known nonmodifiable and modifiable risk factors for AD (Table 7.1). Further information on risk factors is available in previously published reviews [6].

Table 7.1 Modifiable and nonmodifiable risk factors for dementia

Nonmodifiable	Possibly Modifiable
Advanced age	*Increased Risk of AD*
Female gender	Hypertension
Lower educational achievement	Diabetes
Ethnicity	Smoking
Family history	Hypercholesterolemia
Specific genetic mutations (early-onset AD)	Hyperhomocysteinemia
Mild cognitive impairment	
ApoE4 (late-onset AD)	
Down's syndrome	*Decreased Risk*
	Physical exercise
Head injury	Diet

Nonmodifiable risk factors

Age
One of the most consistently identified risk factor for AD is advanced age [7]. In people over the age of 65 years of age, it is estimated that the prevalence of dementia is between 5% and 8% [1], increasing to approximately 30% among adults aged 85 and older [1, 8]. In women over the age of 90 years, the prevalence of dementia appears to continue to roughly double every 5 years [9].

Gender
Compared to men, women have been found be at greater risk of AD [10] even after adjusting for differences in age and level of education. The differences between the sexes in the prevalence of AD may be related to unidentified genetics factors or perhaps hormonal effects.

Education
A higher level of education is associated with a lower incidence of dementia and AD [11]. It is not clear whether the differences demonstrated between groups with different levels of education is a direct result of the protective effect of sustained learning (i.e., increased cognitive reserve) or a marker of other unmeasured factors like socioeconomic status.

Ethnicity
The prevalence of dementia may be increased in African-American men compared to non-Hispanic white men [12]. There may also be differences in the prevalence of other non-AD dementia among different ethnic groups [13]. Additionally, individuals of African and Hispanic backgrounds may have a more prolonged median survival time after diagnosis when compared to Caucasians [14, 15].

Genetic risk factors
A detailed family history of AD and age at onset is helpful in the assessment of genetic risk for AD [16]. The overall risk of AD with a single first-degree relative is 2.6, while the risk is further increased with a family history of two or more first-degree relatives [17]. Genetic risk factors for AD differ for early-onset (age <60–65 years) familial forms of dementia and late-onset AD [18]. Mutations of the amyloid precursor protein (APP) are associated with early-onset familial

forms of AD. The APP gene is located on chromosome 21 and individuals with Down's syndrome are at increased risk for AD [19]. There are three mutations that demonstrate an autosomal dominant pattern of inheritance. Predictive genetic testing, with appropriate pre- and posttesting counseling, may be offered to those individuals with an apparent autosomal dominant inheritance pattern when a specific mutation has been identified [16].

Apolipoprotein (Apo) E4 (ApoE4) has been confirmed as a genetic risk factor for late-onset AD. There are three ApoE polymorphisms: (1) E2, (2) E3, and (3) E4. Homozygous ApoE4 carriers are at highest risk for AD (odds ratio (OR) 11.6, 95% confidence interval (CI) 8.9–15.4) [20]. Unlike the other gene mutations, the presence of ApoE4 is a susceptibility factor that increases the risk for AD, but not all people with ApoE4, even homozygous carriers, will develop the condition. The presence of ApoE4 has been associated with a higher mortality rate [21]. Genetic screening for ApoE genotype in asymptomatic individuals in the general population is not recommended because of the low specificity and sensitivity [16].

Head injury

A history of head injury, especially if associated with loss of consciousness, has been reported to increase a person's risk of developing AD [22]. While discrepancies exist in the literature, there still appears to be evidence to support the hypothesis that traumatic brain injury is a potential risk factor for AD.

Potentially modifiable risk factors

A number of studies have suggested various medical conditions, medications, and lifestyle factors that may affect the risk of AD. Some of these factors have been studied in more rigorous detail in randomized clinical trials, while other associations remain mostly speculative.

Cardiovascular risk factors

Of the potentially modifiable risk factors, the most extensively studied include cardiovascular risk factors including hypertension, hypercholesterolemia, diabetes, and cerebrovascular disease [23]. Vascular risk factors appear to accelerate the rate of progression of AD and treatment of vascular risk factors may be associated with slower cognitive decline in persons with AD [24].

Other studies have not found consistent associations between cardiovascular risk factors and AD [25, 26], highlighting the potential importance of interactions between risk factors.

Hypertension is a well-described risk factor for cardiovascular and cerebrovascular disease. A Cochrane review [27] of treatment for hypertension and subsequent dementia included four randomized trials [28–31]. While some of the individual trials demonstrated a benefit, there was a lack of convincing evidence that treatment of hypertension prevents the development of cognitive impairment in patients without preexisting cerebrovascular disease. A large observational study found that use of any antihypertensive medication was associated with decreased risk of dementia [32]. There is good evidence to support the treatment of hypertension in older individuals in efforts to reduce the risk of stroke and dementia (Level 1b evidence) [16, 33].

Atrial fibrillation has been suggested to have an association with AD as well as vascular dementia [34, 35]. This association may be related both to thromboembolic events and possible effects on cerebral blood flow. Antithrombotic therapy for nonvalvular atrial fibrillation cannot be recommended for the prevention of dementia alone (Level 1b evidence) [16].

Cholesterol plays an essential role in the formation of important components of neuronal membranes and is a risk factor for cerebrovascular disease. Alterations in the balance of cholesterol in the brain may have demonstrable effects on amyloid processing [36]. High levels of serum cholesterol in midlife are associated with an increased risk of AD [37].

Diabetes is also a risk factor for vascular disease, and therefore, it follows that it would be associated with vascular dementia. The Memory in Diabetes (MIND) substudy of the Action to Control Cardiovascular Risk in Diabetes (ACCORD) trial reported higher levels of hemoglobin A1C in persons with poorer performance on cognitive testing [38]. Uncontrolled diabetes or repeated episodes of hypoglycemia may have effects on cognition [39, 40]. Specific medications used to treat diabetes, such as the thiazolidinediones [41] are being reviewed to assess their potential effects on preventing dementia.

High level of homocysteine has been recognized as a risk factor for coronary artery disease and has been implicated as a potential risk factor for AD [42, 43].

Despite multiple reasons for treating type 2 diabetes mellitus, hypercholesterolemia, and hyperhomocysteinemia, there is insufficient evidence to recommend for or against treatment for the specific purpose of reducing the risk of dementia (Level 2b evidence) [16].

Early case-control studies suggest that smoking may protect against the development of dementia [44], although more recent observational studies have consistently demonstrated a positive association between tobacco smoking and increased risk of AD [45, 46]. Even exposure to second-hand smoke has been associated with an increased risk of AD [47].

Mild cognitive impairment and Alzheimer's dementia

Mild cognitive impairment (MCI) is a term used to describe individuals who have demonstrable cognitive deficits that are greater than expected for a person's age but do not significantly interfere with functional abilities and do not meet the diagnostic criteria for dementia [48]. Of persons classified as having MCI, about 10%–15% per year will advance to AD or another form of dementia [49].

Depression and Alzheimer's dementia

There appears to be a relationship between a history of depression and dementia [50] although this relationship is complex [51]. A case-control study suggests that a history of depression is associated with an increased risk of dementia, although the association is less robust with a longer interval between depression onset and dementia diagnosis [52]. Depression may be an early presentation of AD as well as a risk factor.

Possible protective factors

Diet

There is increasing attention placed on nutrition and lifestyle factors as contributing to the risk of AD [40]. At the dietary level, adherence to a Mediterranean-style diet [53, 54] or to diet with high fish consumption [55] and daily fruits and vegetables [56] has been linked to a lower prevalence of dementia. At the micronutrient level, dietary factors such as reduced vitamin B12 levels have been described as associated with a higher frequency of dementia or faster rate of decline [57]. Although dietary factors, like vitamin B12 or folate deficiency, have been shown to be associated with cognitive impairment, their influence on progression

of symptoms is less clear [58]. Prospective trials have not shown a clear cognitive benefit to treating persons with folate, B12 [59] (Level 1a evidence), or polyunsaturated fatty acids (including omega-3) (Level 2b evidence) [60–65]. Given the potential benefits and the biologically plausible mechanism of protection, further clinical trials are in progress [66].

Consumption of coffee in midlife has been reported to be associated with a lower prevalence of dementia/AD compared to those who did not consume coffee (Level 2b evidence) [67]. Drinking alcohol has been suggested to impart benefit, although intake should be moderate (Level 2b evidence) [68, 69]. Clinicians may choose to advise their patients on the potential benefits of increased consumption of fish, decreased dietary fat, and moderate consumption of coffee and wine [16], although a firm recommendation cannot be made based on the available information for primary prevention.

Other lifestyle factors

Increased levels of physical activity have been linked to reduced risk of dementia [70]. Studies have also suggested that those persons who had a higher level of exercise activity/energy expenditure had a lower risk of AD [71, 72]. A recent randomized trial of physical activity showed that in adults with subjective memory problems, a 24-week program of physical activity provided a modest benefit in cognition over the 18-month follow-up period (Level 1b evidence) [73].

Estimating an individual risk for Alzheimer's dementia

There is increasing interest in dementia risk prediction indices to estimate an individual's risk of developing Alzheimer's dementia on the basis of clinical information supplemented by neuroimaging and genetics [74, 75]. Further validation of these indices is required to determine their predictive validity, and indices based on easily obtainable clinical information are required. It is likely that these indices or similar indices will prove useful in predicting the development of AD for individuals at risk.

Clinical Bottom Line

Age, gender, educational achievement, cardiovascular risk factors, genetics, and MCI are strong risk factors for dementia. Treatment of hypertension may reduce the risk of dementia in older adults while role of vitamins, omega-3 fatty acids, alcohol, and caffeine in preventing dementia are unclear.

How can I screen for dementia?

Although there is currently no cure available, the identification of individuals with AD provides the opportunity to offer support and education, initiate future planning, and institute early treatment. The diagnosis of AD remains a clinical diagnosis supported by investigations such as neuroimaging with increasing interest in the use of biomarkers. Dementia assessment integrates a detailed history and physical examination, cognitive testing, and additional tests including laboratory investigations, neuroimaging, and possibly neuropsychological consultation.

Screening tools

Brief cognitive screening tools have been developed to help identify the presence of cognitive impairment and also to give some assessment of the overall severity and possibly the areas of cognitive impairment (Table 7.2). The mini-mental state examination (MMSE) is the most commonly used dementia-screening instrument and is relatively quick and easy to administer (Level 1b evidence) [76, 77]. The sensitivity and specificity of the MMSE in detecting dementia varies depending on the cutoff score used, age of the patient, and educational achievement [78]. It has been suggested that patients with mild dementia usually have a score of 18–26 out of 30, those with moderate dementia a score of 10–28, and those with severe dementia a score of less than 10 [79]. The MMSE is a copyright tool and a "per use" fee is required for any use of the printed version.

The MMSE has also been expanded to the modified mini-mental state examination (3MS), which includes additional measures of cognition such as an assessment of delayed recall [80]. The 3MS appears to have advantages over the MMSE, which may be related to its expanded scoring system [11]. The additional time required to administer the tool is offset by the

Table 7.2 Commonly used dementia screening instruments

Test	Range of Score	Time to Administer (min)	Comments
Mini-Mental State Examination (MMSE) [76]	0–30 points	10–15	• Widely used screening instrument that assesses several cognitive domains • May be susceptible to effects of age, education, and language • Can be insensitive to milder cognitive impairment
Montreal Cognitive Assessment (MoCA) [92]	0–30 points	10–20	• Designed as a rapid screening instrument for mild cognitive dysfunction • Developed in the outpatient setting • Assesses attention and concentration, executive function, memory, language, visuoconstructional skills, conceptual thinking, calculation, and orientation
Clock-Drawing Test [81]	Various scoring systems exist	3–5	• Relatively easy to administer, yet assesses executive function and visuospatial ability • Sensitivity and specificity may vary depending on the scoring system used
Mini-Cog [91]	0–3 points	3–5	• Combines uncued 3-item recall and a clock drawing task • Quick to administer; May be less influenced by differences in language or education
3MS	0–100 points	20–25	• Combines items from MMSE along with additional naming tasks, two trials of delayed recall, naming of four-legged animals, with scoring modifications on certain MMSE items

improved ability of the 3MS to detect dementia (Level 1b evidence) [77].

The clock-drawing test (CDT) is a relatively quick (5 minute) and simple test to administer. Proper performance of the test requires coordination of various cognitive domains, including visuospatial and executive function. Untrained raters can discriminate between normal and abnormal clocks with sufficient accuracy for community screening process [81]. Numerous scoring systems have been developed to aid the identification of dementia and improve the sensitivity and specificity of the CDT [82–85]. However, the key components to scoring include appropriate spatial distribution of the numbers and accurate placement of the clock hands to indicate an abstract concept of time such as 10 past 2. The performance of the CDT and other cognitive screening tools generally show good correlation to other established screening tools (Level 2 evidence). The results on the CDT can be influenced by the effects of age, education, and language [86, 87]. While it appear to be a good screening tool for dementia, by itself, the CDT does not appear to be a sufficient screening method to distinguish between patients with MCI and noncognitively impaired individuals [88–90].

Additional screening tests have been developed with the intention of aiding in the detection and diagnosis of dementia. Some tests, such as the Mini-Cog [91] (Level 2b evidence), are advantageous due to their ease of administration. Other tests attempt to increase their sensitivity to detect dementia and may also identify persons experiencing MCI. For instance, the Montreal Cognitive Assessment (MoCA) [92] assesses memory, executive function, attention, language, and attention (Level 2b evidence). It requires 15–25 minutes to administer, but is more sensitive in the detection of early dementia and MCI in the outpatient setting. There does not appear to be one test that is to be recommended above all others in screening for dementia.

Investigations

Although reversible forms of dementia are uncommon [93], the use of laboratory tests and neuroimaging may help to identify individuals with potentially treatable causes. Current recommendations indicate that basic investigations including a complete blood count, thyroid stimulating hormone, serum calcium, electrolytes, a fasting glucose, and serum B12 level should be performed for all patients, at least once during their evaluation [79]. Selective use of other tests, such as folate levels, rapid plasma regain for syphilis, and HIV testing, should be considered if their medical history suggests that they are at higher risk [16].

Use of neuroimaging studies, like computed tomography or magnetic resonance imaging scans, allows for the exclusion of potentially reversible conditions like mass lesions, subdural hematomas, or hydrocephalus. These investigations may also be helpful in the process of looking for concurrent conditions, like cerebrovascular disease, which may contribute to cognitive impairment. Criteria have been proposed to identify persons in whom neuroimaging may be helpful. Imaging studies should be considered if any of the following are present: age <60 years; rapid cognitive decline (1–2 months); <2 years' duration of dementia; history of recent head trauma; use of anticoagulants or known bleeding disorder; unexplained neurological symptoms or new localizing sign; history of cancer; gait disturbance; urinary incontinence, and change in gait [79, 94].

Specialist referral

In support of primary care physicians, a referral to a geriatrician, geriatric psychiatrist, neurologist, or other professional with specialized skills in the assessment and treatment of patients with dementia can be beneficial. Referrals may be considered in situations such as: continuing uncertainty about the diagnosis; presence of significant depression, especially refractory to initial treatment; need for additional help with management of behavioral problems; treatment problems with medication treatment for AD; access to genetic counseling is desired; research studies are being considered. Support for patients and family may also be obtained through referral to agencies such as the Alzheimer Society [94].

Referral for detailed neuropsychological testing may be made selectively for certain patients. A consultation with a neuropsychologist is beneficial in distinguishing among individuals with MCI, dementia, and those with normal cognitive function [95, 96]. It may also help in assessing the risk of progression of cognitive impairment. Additionally, neuropsychological testing may assist in distinguishing between causes of cognitive impairment, including different subtypes of dementia [16].

Clinical Bottom Line

Cognitive tests such as the MMSE, MoCA, Clock drawing test, or Mini-Cog can be used to screen for dementia and each have benefits and limitations in terms of ease of administration and diagnostic test accuracy. Further evaluation of dementia also involves selective use of blood work, neuroimaging, and specialist referral depending on clinical circumstances.

What are other important areas to assess with caregivers and individuals diagnosed with dementia

For most individuals with early AD, the goals of treatment are to maximize autonomy and delay or prevent institutionalization when possible. Management of AD involves assessing the impact of AD on areas such as capacity to make a variety of decisions, as judgment and higher level cognitive skills are often affected early by the disease. Cognitive difficulties can also pose a risk of unintentional injury such as motor vehicle collisions, wandering, and medication misuse. Finally, supporting the family members and caregivers of individuals with AD is important to delay or prevent institutionalization and decrease the likelihood of the caregiver developing depression or caregiver burnout.

Capacity and advanced care planning

Capacity is defined as the ability to understand and appreciate the consequences of decisions and the ability to communicate a decision. Competency is sometimes used interchangeably with capacity but can also refer to legal concepts that are not determined by physicians. Understanding involves the ability to retain factual information necessary to make decisions, while appreciating involves applying this information to one's circumstances and decisions at hand. There are several areas of capacity that may be compromised by dementia. These include capacity for treatment decisions (or medical decisions), financial decisions, personal care decisions (e.g., decisions around living arrangements), and testamentary capacity (capacity to make a will) [97], among others. The threshold for determining incapacity can vary according to different legal standards [98] and is also dependent upon the complexity of the decision [97], the potential consequences of the decision, stated reasons given for a decision, and likelihood of the individual being coerced. A recent history of questionable decisions or a change in behaviors related to finances or self-care should also be considered when assessing current capacity. Capacity is task and context specific, and individuals may lack capacity for certain tasks while retaining capacity for other tasks. Capacity for all decisions will be affected by increasing severity of dementia. Capacity and its assessment vary by jurisdiction and physicians need to be aware of local requirements and procedures for capacity assessment. It is important to assess capacity and wishes of patients early in the disease process when most people are capable of making decisions. These discussions should also include advanced care planning such as living wills, and powers of attorney for both personal care and finances as applicable. In cases of incapacity, physicians should obtain consent from appropriate substitute decision-makers.

Driving safety

For most older adults, retaining the ability to drive is an important autonomy to preserve and enhance quality of life. Assessment of driving safety is important as older adults with dementia are at an increased risk of motor vehicle collisions when compared to similar populations of older adults without dementia [99]. While many drivers with early or mild dementia are safe to continue driving, all individuals with progressive dementias such as AD will lose the ability to safely operate a motor vehicle at some point in their illness. There is limited information on the predictive ability of office-based cognitive tests to predict driving-related outcomes in dementia and no single cognitive test can be used to predict driving safety [100, 101]. Abnormalities on cognitive screening tests such as the MMSE or other tests are associated with increased likelihood of errors during simulator, on-road testing, or reported driving problems [100, 101]. Abnormalities on cognitive screening tests should alert clinicians to assess driving safety in detail. Most guidelines from professional organizations and medical associations have indicated that dementia of greater than mild severity (i.e., symptoms impacting on multiple IADLS or any ADL) is a contraindication to driving [102–105]. Recent driving history from a reliable, impartial informant is important to obtain and is predictive of on-road test performance [104]. Most guidelines also recommend on-road driving assessment when driving ability is questioned and continued monitoring and reassessment of driving every 6–12 months. There is insufficient evidence at the present time that on-road driving evaluations have any impact on prolonging safe driving for individuals with early dementia [106]. It is also important to assess other medical conditions that may impair driving including reduced vision, mobility, and neurological disorders such as stroke or Parkinson's disease. Many jurisdictions have mandatory reporting for medical conditions that may interfere with driving and each physician must act in accordance with local reporting requirements. Physicians should facilitate the transition to driving cessation and discuss alternatives to driving for transportation needs with their patients.

Caregiver burden and interventions to support dementia caregivers

Caregiver burden is important to assess in the family members of individuals with dementia. Caregivers of individuals with dementia are at increased risk of depression [107]. Caregiver depression is important as it is associated with decreased quality of life and is a significant predictor of long-term care admission. Although caregiver burnout is most commonly associated with individuals living with dementia in the community, substantial caregiver distress can persist even following admission to long-term care. Important patient-related predictors of caregiver distress include younger age, higher functional dependence, and greater number of behavioral symptoms [108]. Caregiver characteristics associated with caregiver distress include being a wife of the individual with dementia, having ADL impairments, low social supports, and number of hours spent caregiving [108, 109].

Community support and respite programs are two groups of interventions for caregivers of older adults with dementia. The goals of these programs are to provide support, education, and resources to patients and caregivers, to improve quality of life, and to delay time until institutionalization. These supports may include referrals to homecare agencies, "Meals on Wheels" programs, dementia organizations such as the Alzheimer Association, local support groups, and referrals to regional geriatric medicine or geriatric psychiatry teams. Two broad categories of community-based interventions have been studied in randomized controlled trials: (1) respite services [110] and (2) information and support interventions [111, 112]. Due to the small number of studies and differences in reported outcomes, conclusions about the effects of psychological interventions on caregivers are difficult to interpret, although there are trends toward decreased caregiver burden in one study. Group-based psychoeducation and support groups may have beneficial effects on caregiver depression (Level 1a evidence) [111] and training caregivers in methods for managing dementia-related behaviors and coping strategies also appear to be beneficial for caregiver's psychological well-being (Level 1b evidence) [112].

Clinical Bottom Line

Management of dementia also must take into account assessment of capacity, driving, and advance care planning. There is limited evidence to support the use of any one cognitive screening test or on-road driving test to evaluate the safety of older adults to operate motor vehicles. Interventions to reduce caregiver stress are also important and include psychoeducation and support groups and strategies to cope with behavioral symptoms of dementia.

Are medications effective in treating the cognitive symptoms of Alzheimer's dementia?

Memory impairment and difficulties with performing activities of daily living are the hallmark symptoms of AD and the target symptoms for most treatments approved for AD. After diagnosing dementia and ensuring patient safety, a discussion of treatment options for AD is the next step in management (Figure 7.2). To date, the best supported medication classes for treating cognitive and functional symptoms are cholinesterase inhibitors and memantine. There are no pharmacological treatments for dementia that have been demonstrated to alter the underlying disease process associated with AD.

Cholinesterase inhibitors

Decreases in acetylcholine pathways in the brain are responsible for many of the memory problems observed in AD and several cholinergic therapies have been developed to treat AD. These medications are classified as cholinesterase inhibitors and increase central nervous system acetylcholine through inhibition of the enzymes that normally degrade acetylcholine. Three cholinesterase inhibitors are available in most countries: (1) donepezil, (2) galantamine, and (3) rivastigmine. All cholinesterase inhibitors are available in oral form and require dose titration over several weeks to minimize the development of adverse events (e.g., gastrointestinal intolerance). Rivastigmine is also available in a transdermal patch preparation that is changed daily. Cholinesterase inhibitors are approved for the treatment of mild-to-moderate AD in most countries, although certain countries have also approved donepezil for severe dementia and rivastigmine for dementia associated with Parkinson's disease.

Efficacy on measures of cognition and functioning

There are several systematic reviews and meta-analyses of cholinesterase inhibitors for treatment of Alzheimer's dementia [113–115]. Statistically significant, although perhaps clinically modest, improvements in cognitive symptoms of mild-to-moderate Alzheimer's dementia have been observed with donepezil [116] (Level 1a evidence), galantamine [117] (Level 1a evidence), and rivastigmine [118] (Level 1a evidence). All cholinesterase inhibitors also produce modest benefits on global clinical ratings and impairment in activities of daily living when compared to placebo [116–118] (galantamine: Level 1a evidence; donepezil and rivastigmine: Level 1b evidence). Higher doses of donepezil are associated with marginal benefits over lower doses of donepezil (10 mg vs. 5 mg), while higher doses of both galantamine ($\geq$16 mg daily vs. lower doses) and rivastigmine ($\geq$6 mg daily vs. <6 mg daily) were more beneficial than lower daily doses. There is limited evidence to suggest that any cholinesterase inhibitor is superior to another in terms of measures of efficacy, although there are relatively few high-quality trials directly comparing different cholinesterase inhibitors. One randomized controlled trial comparing donepezil to rivastigmine found both medications to have similar efficacy with lower rates of adverse events for donepezil compared to rivastigmine [119] (Level 1b evidence). The effects of cholinesterase inhibitors on neuropsychiatric symptoms of dementia are reviewed in a subsequent section of this chapter.

Safety and adverse events associated with cholinesterase inhibitors

Adverse events associated with cholinesterase inhibitors are related to increases in central and peripheral concentrations of acetylcholine. In randomized controlled trials, all cholinesterase inhibitors are associated with nausea, vomiting, and diarrhea when compared to placebo [116–118]. There are relatively few studies directly comparing rates of adverse events with different cholinesterase inhibitors. Donepezil was associated with fewer adverse events than oral rivastigmine in one comparative trial [120] (Level 1b evidence). Transdermal rivastigmine is better tolerated than comparable doses of the oral formulation [118] (Level 1b evidence), while there is no difference in adverse event rate for extended-release galantamine when compared to twice daily immediate-release formulation (Level 1b evidence) [117]. Rates of adverse events are dose-related for donepezil, galantamine, and rivastigmine when compared to lower doses of the same medication. Additional adverse events identified in observational studies have also demonstrated that cholinesterase inhibitors may also be associated with bradyarrhythmias and syncope-related outcomes [121, 122].

Memantine

Memantine is an NMDA (N-methyl-D-aspartate) receptor antagonist that is believed to effect symptoms of AD through decreasing excitotoxicity associated with glutamate in the central nervous system. The efficacy of memantine for treating moderate to severe Alzheimer's dementia has been evaluated in several trials. Overall, memantine is associated with statistically significant improvements in global, cognitive, and functional improvements, although these effects are clinically modest [123, 124] (Level 1a evidence). Memantine may have relatively less benefit when used for mild-to-moderate Alzheimer's dementia or in vascular dementia [123]. Rates of discontinuation and discontinuation due to adverse events were not significantly different for memantine when compared to placebo and it tends to be well tolerated [123, 124].

Other populations

The evidence for cholinesterase inhibitors and memantine in clinical populations other than AD is less well established. Donepezil has been shown to be associated with improvements in cognition and global impression in moderate-to-severe unspecified dementia [116, 125] (Level 1b evidence). Donepezil, galantamine, and rivastigmine have evidence supporting cognitive benefits in vascular dementia with higher rates of adverse events for all medications when compared with placebo [126] (Level 1a evidence). Galantamine may also be beneficial for patients with mixed Alzheimer's and vascular dementia [127] (Level 1b evidence). Rivastigmine is associated with improvements in cognition and functioning in dementia associated with Parkinson's disease [128] (Level 1b evidence). Rivastigmine may improve neuropsychiatric symptoms associated with dementia with Lewy bodies, although there is insufficient evidence to support it or any other cholinesterase inhibitor in this population [129] (Level 1b evidence). There is no evidence to support the use of cholinesterase inhibitors for improving symptoms of MCI or delaying time to development of dementia [117, 130, 131].

Other treatments for Alzheimer's dementia

Huperzine A has cholinesterase inhibitor activity and other potentially beneficial properties that are showing promise as a treatment for Alzheimer's dementia [132] (Level 1a evidence).

A physical exercise program combined with caregiver behavioral management techniques showed benefits in functional outcomes for individuals with dementia [133] (Level 1a evidence). Psychological approaches for rehabilitating or accommodating certain deficits in Alzheimer's are also showing potential promise, although further study is required [134].

Several additional medications have not been shown to have consistent effects on either the prevention or treatment of AD. Prospective trials of statins for cognitive outcomes have been negative [135, 136] (Level 1b evidence). In a meta-analysis of observational studies, a decreased risk of dementia was reported in those persons who were taking NSAIDs (nonsteroidal anti-inflammatory drugs), although beneficial effects were not observed in all subgroups [137] (Level 1a evidence). However, these benefits have not been shown in prospective trials [138, 139] (Level 1b evidence). Randomized clinical trial data suggest an increased risk of harm with estrogens (Level 1b evidence) [140]. No benefit has been observed with studies of vitamin C (Level 2a evidence) or vitamin E (Level 1a evidence) [141–143]. A review of the literature on the use of

Ginkgo biloba found that while generally safe, there is inconsistent and unreliable data to suggest that it is effective for dementia or cognitive impairment [144] (Level 1b evidence). A subsequent large randomized trial did not show a benefit in taking *Gingko biloba* 120 mg twice daily compared to placebo in preventing cognitive decline in older adults with normal cognition or MCI [145] (Level 1b evidence).

Clinical Bottom Line

Evidence-based treatments for AD include the cholinesterase inhibitors—donepezil, galantamine, and rivastigmine—with the greatest support for their use in mild-to-moderate AD. There is some evidence to support the use of certain cholinesterase inhibitors in severe AD, vascular dementia, and Parkinson's disease dementia. There is also evidence to support the use of memantine in moderate-to-severe dementia and vascular dementia. Treatment benefits with both cholinesterase inhibitors and memantine are modest and must be weighed against the risk of side effects. There is limited information to support other pharmacological treatments for treatment of cognitive symptoms of dementia.

What are the best interventions for challenging behaviors associated with dementia?

A wide variety of challenging behavioral and psychological symptoms commonly develop in people with AD and related dementias. This spectrum of neuropsychiatric symptoms is often referred to as behavioral and psychological symptoms of dementia (BPSD). During the course of their illness, more than 90% of people with dementia will develop at least one behavioral or psychiatric symptom [146]. These behavioral manifestations include agitation, aggression, psychosis, and depression. BPSD are associated with a number of poor outcomes, including functional decline, reduced quality of life, institutionalization, and death [147]. Caregivers of people with BPSD also experience adverse outcomes, including reduced quality of life, and an increased sense of burden and depressive symptoms [147]. Evaluating the evidence to support treatments for BPSD is challenging, in part because studies use a number of different assessment scales that are not typically familiar to clinicians. Lee and colleagues and Sink and colleagues describe some of the common outcome measures employed in BPSD trials [148, 149].

Nonpharmacological treatments

Nonpharmacological strategies are often recommended as first-line management for BPSD [149], and a number of different nonpharmacological interventions for BPSD have been evaluated. Many nonpharmacological interventions may be difficult to implement in clinical practice without specific training or specialized resources [150]. There is considerable heterogeneity in how a number of nonpharmacological treatments were defined and operationalized in individual studies, which contributes to ongoing uncertainty about the effectiveness of these treatments. A number of reviews of nonpharmacological interventions for BPSD have been published to help navigate this large and disparate literature [151–153]

Aromatherapy

Aromatherapy uses oils extracted from fragrant plants to relieve health problems. Individual studies of aromatherapy differ in the oils evaluated and their method of delivery (e.g., in oil burners, in bath water, massaged into the skin). Although a 2003 Cochrane review identified four trials of aromatherapy, the authors were only able to analyze data from one relatively small trail [154] (Level 1b evidence). In this trial, aromatherapy using lemon balm showed benefit for people with dementia and agitation.

Music therapy

Music therapy is designed to facilitate and promote communication, relationships, learning, mobilization, expression, organization, and other relevant therapeutic objectives in order to meet physical, emotional, mental, social, and cognitive needs [155]. A Cochrane review evaluated five studies of music therapy for people with dementia and found that reporting quality in these studies made it difficult to draw any meaningful conclusions about effectiveness for BPSD [155] (Level 2b evidence).

Light therapy and melatonin

Older adults with dementia have disruptions in their sleep–wake cycles. Some investigators have proposed light therapy and melatonin to treat these disturbances. A Cochrane review identified eight studies evaluating different forms of light therapy and concluded that there was inadequate evidence of its effectiveness for BPSD [156] (Level 1a evidence). However, one relatively large recent trial (which was included in the Cochrane review) reported findings that suggest light therapy combined with melatonin attenuated aggressive behavior, improved sleep efficiency, and improved nocturnal restlessness [157] (Level 1b evidence). The trial cautioned against use of melatonin without light therapy, as this treatment was found to worsen participants' moods [157] (Level 1b evidence). An earlier Cochrane review of melatonin that does not include the 2008 trial by Riemersma and colleagues was inconclusive [158].

Massage and touch

A Cochrane review identified two small studies that addressed the effectiveness of massage and touch for people with BPSD; one trial evaluated hand massage to reduce agitated behavior (Level 1b evidence), and the second trial evaluated the addition of touch to verbal encouragement to eat in order to improve nutritional intake in participants with dementia (Level 2b evidence) [159]. The review suggests that further research is needed to confirm benefits but simple touch may serve as a quick method of complementing other treatments for BPSD.

Physical activity/exercise

A Cochrane review concluded that there was insufficient evidence to be able to say whether or not physical activity programs improve behavior in people with dementia [160] (Level 1b evidence). Some trials have reported benefits with exercise, but it can be difficult to disentangle the independent effects of exercise in some of these studies because they were offered together with other interventions such as behavioral management [133].

Reality orientation and cognitive stimulation

Reality orientation therapy is based on the concept that impairments in orientating information prevents patients with dementia from functioning well and that reminders can improve functioning [161]. Cognitive stimulation therapy is related to reality orientation therapy, but uses information processing rather than factual knowledge to address problems in functioning in patients with dementia. Three of the four randomized controlled trials of cognitive stimulation therapy identified by Livingston and colleagues showed some positive results, but the early benefits did not persist to 9 months postintervention [151] (Level 2b evidence).

Reminiscence therapy

Reminiscence therapy involves discussion of past activities and events, usually with the aid of prompts (e.g., photographs, videos, household items) to stimulate memories and enable patients to share and reflect on their life experiences. A Cochrane review evaluating reminiscence therapy for dementia suggested that this therapy appeared to have modest benefits on cognition, mood, and a measure of general behavior. In addition, reminiscence therapy reduced caregiver strain [162] (Level 1b evidence).

Validation therapy

Validation therapy is intended to give an opportunity to resolve unfinished conflicts by encouraging and validating the patient's expression of feelings. It is based upon the general principle of validation, which involves accepting and respecting the patient's reality and the truth of their experiences [163]. Validation therapy is usually delivered in a group setting, and can involve reminiscence, music, and movement. A Cochrane review suggested data from three trials of validation therapy were insufficient to permit any definitive conclusions about the effectiveness of this treatment for people with dementia [163] (Level 2b evidence).

Snoezelen (multisensory stimulation)

Snoezelen provides sensory stimuli to the primary senses through the use of lights, tactile stimulation, sounds, and smells. Snoezelen is used to manage maladaptive behaviors and to promote positive mood of older people with dementia. An updated Cochrane review concluded that snoezelen failed to demonstrate any significant effects on the behavior, interaction, or mood of people with dementia [164] (Level 2b evidence).

Changes to physical environment for wandering and care

Two Cochrane reviews discuss interventions designed to manage wandering by people with dementia. One review found no trials of nonpharmacological interventions to manage wandering in the domestic setting [165], while the second Cochrane review also failed to identify any randomized trials of visual or other selective barriers (e.g., mirrors, camouflage) that might reduce wandering [166]. Further research is needed to better evaluate strategies to manage wandering in both community and institutional settings.

A third Cochrane review examining the effectiveness of special care units for individuals with dementia and BPSD was unable to identify any relevant randomized controlled trials [167].

Other forms of nonpharmacological therapy

Aside from the interventions discussed above, a number of other nonpharmacological treatments have been evaluated to manage BPSD, including animal-assisted (pet) therapy, acupuncture, cognitive stimulation therapy, dementia-care mapping, and person-centered care [151–153]. Like many of the interventions discussed earlier, these other interventions also require further evaluation to clarify their effectiveness in treating BPSD. Randomized trials indicate that intensive 6–12 month programs to educate staff in person-centered care can reduce the use of psychotropic medication in long-term care, without a negative influence on levels of agitated or disruptive behavior [168] (Level 1b evidence).

Clinical Bottom Line

Nonpharmacological treatments for dementia should be used whenever available and feasible. There is some limited evidence to support the use of some nonpharmacological treatments such as aromatherapy, reminiscence therapy, and person-centered care in long-term care residents with other potential treatments having less evidence to support their use.

Pharmacological treatments

Antipsychotics

Antipsychotic drugs are the best-studied pharmacological interventions for BPSD, but the attention they have received has led to important concerns about their adverse effects. A large number of reviews examining the role of antipsychotic drugs to manage BPSD have been published; earlier reviews focused on the older typical antipsychotics (e.g., haloperidol, thioridazine) [169–172], while more recent reviews have focused on the atypical antipsychotic drugs (e.g., risperidone, olanzapine, quetiapine, aripiprazole) [173, 174].

Typical antipsychotic drugs

Schneider and colleagues performed a meta-analysis of typical antipsychotic drugs to manage BPSD, which concluded that these agents provided modest benefits (i.e., 18 of every 100 people with dementia who received a typical antipsychotic rather than placebo would benefit) [168] (Level 1a evidence). Comparisons of several typical antipsychotic drugs suggested that no particular typical antipsychotic was clearly superior to other agents in this class and there are high rates of adverse events associated with these drugs [169–172] (Level 1a evidence).

Atypical antipsychotic drugs

Atypical antipsychotic drugs have become increasingly popular, and they have now largely replaced typical antipsychotic drugs as treatments for BPSD. Schneider and colleagues reviewed 15 trials of atypical antipsychotic drugs (risperidone, olanzapine, quetiapine, aripiprazole), including nine unpublished trials, and found small but statistically significant improvements in symptoms with aripiprazole and risperidone over placebo [173] (Level 1a evidence). Incomplete reporting limited the ability to draw conclusions about the clinical relevance of these findings.

The review also emphasize the adverse events associated with atypical antipsychotic drugs; aside from somnolence and worsening cognitive test scores, the review highlights concerns about the higher risk of cerebrovascular adverse events observed with atypical antipsychotic drugs. Observational studies have also supported the association between antipsychotics and stroke [175], death [176], and other adverse events [177]. A separate but related meta-analysis by Schneider and colleagues details higher overall mortality in patients who received atypical antipsychotic drugs (OR 1.54; 95% CI 1.06–2.23) [178]. Sensitivity analyses did not demonstrate any differential risk for individual atypical antipsychotic drugs. Other reviews have arrived at similar conclusions [148, 174].

A relatively large randomized controlled trial was published after these reviews to compare the effects of risperidone, olanzapine, quetiapine, and placebo in 421 subjects with BPSD for up to 36 weeks [179] (Level 1b evidence). This trial concluded that the ad-verse effects of atypical antipsychotic drugs often offset their modest benefits over placebo. Because of adverse events (e.g., extrapyramidal symptoms, somnolence), improvements in behavioral symptoms observed with antipsychotic drug treatment do not necessarily lead to improvements in overall clinical status or the patient's quality of life.

Antidepressants

Concerns about the adverse effects of antipsychotic drugs have promoted efforts to identify safer pharmacological treatments for BPSD. A few randomized controlled trials have evaluated antidepressants. One trial compared the selective serotonin reuptake inhibitor (SSRI) citalopram with the typical antipsychotic perphenazine and placebo in 85 nondepressed, hospitalized patients with dementia who had psychosis or other behavioral disturbances [180]. Compared to those receiving placebo, patients treated with only citalopram showed significant improvement in their behavior scores (Level 1b evidence). Adverse events were similar among the three treatment groups. Another trial by the same investigators comparing citalopram and the atypical antipsychotic risperidone for the treatment of psychotic symptoms and agitation associated with dementia failed to demonstrate the superiority of risperidone [181] (Level 1b evidence). A Cochrane review concluded that there was insufficient evidence from randomized controlled trials to support the common clinical use of antidepressant trazodone for BPSD [182].

The use of antidepressants for patients with dementia accompanied by depressive symptoms is widespread. A 2002 Cochrane review evaluated studies of antidepressants for depressive symptoms in dementia [183]. The review found several trials of older tricyclic antidepressants but only one small trial ($N = 44$) supporting the use of the SSRI serotonin [184]. A more recent meta-analysis of both SSRI and tricyclic antidepressants found that antidepressants were more likely to produce remission of depression when compared to placebo [185]. More recently, results from a larger trial of serotonin ($N = 131$) have been published [186, 187]. In contrast to the findings of the earlier trial, the larger trial of sertraline found that it was not effective in treating depressive symptoms in dementia and its use was associated with adverse effects [186, 187].

Cholinesterase inhibitors

Although cholinesterase inhibitors are prescribed primarily for their influence on cognitive outcomes, several reviews suggested that these agents might also have modest benefits in treating BPSD based on secondary endpoint data in earlier trials [188, 189]. More recent data have not supported this view. In particular, a trial by Howard and colleagues randomized 272 patients with AD who had clinically significant agitation to either donepezil or placebo for 12 weeks. Donepezil failed to demonstrate any benefits over placebo on multiple behavioral outcome measures in this trial (Level 1b evidence). These findings may indicate that cholinesterase inhibitors can reduce the chance of BPSD developing in patients who do not have agitation at the outset, but these drugs do not appear to be effective to manage active BPSD.

Anticonvulsants

Valproic acid derivatives have been used for many years to treat BPSD, but evidence to support this practice is inconsistent. A Cochrane review examined five trials that evaluated valproic acid derivatives and recommended against valproic acid derivatives, as their use appears to be ineffective and is associated with high rates of adverse effects [190] (Level 2b evidence).

Carbamazepine has been studied in randomized controlled trials for the treatment of agitation associated with dementia. Three relatively small trials found improvements in measures of agitation and aggressive behaviors for low-dose carbamazepine when compared to placebo [191–193] (Level 1b evidence).

Memantine

A Cochrane review has evaluated the NMDA receptor antagonist memantine in patients with dementia and found patients taking memantine were less likely to develop agitation, with the effect more evident in moderate-to-severe dementia (Level 1a evidence). Further research is needed to determine whether memantine is effective in treating active behavioral disturbances in dementia.

Clinical Bottom Line

There is evidence to support the use of some atypical antipsychotics for the treatment of agitation and psychosis, although benefits need to be balanced against risks of serious adverse events and their use should be restricted to instances of severe behavioral problems that do not respond to nonpharmacological treatments. Other medications that may be helpful for these symptoms include the antidepressant citalopram, carbamazepine, and possibly memantine. There is no evidence to support the use of cholinesterase inhibitors in treating agitation in dementia.

Chapter summary

In this chapter, we reviewed the evidence for AD risk factors, screening tools for dementia, and interventions for behavioral and cognitive symptoms of dementia. A number of nonmodifiable risk factors were identified that may be helpful in identifying individuals at high risk of dementia who may benefit from monitoring for disease development and screening. Identification of potentially modifiable risk factors may also help to reduce the risk of developing Alzheimer's for individuals affected. Currently, there are a number of office-based screening tools that can be helpful to quantify cognitive changes and identify individuals who may have dementia. Evidence-based treatments for AD include cholinesterase inhibitors and memantine, although therapies for AD have clinically modest effects and appear to be best supported in mild-to-moderate stages of dementia. A number of nonpharmacological and medication-based interventions for behavioral symptoms associated with dementia exist and treatment decisions need to consider patient preference, availability of treatments, and safety. Finally, ensuring safety and providing support for dementia caregivers is an integral part of management that must be integrated into the overall treatment plan.

Acknowledgments

Dr. Seitz is supported by a Postdoctoral Fellowship Award from the Alzheimer Society of Canada. Dr. Gill is supported by an Early Career Investigator Award from the Canadian Institute of Health Research (CIHR). Dr. Lee is supported by the Ralph Fisher Professorship and Alzheimer Society of British Columbia. This work was supported by an Interdisciplinary Capacity Enhancement Grant (HOA-80075) from the CIHR Institute of Gender and Health and the CIHR Institute of Aging.

References

1. Canadian Study of Health and Aging Study Group (1994) Canadian study of health and aging: study methods and prevalence of dementia. *Can Med Assoc J* 150: 899–913.

2. Tschanz JT, et al (2004) Dementia: the leading predictor of death in a defined elderly population: the cache county study. *Neurology* 62: 1156–1162.

3. Alzheimer Society of Canada (2010) Rising tide: the impact of dementia on Canadian society. *Alzheimer Society*.

4. Ferri CP, et al (2005) Global prevalence of dementia: a Delphi consensus study. *Lancet* 366: 2112–2117.

5. Brookmeyer R, Gray S, Kawas C (1998) Projections of Alzheimer's disease in the United States and the public health impact of delaying disease onset. *Am J Public Health* 88: 1337–1342.

6. Scalco MZ, van Reekum R (2006) Prevention of Alzheimer's disease. *Can Fam Physician* 52: 200–207.

7. Rockwood K, Stadnyk K (1994) The prevalence of dementia in the elderly: a review. *Can J Psychiatry* 39: 253–257.

8. Ebly EM, Parhad IM, Hogan DB, Fung TS (1994) Prevalence and types of dementia in the very old: results from the Canadian Study of Health and Aging. *Neurology* 44: 1593–1600.

9. Corrada MM, Brookmeyer R, Paganini-Hill A, Berlau D, Kawas CH (2010) Dementia incidence continues to increase with age in the oldest old: the 90+ study. *Ann Neurol* 67: 114–121.

10. Tariman JD (2009) Men and Alzheimer's disease. Sex differences in risk. *Adv Nurse Pract* 17: 23.

11. McDowell I, Kristjansson B, Hill GB, Hebert R (1997) Community screening for dementia: the Mini Mental State Exam (MMSE) and modified mini-mental State Exam (3MS) compared. *J Clin Epidemiol* 50: 377–383.

12. Demirovic J, et al (2003) Prevalence of dementia in three ethnic groups: the South Florida program on aging and health. *Ann Epidemiol* 13: 472–478.

13. Hou CE, Yaffe K, Perez-Stable EJ, Miller BL (2006) Frequency of dementia etiologies in four ethnic groups. *Dement Geriatr Cogn Disord* 22: 42–47.

14. Mehta KM, et al (2008) Race/ethnic differences in AD survival in US Alzheimer's disease centers. *Neurology* 70: 1163–1170.

15. Helzner EP, Scarmeas N, Cosentino S, Tang MX, Schupf N, Stern Y (2008) Survival in Alzheimer disease: a multiethnic, population-based study of incident cases. *Neurology* 71: 1489–1495.

16. Patterson C, Feightner JW, Garcia A, Hsiung GY, MacKnight C, Sadovnick AD (2008) Diagnosis and treatment of dementia: 1. Risk assessment and primary prevention of Alzheimer disease. *Can Med Assoc J* 178: 548–556.

17. van Duijn E, et al (2008) Cross-sectional study on prevalence of psychiatric disorders in mutation carriers of Huntington's disease compared with mutation-negative first-degree relatives. *J Clin Psychiatry* 69: 1804–1810.

18. Sleegers K, et al (2004) Familial clustering and genetic risk for dementia in a genetically isolated Dutch population. *Brain* 127: 1641–1649.

19. Lai F, Williams RS (1989) A prospective study of Alzheimer disease in Down syndrome. *Arch Neurol* 46: 849–853.

20. Hsiung GY, Sadovnick AD, Feldman H (2004) Apolipoprotein E epsilon4 genotype as a risk factor for cognitive decline and dementia: data from the Canadian Study of Health and Aging. *Can Med Assoc J* 171: 863–867.

21. Rosvall L, Rizzuto D, Wang HX, Winblad B, Graff C, Fratiglioni L (2009) APOE-related mortality: effect of dementia, cardiovascular disease and gender. *Neurobiol Aging* 30: 1545–1551.

22. Plassman BL, et al (2000) Documented head injury in early adulthood and risk of Alzheimer's disease and other dementias. *Neurology* 55: 1158–1166.

23. de la Torre JC (2009) Cerebrovascular and cardiovascular pathology in Alzheimer's disease. *Int Rev Neurobiol* 84: 35–48.

24. Deschaintre Y, Richard F, Leys D, Pasquier F (2009) Treatment of vascular risk factors is associated with slower decline in Alzheimer disease. *Neurology* 73: 674–680.

25. Abellan van Kan G, Rolland Y, Nourhashemi F, Coley N, Andrieu S, Vellas B (2009) Cardiovascular disease risk factors and progression of Alzheimer's disease. *Dement Geriatr Cogn Disord* 27: 240–246.

26. Purnell C, Gao S, Callahan CM, Hendrie HC (2009) Cardiovascular risk factors and incident Alzheimer disease: a systematic review of the literature. *Alzheimer Dis Assoc Disord* 23: 1–10.

27. McGuinness B, Todd S, Passmore P, Bullock R (2009) Blood pressure lowering in patients without prior cerebrovascular disease for prevention of cognitive impairment and dementia. *Cochrane Database Syst Rev* 004034.

28. Seux ML, et al (1998) Correlates of cognitive status of old patients with isolated systolic hypertension: the Syst-Eur Vascular Dementia Project. *J Hypertens* 16: 963–969.

29. Di Bari M, et al (2001) Dementia and disability outcomes in large hypertension trials: lessons learned from the systolic hypertension in the elderly program (SHEP) trial. *Am J Epidemiol* 153: 72–78.

30. Tzourio C, et al (2003) Effects of blood pressure lowering with perindopril and indapamide therapy on dementia and cognitive decline in patients with cerebrovascular disease. *Arch Intern Med* 163: 1069–1075.

31. Peters R, et al (2009) Cardiovascular and biochemical risk factors for incident dementia in the hypertension in the very elderly trial. *J Hypertens* 27: 2055–2062.

32. Haag MD, Hofman A, Koudstaal PJ, Breteler MM, Stricker BH (2009) Duration of antihypertensive drug use and risk of dementia: a prospective cohort study. *Neurology* 72: 1727–1734.

33. Forette F, et al (1998) Prevention of dementia in randomized double-blind placebo-controlled systolic hypertension in Europe (Syst-Eur) trial. *Lancet* 352: 1347–1351.

34. Formiga F, Fort I, Reig L, Robles MJ, Espinosa MC, Rodriguez D (2009) Atrial fibrillation in elderly patients with dementia. *Gerontology* 55: 202–204.

35. Ettorre E, et al (2009) A possible role of atrial fibrillation as a risk factor for dementia. *Arch Gerontol Geriatr* 49: 71–76.

36. Querfurth HW, LaFerla FM (2010) Alzheimer's disease. *N Engl J Med* 362: 329–344.

37. Panza F, et al (2006) Lipid metabolism in cognitive decline and dementia. *Brain Res* 51: 275–292.

38. Cukierman-Yaffe TGHCWJDLRMLLMMECLHMASM (2009) Relationship between baseline glycemic control and cognitive function in individuals with type 2 diabetes and other cardiovascular risk factors: the action to control cardiovascular risk in diabetes-memory in diabetes (ACCORD-MIND) trial. *Diabetes care* 32: 221–226.

39. Xu WL, von Strauss E, Qiu CX, Winblad B, Fratiglioni L (2009) Uncontrolled diabetes increases the risk of Alzheimer's disease: a population-based cohort study. *Diabetologia* 52: 1031–1039.

40. Weih M, Wiltfang J, Kornhuber J (2007) Non-pharmacologic prevention of alzheimer's disease: nutritional and life-style risk factors. *J Neural Transm* 114: 1187–1197.

41. Zhou Y, Yang M, Liu GJ, Dong BR (2009) Thiazolidinediones for dementia and mild cognitive impairment. *Cochrane Database Syst Rev* 1.

42. Kivipelto M, et al (2009) Homocysteine and holo-transcobalamin and the risk of dementia and Alzheimer's disease: a prospective study. *Eur J Neurol* 16: 808–813.

43. Van Dam F, Van Gool WA (2009) Hyperhomocysteinemia and Alzheimer's disease: a systematic review. *Arch Gerontol Geriatr* 48: 425–430.

44. van Duijn CM, Hofman A (1991) Relation between nicotine intake and Alzheimer's disease. *BMJ* 302: 1491–1494.

45. Reitz C, den Heijer T, van Duijn C, Hofman A, Breteler MM (2007) Relation between smoking and risk of dementia and Alzheimer disease: the Rotterdam Study. *Neurology* 69: 998–1005.

46. Peters R, Poulter R, Warner J, Beckett N, Burch L, Bulpitt C (2008) Smoking, dementia and cognitive decline in the elderly, a systematic review. *BMC geriatr* 8: 36.

47. Barnes DE, Haight TJ, Mehta KM, Carlson MC, Kuller LH, Tager IB (2010) Secondhand smoke, vascular disease, and dementia incidence: findings from the cardiovascular health cognition study. *Am J Epidemiol* 171: 292–302.

48. Petersen RC (2000) Aging, mild cognitive impairment, and Alzheimer's disease. *Neurol Clin* 18: 789–806.

49. Petersen RC, et al (2001) Current concepts in mild cognitive impairment. *Arch Neurol* 58: 1985–1992.

50. Tsuno N, Homma A (2009) What is the association between depression and Alzheimer's disease? *Expert Rev Neurother* 9: 1667–1676.

51. Korczyn AD, Halperin I (2009) Depression and dementia. *J Neurol Sci* 283: 139–142.

52. Brommelhoff JA, Gatz M, Johansson B, McArdle JJ, Fratiglioni L, Pedersen NL (2009) Depression as a risk factor or prodromal feature for dementia? Findings in a population-based sample of Swedish twins. *Psychol Aging* 24: 373–384.

53. Feart C, et al (2009) Adherence to a Mediterranean diet, cognitive decline, and risk of dementia. *JAMA* 302: 638–648.

54. Scarmeas N, et al (2009) Physical activity, diet, and risk of Alzheimer disease. *JAMA* 302: 627–637.

55. Fotuhi M, Mohassel P, Yaffe K (2009) Fish consumption, long-chain omega-3 fatty acids and risk of cognitive decline or Alzheimer disease: a complex association. *Nature Clinical Practice Neurology* 5: 140–152.

56. Barberger-Gateau P, et al (2007) Dietary patterns and risk of dementia: the three-city cohort study. *Neurology* 69: 1921–1930.

57. Clarke R, et al (2007) Low vitamin B-12 status and risk of cognitive decline in older adults. *Am J Clin Nutr* 86: 1384–1391.

58. Siuda J, et al (2009) From mild cognitive impairment to Alzheimer's disease – influence of homocysteine, vitamin B12 and folate on cognition over time: results from one-year follow-up. *Neurol Neurochir Pol* 43: 321–329.

59. Malouf R, Grimley Evans J (2008) Folic acid with or without vitamin B12 for the prevention and treatment of healthy elderly and demented people. *Cochrane Database Syst Rev* (4): CD004514.

60. Devore EE, et al (2009) Dietary intake of fish and omega-3 fatty acids in relation to long-term dementia risk. *Am J Clin Nutr* 90: 170–176.

61. Lim W, Gammack JK, Van Niekerk JK, Dangour A (2009) Omega 3 fatty acid for the prevention of dementia. *Cochrane Database Syst Rev* (1): CD005379.

62. Kroger E, et al (2009) Omega-3 fatty acids and risk of dementia: the Canadian study of health and aging. *Am J Clin Nutr* 90: 184–192.

63. Laurin D, Verreault R, Lindsay J, Dewailly E, Holub BJ (2003) Omega-3 fatty acids and risk of cognitive impairment and dementia. *J Alzheimers Dis* 5: 315–322.

64. Freund-Levi Y, et al (2006) Omega-3 fatty acid treatment in 174 patients with mild to moderate Alzheimer disease: OmegAD study: a randomized double-blind trial. *Arch Neurol* 63: 1402–1408.

65. Issa AM, et al (2006) The efficacy of omega-3 fatty acids on cognitive function in aging and dementia: a systematic review. *Dement Geriatr Cogn Disord* 21: 88–96.

66. Cole GM, Ma QL, Frautschy SA (2009) Omega-3 fatty acids and dementia. *Prostaglandins Leukot Essent Fatty Acids* 81: 213–221.

67. Eskelinen MH, Ngandu T, Tuomilehto J, Soininen H, Kivipelto M (2009) Midlife coffee and tea drinking and the risk of late-life dementia: a population-based CAIDE study. *J Alzheimers Dis* 16: 85–91.

68. Ngandu T, et al (2007) Alcohol drinking and cognitive functions: findings from the cardiovascular risk factors aging and dementia (CAIDE) study. *Dement Geriatr Cogn Disord* 23: 140–149.

69. Xu G, Liu X, Yin Q, Zhu W, Zhang R, Fan X (2009) Alcohol consumption and transition of mild cognitive impairment to dementia. *Psychiatry Clin Neurosci* 63: 43–49.

70. Lindsay J, et al (2002) Risk factors for alzheimer's disease: a prospective analysis from the Canadian study of health and aging. *Am J Epidemiol* 156: 445–453.

71. Laurin D, Verreault R, Lindsay J, MacPherson K, Rockwood K (2001) Physical activity and risk of cognitive impairment and dementia in elderly persons. *Arch Neurol* 58: 498–504.

72. Podewils LJ, et al (2005) Physical activity, APOE genotype, and dementia risk: findings from the cardiovascular health cognition study. *Am J Epidemiol* 161: 639–651.

73. Lautenschlager NT, et al (2008) Effect of physical activity on cognitive function in older adults at risk for Alzheimer disease: a randomized trial. *JAMA* 300: 1027–1037.

74. Barnes DE, Covinsky KE, Whitmer RA, Kuller LH, Lopez OL, Yaffe K (2009) Predicting risk of dementia in older adults: the late-life dementia risk index. *Neurology* 73(3): 173–179.

75. Kivipelto M, Ngandu T, Laatikainen T, Winblad B, Soininen H, Tuomilehto J (2006) Risk score for the prediction of dementia risk in 20 years among middle aged people: a longitudinal, population-based study. *Lancet Neurol* 5: 735–741.

76. Folstein MF, Folstein SE, McHugh PR (1975) "Mini-mental state." A practical method for grading the cognitive state of patients for the clinician. *J Psychiatric Res* 12: 189–198.

77. Holsinger T, Deveau J, Boustani M, Williams JW, Jr (2007) Does this patient have dementia? *JAMA* 297: 2391–2404.

78. Crum RM, Anthony JC, Bassett SS, Folstein MF (1993) Population-based norms for the mini-mental state examination by age and educational level. *JAMA* 269: 2386–2391.

79. Feldman HH, et al (2008) Diagnosis and treatment of dementia: 2. diagnosis. *Can Med Assoc J* 178: 825–836.

80. Teng EL, Chui HC (1987) The modified mini-mental state (3MS) examination. *J Clin Psychiatry* 48: 314–318.

81. Scanlan JM, Brush M, Quijano C, Borson S (2002) Comparing clock tests for dementia screening: naive judgments vs formal systems–what is optimal? *Int J Geriatr Psychiatry* 17: 14–21.

82. Mendez MF, Ala T, Underwood KL (1992) Development of scoring criteria for the clock drawing task in Alzheimer's disease. *J Am Geriatr Soc* 40: 1095–1099.

83. Sunderland T, et al (1989) Clock drawing in Alzheimer's disease. A novel measure of dementia severity. *J Am Geriatr Soc* 37: 725–729.

84. Rouleau I, Salmon DP, Butters N, Kennedy C, McGuire K (1992) Quantitative and qualitative analyses of clock drawings in Alzheimer's and Huntington's disease. *Brain Cogn* 18: 70–87.

85. Shulman KI (2000) Clock-drawing: is it the ideal cognitive screening test? *Int J Geriatr Psychiatry* 15: 548–561.

86. Pinto E, Peters R (2009) Literature review of the clock drawing test as a tool for cognitive screening. *Dement Geriatr Cogn Disord* 27: 201–213.

87. Lourenco RA, Ribeiro-Filho ST, Moreira Ide F, Paradela EM, Miranda AS (2008) The clock drawing test: performance among elderly with low educational level. *Rev Bras Psiquiatr* 30: 309–315.

88. Ehreke L, Luppa M, Konig HH, Riedel-Heller SG (2010) Is the clock drawing test a screening tool for the diagnosis of mild cognitive impairment? A systematic review. *Int Psychogeriatr* 22: 56–63.

89. Lee KS, Kim EA, Hong CH, Lee DW, Oh BH, Cheong HK (2008) Clock drawing test in mild cognitive impairment: quantitative analysis of four scoring methods and qualitative analysis. *Dement Geriatr Cogn Disord* 26: 483–489.

90. Storey JE, Rowland JT, Basic D, Conforti DA (2002) Accuracy of the clock drawing test for detecting dementia in a multicultural sample of elderly Australian patients. *Int Psychogeriatr/IPA* 14: 259–271.

91. Borson S, Scanlan JM, Chen P, Ganguli M (2003) The mini-cog as a screen for dementia: validation in a population-based sample. *J Am Geriatr Soc* 51: 1451–1454.

92. Nasreddine ZS, et al (2005) The Montreal Cognitive Assessment, MoCA: a brief screening tool for mild cognitive impairment. *J Am Geriatr Soc* 53: 695–699.

93. Clarfield AM (1988) The reversible dementias: do they reverse? *Ann Intern Med* 109: 476–486.

94. Patterson CJ, Gass DA (2001) Screening for cognitive impairment and dementia in the elderly. *Can J Neurol Sci* 28: S42–S51.

95. Lambon Ralph MA, Patterson K, Graham N, Dawson K, Hodges JR (2003) Homogeneity and heterogeneity in mild cognitive impairment and Alzheimer's disease: a cross-sectional and longitudinal study of 55 cases. *Brain* 126: 2350–2362.

96. Backman L, Jones S, Berger AK, Laukka EJ, Small BJ (2005) Cognitive impairment in preclinical Alzheimer's disease: a meta-analysis. *Neuropsychology* 19: 520–531.

97. Shulman KI, et al (2007) Assessment of testamentary capacity and vulnerability to undue influence. *Am J Psychiatry* 164: 722–727.

98. Marson DC, Ingram KK, Cody HA, Harrell LE (1995) Assessing the competency of patients with Alzheimer's disease under different legal standards. A prototype instrument. *Arch Neurol* 52: 949–954.

99. Ott BR, et al (2008) A longitudinal study of drivers with Alzheimer disease. *Neurology* 70: 1171–1178.

100. Molnar FJ, et al (2006) Clinical utility of office-based cognitive predictors of fitness to drive in persons with dementia: a systematic review. *J Am Geriatr Soc* 54: 1809–1824.

101. Mathias JL, Lucas LK (2009) Cognitive predictors of unsafe driving in older drivers: a meta-analysis. *Int Psychogeriatr* 21: 637–653.

102. Canadian Medical Association (2006) *Determining Medical Fitness to Operate Motor Vehicles: CMA Driver's Guide.* 7th edn. Ottawa, ON: Canadian Medical Association.

103. Carr DB, Schwartzberg JG, Manning L, Sempek J (2010) *Physician's Guide to Assessing and Counseling Older Drivers.* Washington, D.C.: National Highway Traffic Safety Administration.

104. Iverson DJ, Gronseth GS, Reger MA, Classen S, Dubinsky RM, Rizzo M (2010) Practice parameter update: evaluation and management of driving risk in dementia. *Neurology* 74: 1316–1324.

105. Hogan DB, et al (2007) Management of mild to moderate Alzheimer's disease and dementia. *Alzheimer's & Dementia* 3: 355–384.

106. Martin AJ, Marottoli R, O'Neill D, Martin AJ, Marottoli R, O'Neill D (2009) Driving assessment for maintaining mobility and safety in drivers with dementia. *Cochrane Database Syst Rev* (1): CD006222.

107. Cuijpers P (2005) Depressive disorders in caregivers of dementia patients: a systematic review. *Aging & mental health* 9: 325–330.

108. Covinsky KE, et al (2003) Patient and caregiver characteristics associated with depression in caregivers of patients with dementia. *J Gen Intern Med* 18: 1006–1014.

109. Clyburn LD, Stones MJ, Hadjistavropoulos T, Tuokko H (2000) Predicting caregiver burden and depression in Alzheimer's disease. *J Gerontol B Psychol Sci Soc Sci* 55: S2–S13.

110. Lee H, Cameron M (2004) Respite care for people with dementia and their carers. *Cochrane Database Syst Rev* (2): CD004396.

111. Thompson CA, et al (2007) Systematic review of information and support interventions for caregivers of people with dementia. *BMC geriatr* 7: 18.

112. Selwood A, Johnston K, Katona C, Lyketsos C, Livingston G (2007) Systematic review of the effect of psychological interventions on family caregivers of people with dementia. *J Affect Disord* 101: 75–89.

113. Lanctot KL, et al (2003) Efficacy and safety of cholinesterase inhibitors in Alzheimer's disease: a meta-analysis.[see comment]. *Can Med Assoc J* 169: 557–564.

114. Kaduszkiewicz H, et al (2005) Cholinesterase inhibitors for patients with Alzheimer's disease: systematic review of randomised clinical trials. *BMJ* 331: 321–327.

115. Birks J (2009) Cholinesterase inhibitors for Alzheimer's disease. *Cochrane Database Syst Rev* (2): CD001191.

116. Birks J, Harvey RJ (2009) Donepezil for dementia due to Alzheimer's disease. *Cochrane Database Syst Rev* (1): CD001190.

117. Loy C, Schneider L (2009) Galantamine for Alzheimer's disease and mild cognitive impairment. *Cochrane Database Syst Rev* (1): CD001747.

118. Birks J, Grimley Evans J, Iakovidou V, Tsolaki M (2009) Rivastigmine for Alzheimer's disease. *Cochrane Database Syst Rev* (4): CD001191.

119. Hogan DB, et al (2004) Comparison studies of cholinesterase inhibitors for Alzheimer's disease. *Lancet Neurol* 3: 622–626.

120. Wilkinson DG, et al (2002) A multinational, randomised, 12-week, comparative study of donepezil and rivastigmine in patients with mild to moderate Alzheimer's disease. *Int J Clin Pract* 56: 441–446.

121. Gill SS, et al (2009) Syncope and its consequences in patients with dementia receiving cholinesterase inhibitors: a population-based cohort study. *Arch Intern Med* 169(9): 867–873.

122. Park-Wyllie LY, Mamdani MM, Li P, Gill SS, Laupacis A, Juurlink DN (2009) Cholinesterase inhibitors and hospitalization for bradycardia: a population-based study. *PLoS Med* 6: e1000157.

123. McShane R, Areosa Sastre A, Minakaran N (2006) Memantine for dementia. *Cochrane Database Syst Rev* (2): CD003154.

124. Winblad B, et al (2007) Memantine in moderate to severe Alzheimer's disease: a meta-analysis of randomised clinical trials. *Dement Geriatr Cogn Disord* 24: 20–27.

125. Black SE, et al (2007) Donepezil preserves cognition and global function in patients with severe Alzheimer disease. *Neurology* 69: 459–469.

126. Kavirajan H, Schneider LS, Kavirajan H, Schneider LS (2007) Efficacy and adverse effects of cholinesterase inhibitors and memantine in vascular dementia: a meta-analysis of randomised controlled trials. *Lancet Neurol* 6: 782–792.

127. Erkinjuntti T, et al (2002) Efficacy of galantamine in probable vascular dementia and Alzheimer's disease combined with cerebrovascular disease: a randomised trial. *Lancet* 359: 1283–1290.

128. Maidment I, Fox C, Boustani M (2006) Cholinesterase inhibitors for Parkinson's disease dementia. *Cochrane Database Syst Rev (Online)*. (1): CD004747.

129. Wild R, Pettit TACL, Burns A. (2009) Cholinesterase inhibitors for dementia with Lewy bodies. *Cochrane Database Syst Rev*. (3): CD003672.

130. Birks J, Flicker L . (2009) Donepezil for mild cognitive impairment. *Cochrane Database Syst Rev* 3: CD006104.

131. Raschetti R, et al (2007) Cholinesterase inhibitors in mild cognitive impairment: a systematic review of randomised trials. *PLoS Med* 4: e338.

132. Li J, Wu HM, Zhou RL, Liu GJ, Dong BR. (2008) Huperzine A for Alzheimer's disease. *Cochrane Database Syst Rev* (2): CD005592.

133. Teri L, et al (2003) Exercise plus behavioral management in patients with Alzheimer disease: a randomized controlled trial. *JAMA* 290: 2015–2022.

134. Sitzer DI, Twamley EW, Jeste DV (2006) Cognitive training in Alzheimer's disease: a meta-analysis of the literature. *Acta Psychiatr Scand* 114: 75–90.

135. Rockwood K (2006) Epidemiological and clinical trials evidence about a preventive role for statins in Alzheimer's disease. *Acta Neurol Scand* 185: 71–77.

136. Panza F, et al (2009) Higher total cholesterol, cognitive decline, and dementia. *Neurobiol Aging* 30: 546–548.

137. de Craen AJ, Gussekloo J, Vrijsen B, Westendorp RG (2005) Meta-analysis of nonsteroidal anti-inflammatory drug use and risk of dementia. *Am J Epidemiol* 161: 114–120.

138. ADAPT Research Group (2008) Cognitive function over time in the Alzheimer's disease anti-inflammatory prevention trial (ADAPT). *Arch Neurol* 65: 896–905.

139. Aisen PS, et al (2003) Effects of rofecoxib or naproxen vs placebo on Alzheimer disease progression: a randomized controlled trial. *JAMA* 289: 2819–2826.

140. Shumaker SA, et al (2004) Conjugated equine estrogens and incidence of probable dementia and mild cognitive impairment in postmenopausal women: women's health initiative memory study. *JAMA* 291: 2947–2958.

141. Boothby LA, Doering PL (2005) Vitamin C and vitamin E for Alzheimer's disease. *Ann Pharmacother* 39: 2073–2080.

142. Fillenbaum GG, et al (2005) Dementia and Alzheimer's disease in community-dwelling elders taking vitamin C and/or vitamin E. *Ann Pharmacother* 39: 2009–2014.

143. Isaac MG, Quinn R, Tabet N (2008) Vitamin E for Alzheimer's disease and mild cognitive impairment. *Cochrane Database Syst Rev* (3): 002854.

144. Birks J, Grimley Evans J (2009) Ginkgo biloba for cognitive impairment and dementia. *Cochrane Database Syst Rev* (1): 003120.

145. Snitz BEOMESCMCAAMIDGRSRSJLOL (2009) Ginkgo biloba for preventing cognitive decline in older adults: a randomized trial. *JAMA* 302: 2663–2670.

146. Steinberg M, et al (2008) Point and 5-year period prevalence of neuropsychiatric symptoms in dementia: the Cache County Study. *Int J Geriatr Psychiatry* 23: 170–177.

147. McKeith I, Cummings J, McKeith I, Cummings J (2005) Behavioural changes and psychological symptoms in dementia disorders. *Lancet Neurol* 4: 735–742.

148. Lee PE, Gill SS, Freedman M, Bronskill SE, Hillmer MP, Rochon PA (2004) Atypical antipsychotic drugs in the treatment of behavioural and psychological symptoms of dementia: systematic review. See comment. *BMJ* 329: 75.

149. Sink KM, Holden KF, Yaffe K (2005) Pharmacological treatment of neuropsychiatric symptoms of dementia: a review of the evidence. *JAMA* 293: 596–608.

150. Covinsky KE, Johnston CB, Covinsky KE, Johnston CB (2006) Envisioning better approaches for dementia care. *Ann Intern Med* 145: 780–781.

151. Livingston G, Johnston K, Katona C, Paton J, Lyketsos CG (2005) Old age task force of the world federation of biological P. Systematic review of psychological approaches to the management of neuropsychiatric symptoms of dementia. *Am J Psychiatry* 162: 1996–2021.

152. Ayalon L, Gum AM, Feliciano L, Arean PA (2006) Effectiveness of nonpharmacological interventions for the management of neuropsychiatric symptoms in patients with dementia: a systematic review. *Arch Intern Med* 166: 2182–2188.

153. Hulme C, Wright J, Crocker T, Oluboyede Y, House A (2010) Non-pharmacological approaches for dementia that informal carers might try or access: a systematic review. *Int J Geriatr Psychiatry.* 25(7): 756–763.

154. Thorgrimsen L, Spector A, Wiles A, Orrell M (2003) Aroma therapy for dementia. *Cochrane Database Syst Rev* (3): CD003150.

155. Vink AC, Birks JS, Bruinsma MS, Scholten RJ, Scholten RJS (2004) Music therapy for people with dementia. *Cochrane Database Syst Rev* (3): CD003477.

156. Forbes D, et al (2009) Light therapy for managing cognitive, sleep, functional, behavioural, or psychiatric disturbances in dementia. *Cochrane Database Syst Rev* (4): CD003946.

157. Riemersma-van der Lek RF, et al (2008) Effect of bright light and melatonin on cognitive and noncognitive function in elderly residents of group care facilities: a randomized controlled trial. *JAMA* 299: 2642–2655.

158. Jansen SL, Forbes DA, Duncan V, Morgan DG (2006) Melatonin for cognitive impairment. *Cochrane Database Syst Rev* (1): CD003802.

159. Viggo Hansen N, Jorgensen T, Ortenblad L (2006) Massage and touch for dementia. *Cochrane Database Syst Rev* (4): CD004989.

160. Forbes D, Forbes S, Morgan DG, Markle-Reid M, Wood J, Culum I (2008) Physical activity programs for persons with dementia. *Cochrane Database Syst Rev* 16: CD006489.

161. Livingston G, Johnston K, Katona C, Paton J, Lyketsos CG (2005) Old age task force of the world federation of biological P. systematic review of psychological approaches to the management of neuropsychiatric symptoms of dementia. *Am J Psychiatry* 162: 1996.

162. Woods B, Spector A, Jones C, Orrell M, Davies S (2005) Reminiscence therapy for dementia. *Cochrane Database Syst Rev* (2): CD001120.

163. Neal M, Briggs M (2003) Validation therapy for dementia. *Cochrane Database Syst Rev* (3): CD001394.

164. Chung JC, Lai CK, Chung PM, French HP (2002) Snoezelen for dementia. *Cochrane Database Syst Rev (Online)* (4): CD003152.

165. Hermans DG, Htay UH, McShane R, Htay UH (2007) Non-pharmacological interventions for wandering of people with dementia in the domestic setting. *Cochrane Database Syst Rev* (1): CD005994.

166. Price JD, Hermans DG, Grimley Evans J (2000) Subjective barriers to prevent wandering of cognitively impaired people. *Cochrane Database Syst Rev* (4): CD001932.

167. Lai CK, et al (2009) Special care units for dementia individuals with behavioural problems. *Cochrane Database Syst Rev* (4): CD006470.

168. Fossey J, et al (2006) Effect of enhanced psychosocial care on antipsychotic use in nursing home residents with severe dementia: cluster randomised trial. *BMJ* 2006; 332: 756–761. [Erratum in *BMJ.* 2006 Apr 1; 332(7544): 61]

169. Schneider LS, Pollock VE, Lyness SA (1990) A meta-analysis of controlled trials of neuroleptic treatment in dementia. *J Am Geriatr Soc* 38: 553.

170. Lonergan E, Luxenberg J, Colford J (2002) Haloperidol for agitation in dementia. *Cochrane Database Syst Rev (Online)* (2): CD002852.

171. Lanctot KL, et al (1998) Efficacy and safety of neuroleptics in behavioral disorders associated with dementia. *J Clin Psychiatry* 59: 550–561; quiz 562–553.

172. Kirchner V, Kelly CA, Harvey RJ (2001) Thioridazine for dementia. *Cochrane Database Syst Rev* (4): CD000464.

173. Schneider LS, Dagerman K, Insel PS (2006) Efficacy and adverse effects of atypical antipsychotics for dementia:

meta-analysis of randomized, placebo-controlled trials. *Am J Geriatr Psychiatry* 14: 191–210.

174. Ballard C, Waite J (2006) The effectiveness of atypical antipsychotics for the treatment of aggression and psychosis in Alzheimer's disease. *Cochrane Database Syst Rev (Online).* (1): CD003476.

175. Gill SS, et al (2005) Atypical antipsychotic drugs and risk of ischaemic stroke: population based retrospective cohort study. *BMJ (Clinical research ed)* 330: 445.

176. Gill SS, et al (2007) Antipsychotic drug use and mortality in older adults with dementia. *Ann Intern Med* 146: 775–786.

177. Rochon PA, et al (2008) Antipsychotic therapy and short-term serious events in older adults with dementia. *Arch Intern Med* 168: 1090–1096.

178. Schneider LS, Dagerman KS, Insel P (2005) Risk of death with atypical antipsychotic drug treatment for dementia: meta-analysis of randomized placebo-controlled trials. *JAMA* 294: 1934–1943.

179. Schneider LS, et al (2006) Effectiveness of atypical antipsychotic drugs in patients with Alzheimer's disease. *N Engl J Med* 355: 1525–1538.

180. Pollock BG, et al (2002) Comparison of citalopram, perphenazine, and placebo for the acute treatment of psychosis and behavioral disturbances in hospitalized, demented patients. *Am J Psychiatry* 159: 460–465.

181. Pollock BG, et al (2007) A double-blind comparison of citalopram and risperidone for the treatment of behavioral and psychotic symptoms associated with dementia. *Am J Geriatr Psychiatry* 15: 942–952.

182. Martinon-Torres G, Fioravanti M, Grimley EJ (2004) Trazodone for agitation in dementia. *Cochrane Database Syst Rev (Online)* (4): CD004990.

183. Bains J, Birks JS, Dening TR (2002) The efficacy of antidepressants in the treatment of depression in dementia. *Cochrane Database Syst Rev* (4): CD003944.

184. Lyketsos CG, et al (2000) Randomized, placebo-controlled, double-blind clinical trial of sertraline in the treatment of depression complicating Alzheimer's disease: initial results from the depression in Alzheimer's disease study. *Am J Psychiatry* 157: 1686–1689.

185. Thompson S, et al (2007) Efficacy and safety of antidepressants for treatment of depression in Alzheimer's disease: a meta-analysis. *Can J Psychiatry* 52: 248–255.

186. Rosenberg PB, et al (2010) Sertraline for the treatment of depression in Alzheimer's disease. *Am J Geriatr Psychiatry* 18: 136–145.

187. Weintraub D, et al (2010) Sertraline for the treatment of depression in Alzheimer disease: week-24 outcomes. *Am J Geriatr Psychiatry* 18: 332–340.

188. Trinh NH, Hoblyn J, Mohanty S, Yaffe K (2003) Efficacy of cholinesterase inhibitors in the treatment of neuropsychiatric and functional impairment in Alzheimer disease. *JAMA* 289: 210–216.

189. Birks J (2006) Cholinesterase inhibitors for Alzheimer's disease. *Cochrane Database Syst Rev (Online).* (1): CD005593.

190. Lonergan E, Luxenberg J (2009) Valproate preparations for agitation in dementia. *Cochrane Database Syst Rev (Online).* (3): CD003945.

191. Tariot PN, et al (1994) Carbamazepine treatment of agitation in nursing home patients with dementia: a preliminary study. *J Am Geriatr Soc* 42: 1160–1166.

192. Olin JT, Fox LS, Pawluczyk S, Taggart NA, Schneider LS (2001) A pilot randomized trial of carbamazepine for behavioral symptoms in treatment-resistant outpatients with Alzheimer disease. *Am J Geriatr Psychiatry* 9: 400–405.

193. Tariot PN, et al (1998) Efficacy and tolerability of carbamazepine for agitation and aggression in dementia. *Am J Psychiatry* 155: 54–61.

CHAPTER 8

Enjoying the golden years: diagnosing and treating depression

Jane Pearce[1,2] & Stuart Carney[3]
[1]*University of Oxford, Oxford, UK*
[2]*Fulbrook Centre, Churchill Hospital, Oxford, UK*
[3]*UK Foundation Programme Office, Cardiff Bay, UK*

Introduction

What is depression?

Depression is a psychiatric disorder of mood. Diagnosis is made on the basis of characteristic symptoms in the presence of clinically significant distress or functional impairment. Depressive episodes in older adults can either occur in the absence of a psychiatric history (late-onset depression) or can be part of a recurrent depressive disorder. A diagnosis of recurrent depressive disorder is made when there have been at least two depressive episodes with several months of being well in between.

There are two main sets of diagnostic criteria: (1) the DSM-IV (*Diagnostic and Statistical Manual of Mental Disorders*, 4th Edition) and (2) ICD-10 (*International Statistical Classification of Diseases and Related Health Problems*, 10th Revision) [1, 2]. DSM-IV criteria predominate in the research we reviewed. We have focused on the identification and initial treatment of major depression for which symptoms should be present for over 2 weeks, for most of every day and of sufficient severity. A DSM-IV "major depressive episode" would be diagnosed if the person has at least five out of nine characteristic symptoms of which at least either (1) depressed mood or (2) loss of interest/pleasure in activities are present. These two are regarded as "core" symptoms. Other possible symptoms include: fatigue or loss of energy, worthlessness or inappropriate guilt, suicidal ideation, indecisiveness/impaired concentrations, agitation or retardation, insomnia or increased sleep, and loss of appetite often with weight loss.

Major depressive episodes can be further divided into mild, moderate, severe without psychotic features and severe with psychotic features. Severity is judged on the basis of the number of symptoms, the severity of the symptoms, and the degree of functional disability and distress. A "minor depressive episode" is diagnosed if only two to four out of nine characteristic symptoms are present, with at least one of these a core symptom. A further update to the DSM criteria is expected soon.

In this chapter, we refer to depressive disorders as those in which depressed mood and/or loss of pleasure in most activities is a central feature.

Burden of disease

There are variable cutoffs used to define the status of "older adult." The nonpsychiatric medical literature frequently takes the perspective of age-related physical burdens and hence uses cutoffs of 70 or 80 years. In the psychiatric literature, it is more common to use the cutoff age of 65 years, although some researchers have set the bar much lower at 41 years of age. Here and for the rest of this chapter, we have adopted the practice of routinely using a cutoff of 65 years to define an "older adult," with the exception of some psychiatric

Evidence-Based Geriatric Medicine: A Practical Clinical Guide, First Edition. Edited by Jayna M. Holroyd-Leduc and Madhuri Reddy.
© 2012 Blackwell Publishing Ltd. Published 2012 by Blackwell Publishing Ltd.

treatment studies in which we justify the relevance of a younger age cutoff.

Depression is the fourth leading cause of disease burden worldwide, accounting for 4.4% of total disability-adjusted life years (DALYs) in the year 2000, and represents an even larger burden in high-income countries. It causes the largest amount of nonfatal burden, accounting for almost 12% of all total years lived with disability (YLDs) worldwide [3].

In England and Wales, depression is the most common mental illness in older people. The MRC (Medical Research Council) Cognitive Function and Ageing Study found a prevalence of 8.7%, (95% confidence interval (CI) 7.3–10.2) among people aged 65 and over, rising to 9.7% (95% CI 8.2–11.1) if patients with concurrent dementia were included [4]. Prevalence of severe depression was 2.7% (95% CI 1.9–3.5). There were associations with female gender, functional disability, high deprivation, and medical comorbidity, with disability being the most strongly associated factor. The prevalence in long-term care was high at 27.1% (95% CI 17.8–36.3) [5]. There is variation in prevalence of depression among countries, regions, ethnic groups, and study centers. The EURODEP study provides comparative data on people over 65 years for cities in nine European countries with major and minor depression prevalence ranging from 8.8% (Iceland) to 23.6% (Munich), with a mean level of depression of 12.3% (95% CI 11.8–12.9) [6]. The US Health and Retirement Study found a prevalence of major depression of 6.6% in people over the age of 50 (95% CI 6.1–7.1) [7].

Causation and risk factors

There are different causative factors for late-onset depressive disorders compared to depressive disorder recurring in older age. These illnesses differ in prognosis, symptoms, and neurocognitive characteristics. Late-onset depressive disorders most likely have a relatively greater contribution from vascular and cerebrovascular disorders and associated cognitive impairment [8, 9]. In recurrence of earlier age-onset depression, genetic factors are thought to be relatively more important.

Debate continues about whether there is a subtype of depression comorbid with cerebrovascular disease, based on the hypothesis of a vascular depression [10]. Early associations reported include subcortical lesions (silent lacunar infarctions or hyperintense lesions). However, there is heterogeneity in later life presentations, variability in the presence of brain lesions, and variability in the size of the lesion. Separating these risk effects from other etiological factors, including the overall medical burden in older patients, is not yet possible. Current research is applying functional magnetic resonance imaging and DTI (diffusion tensor imaging) to test these links.

Psychosocial factors such as social isolation, bereavement, and poor social support are reported as risk factors for depression at all ages. In older adults, when depression presents, social isolation may be either a consequence of depression or a cause, or both. Socioeconomic deprivation further compounds the effects of physical illness on functional impairment and social isolation. Psychosocial factors may also be the trigger for an episode even when the underlying predisposition lies in chronic physical illness. Importantly, sadness should neither be attributed solely to the isolation nor viewed as an understandable consequence of negative life events that will resolve without intervention.

Comorbidity and outcomes

In older people, chronic physical health problems and symptoms of depression frequently coexist, adversely affecting outcomes such as higher functional impairment and shortening life expectancy. Although suicide is a serious risk and must be considered (see Figure 8.1) within management, in this chapter we focus on mortality due to other causes.

There is an association across all ages between chronic physical illness and depression. A cross-sectional study of people in 60 countries found that between 9.3% and 23.0% of participants with one or more chronic physical diseases (e.g., angina, arthritis, asthma, and diabetes) had comorbid depression [11]. This result was significantly higher than the likelihood of having depression in the absence of a chronic physical disease ($p < 0.0001$). After adjustment for socioeconomic factors and health conditions, depression had the strongest association with worsening mean health scores compared with the other chronic conditions. Similar results were found in a cross-sectional study of older people living in long-term care with an association between depression and dementia or functional impairment [5]. A prospective, population-based,

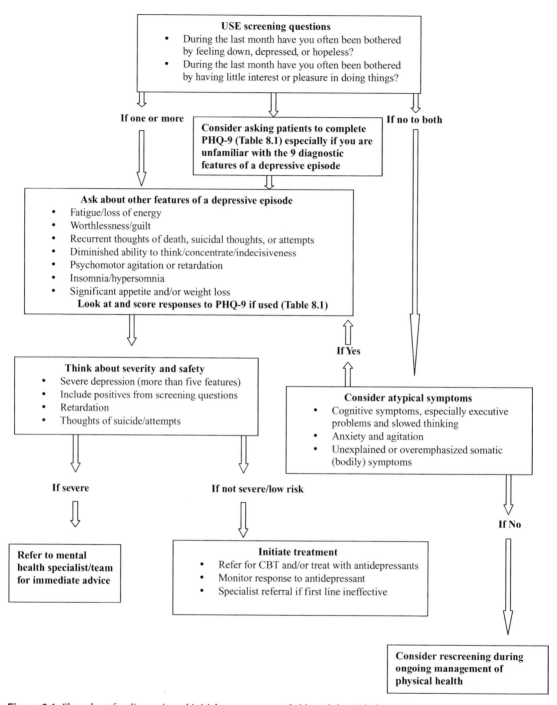

Figure 8.1 Flow chart for diagnosis and initial management of older adults with depressive symptoms.

longitudinal study of adults 65 years or older residing in an Italian municipality (baseline data for 595 subjects with no cognitive impairment with 4-year follow-up for incident mild cognitive impairment (MCI)) found that baseline depressive symptoms were associated with increased risk of MCI at follow-up, although only for subjects on antidepressant drugs at baseline [12]. Incident cases were 72.7% compared with 24.0% incident cases for those without depressive symptoms and not on antidepressant therapy. The association was independent of other confounders, sociodemographic factors, and vascular risk factors. The association was stronger for the MCI subtype without memory impairment.

Depression is also associated with higher mortality—both alone and when comorbid. For example, one prospective, representative study of people aged 70 years and older living in the community found that depressive symptoms reduced active life expectancy (ALE) by 6.5 years in men aged 70 and total life expectancy (TLE) by 3.5 years; for women aged 70 ALE was reduced by 4.2 years and TLE by 2.9 years. Effects were smaller among the oldest old (85+ years) [13]. Effects on ALE generally remained significant after controlling for chronic physical disorder (e.g., cancer, diabetes, heart disease, and stroke), although controls for some chronic diseases eliminated the effect on TLE. A further longitudinal study (up to 15 years' duration) of the relationship between depression and mortality among participants aged 70–103 years in Berlin identified strong predictive effects of diagnoses of depression on mortality among the young old, aged 70–84 years (relative risk (RR) 1.60; 95% CI 1.13–2.26) that were not due to the effects of other mortality predictors [14]. Among the oldest old (85+ years), no association was found between depression and mortality. Depression is, therefore, a significant risk factor for all-cause mortality in old age although the risk conveyed by depression may not hold in very old age.

Depression is a risk factor in the development of cardiovascular disease. The relationship between the onset of cardiovascular disease and depression has been of interest for several years. A systematic review and meta-analysis of longitudinal case-control or cohort studies has confirmed an association between depression and the subsequent development of cardiovascular-related disorders [15]. The study used meta-regression methods and included myocardial infarction, coronary heart disease, and cerebrovascular disease. It is of interest that depressed mood was found to moderately increase risk for these disorders. However, the greatest risk for the development of cardiovascular disease was in patients with a clinically diagnosed major depressive disorder. This risk was found equal to that of smoking and diabetes.

Prognosis

Major depression appears to have a poor prognosis. In a 2-year observational cohort study of 392 primary care attenders in the United States aged over 65, the trajectories of patients with more severe depressive symptoms (e.g., major depression or the more highly symptomatic cases of minor depression) were strikingly poor, with the cluster of subjects with Psychiatric Status Ratings initially near the major depression level remaining at that level throughout the follow-up period [16]. At the same time, the outcomes of those with subsyndromal to more mild forms of minor depression were diverse, with substantial numbers improving under "usual care" from their general practitioner (GP) and others remaining symptomatic or worsening over time. Antidepressant treatment was not independently associated with outcome, perhaps due to the low doses prescribed on average. Consistent predictors of depression trajectory were baseline depressive symptom severity, medical burden, and psychiatric functional status.

In a 6-year observational cohort study in the Netherlands of community dwelling elderly persons aged 55–85 years, prognosis was also found to be poor [17]. The average level of symptoms remained elevated throughout the study with 32% remaining chronically depressed, 12% had remission with recurrence, 32% had a chronic–intermittent course, and 23% had true remissions. While DSM severity categories at baseline predicted the severity and duration of episodes, subjects with subthreshold depression on DSM criteria at baseline experienced outcomes that were more similar to the DSM disorders than to a similarly followed-up group of nondepressed persons. This prognostic evidence supports a view that a range of clinically relevant depressive symptoms that do not meet diagnostic criteria are relevant in older patients.

Thus far, we have described the burden of depression and focused on associations between physical risk factors and outcomes for older people who have depression. We now address two main clinical questions pertinent to clinicians practicing in both hospital and community-based settings. These are as follows:

1 Is this older adult depressed?

2 What are the best options for the initial treatment of this depressed older adult?

Search strategy

For question 1, "Is this older adult depressed?", we searched the Cochrane Library, EMBASE, MEDLINE, and PsychINFO between February 2000 and February 2010 for systematic reviews, meta-analyses, and cross-sectional studies. Search terms included: "depress*," "diagnosis," "Geriatric Depression Scale (GDS)" or "Center for Epidemiology Studies Depression (CES-D)" or "Patient Health Questionnaire" or "screening" or "screening tools," "sensitivity" or "specificity" or "likelihood ratios" or "odds ratio." We included studies of persons over 65 years of age or that identified "geriatric patients," and the studies that took place within the community, primary, or secondary care settings, and/or long-term care. Only English language articles were included.

For question 2, "What are the best options for the initial treatment of this depressed older adult?," we searched Cochrane Library, EMBASE, MEDLINE, and PsychINFO between January 2005 and February 2010 for systematic reviews, meta-analyses, and randomized controlled trials. Search terms included: "depress*" or "bipolar" or "unipolar," "intervention*" or "manage*" or "cognitive behaviour therapy" or "cbt" or "interpersonal therapy" or "ipt" or "antidepressant*" or "electroconvulsive therapy" or "ect" or "sleep hygiene" or "exercise," "outcome*" or "result*" or "effect*" or "remission" or "recovery" or "quality of life". The search was limited to persons over 45 years of age with depression. Only English language articles were included.

For this chapter, we graded relevant clinical studies using the Oxford Centre for Evidence-based Medicine Levels of Evidence.

Is this older adult depressed?

Diagnosis

Depression in the older adult is associated with physical symptoms and cognitive difficulties (slowed thinking and problems in abstract thinking, sequencing, and planning). Hence, it is possible that older people with depression may not display prominent symptoms as described within the diagnostic criteria at the beginning of this chapter. Older adults may present with emphasis on either the physical or cognitive difficulties. Atypical presentations are possible with features such as oversleeping and overeating, or with dominant anxiety. When depression is severe, extremes of either distress and agitation or retardation even to the extent of stupor can predominate.

The search yielded only one secondary study identifying older adults with the outcome of diagnosis of depression: a systematic search conducted within a treatment guideline [18]. Two other systematic reviews focused on adults over 18 years with the outcome measure of management of depression and depression outcomes [19, 20]. The search was then broadened to cross-sectional studies to form the basis of discussion of best clinical practice.

Underdiagnosis of depression

Given the risk of atypical presentations mentioned above, there is a significant risk of underdiagnosis. A study of patients attending outpatient clinics and family practices in Germany found that the diagnoses by physicians (without psychiatric training) had low sensitivity (40%), although higher specificity (87%) for major depressive disorder was observed when compared with structured clinical interviews using the DSM-IV criteria (Level 1b evidence) [21]. It is likely that comorbidity of physical and depressive disorders raises difficulties with attribution of presenting symptoms to physical illness, and clinicians may regard the symptoms simply as understandable reactions to morbidity or to a (possibly coexisting) depressive disorder in its own right. Atypical presentations may also be more common with older patients.

Screening questions for depression are increasingly widely used and recommended by the National Institute for Health and Clinical Excellence in England and Wales (NICE). Screening questions may take the form of brief questionnaires either completed by patients or alternatively by physicians, or in the case of the elderly may be completed by caregivers.

There is evidence in the general adult population that the following two screening questions may be of use in increasing the identification of depression

Table 8.1 The patient health questionnaire-9 (PHQ-9)

Over the *Last 2 Weeks*, have You been Bothered by any of the Following Problems?[a]

1 Little interest or pleasure in doing things

2 Feeling down, depressed, or hopeless

3 Trouble falling or staying asleep, or sleeping too much

4 Feeling tired or having little energy

5 Poor appetite or overeating

6 Feeling bad about yourself—or that you are a failure or have let yourself or your family down

7 Trouble concentrating on things, such as reading the newspaper or watching television

8 Moving or speaking so slowly that other people could have noticed? Or, the opposite—being so fidgety or restless that you have been moving around a lot more than usual

9 Thoughts that you would be better off dead or of hurting yourself in some way

If you checked off *any* problems, how *difficult* have these problems made it for you to do your work, to take care of things at home, or get along with other people? Not difficult at all; Somewhat difficult; Very difficult; extremely difficult.

---

[a]For each of the nine items, patients are asked to state whether they had been bothered "not at all," "several days," "more than half the days," or "nearly every day." These are scored 0,1,2,3, respectively.

A tentative diagnosis requires a total score of 5 or more; 2 and 3s for questions 1–8; or 1–3 for question 9, INCLUDING one or both questions 1 and 2, PLUS a "somewhat difficult" or greater for the "difficulty" question.

Severity can also be described using total scores: 10–14 suggests major depression—mild; 15–19 major depression—moderate; ≥20 suggests major depression—severe.

The PHQ-9 is freely available. Users can download the questionnaire in a table format from the Pfizer website at: www.phqscreeners.com

during consultations in primary care (Level 1b evidence) [22]:

1 During the last month, have you often been bothered by feeling down, depressed, or hopeless?

2 During the last month, have you often been bothered by having little interest or pleasure in doing things?

These two questions correspond to the two core DSM criteria (Table 8.1). A "yes" response to one of the two questions was found to have high sensitivity for depression (0.95, 95% CI 0.91–0.97) but low specificity (0.66, 95% CI 0.55–0.76) (Level 1b evidence) [23]. This two-question screen has been recommended in guidelines for detection of depression in chronic physical illness and older adults [18, 24].

Another approach has been to use the Patient Health Questionnaire-9 (PHQ-9) screening tool (Table 8.1) for use in primary care, which assesses severity, duration, and impact on function of emotional difficulties (Level 1b evidence) [25]. The questions directly reflect the criteria of DSM-IV and the tool is completed by the patient. In medical settings for the general population of all ages, sensitivity was found to be very high at 98% (95% CI 92–100), with specificity of 80% (95% CI 76–83) (Level 1b evidence) [21].

However, the diagnostic effectiveness of screening tools among older populations does not appear to be as high as that for younger people. A cross-sectional study of older people (aged 50 and over), with musculoskeletal pain presenting in primary care, found that when GPs administered the two screening questions a large number of patients with depressive symptoms were missed (Level 1b evidence) [26]. Screening based on the Hospital Anxiety and Depression Scale (HAD) showed that 35.5% of study participants had evidence of depressive symptoms while GP screening detected only 20.8%. The authors concluded that ultrashort screening questions miss a large number of those with depressive symptoms, including six out of eight patients with severe symptoms, and they suggest that the presence of pain may reduce the recognition of depression, a problem that may be further exacerbated by multimorbidity in older age.

Longer screening instruments also appear to have lower sensitivity for older patients. A number of tools such as CES-D and HAD have been validated on older populations, and GDS was developed for screening older people (Level 1a evidence) [18]. Subsequently, several versions of GDS of differing length have been validated in a variety of physical care settings and a range of different physical disorders. In one recent study, the 15-item version was administered to 526 subjects aged 65 and older in Eastern United States who had been admitted to a large visiting nurse service agency. Using the optimal cutoff of 5, the sensitivity was 71.8% and specificity 78.2% (Level 1b evidence) [27].

There are unique difficulties when the screening instruments are used by caregivers. A small-scale study in long-term care in Southeast United States found that, when using a 19-item screening instrument (a modified version of the Cornell Scale for Depression in Dementia (CSDD)), caregivers failed to detect depression (Level 1b evidence) [28]. The sensitivity of the instrument was low at 47% (95% CI 21–73), although specificity was better at 65% (95% CI 55–75). The authors concluded that the findings might reflect that caregivers were not in tune with residents' depressive behaviors, or was due to variations in how well the residents were known by different caregivers.

While screening may be useful, the risk of underdiagnosis remains. This may be a particular risk when there is comorbidity. Any screening tool needs to be followed by fuller assessment. After treatment begins the functional status can be used to assess patient improvement and the PHQ-9, discussed earlier, can be used to review progress (Level 1b evidence) [21].

Part of the impact of advice and feedback may lie in the continued difficulty of distinguishing which physical symptoms are attributable to depression. Psychiatrists share this dilemma in screening. It can be argued that there will be fewer missed cases if somatic symptoms are included regardless of whether the clinician judges them to be of medical or psychological cause [29]. The other approach has been to use further screening questions that exclude somatic symptoms, hence reducing false positives [30]. However, this is less reliable for milder cases of depression.

An entirely different approach to improving the sensitivity of case finding has been tested in a randomized multicenter clinical trial involving 14 geriatric outpatient clinics in Italy (Level 1b evidence) [31]. Geriatricians in the treatment arm received a 3-day educational program of lectures and simulated clinical cases of depression. Sensitivity of diagnosis using DSM-IV increased from 35% in the untrained arm to 49% in the trained arm, with respective specificities of 88% and 91%.

Clinical bottom line

Brief screening tools may have low sensitivity for elderly patients. Use clinical judgment in addition to the screening tool when excluding the diagnosis of depression.

The patient-completed PHQ-9 may be helpful clinically (see Table 8.1). The questions map clearly onto the diagnostic criteria for depression in DSM-IV, and include the two-question screen. This tool would fit within our flow chart (Figure 8.1), strengthening the clinical evidence for detection of the key features for diagnosis and contributing to an assessment of severity, which, in turn, guides treatment. The flow chart reminds the clinician of the need to consider the atypical features in anyone with a positive response to the two screening questions. In addition, the PHQ-9 is a tool that can readily be used for shared care monitoring of treatment response in primary care. Reviewing the responses to the PHQ-9 will help the clinician become more familiar with the full range of symptoms of depression, increase the likelihood of making a correct diagnosis, and quantifying the severity of depression.

People with impaired function, chronic illnesses, or past history of depression are at highest risk of a depressive episode. Dominant presenting symptoms may not correspond to the classic symptoms (as defined in diagnostic criteria), which are more likely to be observed in younger people. In cases where there is chronic illness or neurocognitive problems (such as difficulty with abstract thinking, sequencing, and planning) or predominant anxiety, consideration should be given to a diagnosis of comorbid depression.

What are the best options for the initial treatment of this depressed older adult?

The management of depression in older adults depends on a number of factors. These include the severity of depression (typically described as: either mild-to-moderate or severe), risk (most commonly: self-harm/suicide, self-neglect, abuse, and coexistent physical health problems), patient preference, and what has worked in the past if the patient has a history of depressive disorder.

We have divided the therapeutic options for the management of patients with depression into talking therapies, antidepressants, and electroconvulsive therapy (ECT). Our search yielded no systematic reviews or randomized controlled trials investigating more conservative strategies such as exercise or sleep hygiene.

Talking therapies for mild to moderate depression in older adults

One 2006 Cochrane Systematic Review identified nine randomized controlled trials of psychotherapeutic treatments for older adults with depression (Level 1a evidence) [32]. The review investigated four types of psychotherapeutic interventions: (1) cognitive behavioral therapy (CBT), (2) psychodynamic therapy, (3) interpersonal therapy, and (4) supportive therapies (e.g., counseling) compared with either controls or each other. All trials were of a parallel design and excluded patients with cognitive impairment.

Five trials, with 153 participants, compared a cognitive behavioral approach (cognitive therapy, cognitive bibliotherapy, and problem-solving therapy) with waiting list controls. Cognitive behavioral therapies were statistically and clinically more effective than waiting list controls when measured using the Hamilton Depression Rating Scale (WMD −9.85; 95% CI −11.97, −7.73). One trial (231 participants), which used a dichotomous outcome, did not identify a statistically significant improvement of problem-solving therapy compared to a nonactive drug placebo group (odds ratio (OR) 0.88; 95% CI 0.24, 0.69). Six trials (462 participants) provided data on dropouts and there were more dropouts in control groups compared to CBT in the six trials (OR 0.43; 95% CI 0.27, 0.68), although there were a large number of dropouts in both groups: 180/243 in the CBT group and 193/221 in the control group. There were no trials comparing psychodynamic psychotherapies, interpersonal therapies, or supportive/counseling therapies with controls.

Three trials compared CBT with psychodynamic therapy. There was no statistically significant difference in the two trials (57 participants) that assessed reduction in symptoms or in the third trial (52 participants), which considered a dichotomous outcome of clinical response.

Antidepressants for older adults with depression

Three systematic reviews were identified, of which two compared antidepressants with placebo (Level 1a evidence) [33, 34] and one compared different classes of antidepressants (Level 1a evidence) [35].

One systematic review identified 17 trials with just under 2000 participants comparing antidepressants with placebo in older adults, who were aged 60 and over [33]. Participants with concomitant physical illness were included but those with an explicit diagnosis of dementia were excluded. Meta-analysis of 11 trials (468 participants) found that tricyclic antidepressants (TCAs) were more effective than placebo (OR: 0.32; 95% CI 0.21, 0.47). The number needed to treat (NNT) was 4 (95% CI 3.9, 4.05), suggesting that four older adults with depression would need to be treated to see one additional patient recovering. Two trials (737 participants) compared serotonin selective reuptake inhibitors (SSRIs) with placebo and found that more patients recovered with SSRIs (OR 0.51; 95% CI 0.36, 0.72). The NNT was 9 (95% CI 8.38, 8.53). Finally, two trials (121 participants) found evidence in favor of monoamine oxidase inhibitors (MAOIs) (OR 0.17; 95% CI 0.07, 0.39) with an NNT of 4 (3.14; 95% CI 2.99, 3.29). Similar results were found for atypical antidepressants (minaprine, mirtazapine, and medifoxamine). All four classes of antidepressants had similar discontinuation rates compared to placebo.

Another systematic review identified ten trials of nontricyclic or non-MAOI antidepressants in patients aged 60 or above living with nonpsychotic depression in a community setting [34]. Trials investigating depression secondary to a medical disorder were excluded. Treatments considered included: SSRIs (citalopram escitalopram, fluoxetine, paroxetine and sertraline), serotonin norepinephrine reuptake inhibitors (duloxetine and venlafaxine), and dopamine norepinephrine reuptake inhibitors (bupropion). All classes of antidepressants were more effective than placebo. The longer treatment was continued, the more likely participants were to respond to medication. However, there were more discontinuations for any reason and adverse events among participants allocated to antidepressants.

Finally, the third systematic review examined the efficacy and side effects of different antidepressant classes

[35]. A total of 32 trials were included. There was no statistically significant difference in efficacy of the different classes of antidepressants (MAOIs, TCAs, SSRIs, and atypical antidepressants). Participants receiving classical TCAs (amitriptyline, clomipramine, doxepin, and dothiepin) were more likely to withdraw from the study (ten studies; 1154 participants, RR 1.24; 95% CI 1.05, 1.46). However, there was no statistically significant difference in the four trials (174 participants) comparing TCA-related antidepressants (mianserin and trazodone) with SSRIs.

The choice of antidepressant medication should be based on the patient's preferences, coexistent illness and treatment, suicide risk, and previous response to antidepressant treatment [36]. As noted earlier, SSRIs are better tolerated than TCAs. They are relatively safe in overdose and are recommended as first-line antidepressants. The most common side effects of SSRIs include nausea, vomiting, abdominal pain, diarrhea, possible short-term exacerbation of anxiety and less commonly constipation, loss of appetite, and weight loss. TCAs can cause sedation, constipation, and postural hypotension, occasionally cause cardiac arrhythmias and heart block and are more toxic in overdose than SSRIs. The sedative properties of some of the TCAs can be useful in patients with difficulty sleeping; however, they can increase risk of falls. MAOIs have dangerous interactions with some foods, for example, cheese, and should only be prescribed by specialists. Each of the atypical antidepressants has its own side effect profile. Antidepressants should not be used if the patient enters a manic phase. Readers should consult a drug database or compendium for more information.

ECT for severe depression in older adults

A 2006 Cochrane Systematic Review assessed the efficacy and safety of ECT compared to simulated ECT or antidepressants in older adults aged 60 or over with depression (Level 1b evidence) [37]. Only one trial was identified comparing ECT with simulated ECT. This trial included patients referred for ECT who had been diagnosed with major depression according to DSM-III but did not specify severity of depression or previous treatment with antidepressants. Although ECT was found to be more effective than simulated ECT, these results must be interpreted with caution as it was based on reexamination of findings from an ear-lier study and only included 35 participants. No randomized evidence that included depressed older adults with coexisting physical conditions such as dementia, Parkinson's disease, and cerebrovascular disorders was identified.

Clinical bottom line

CBT can be effective for the treatment of older adults with a mild-to-moderate depressive episode. The evidence is not strong enough to rule out other psychological treatments, which may be more appropriate to the patient's wishes and circumstances.

Antidepressants are effective in the initial treatment of older adults with depression in community or hospital settings including those with coexistent physical illness. When choosing an antidepressant, clinicians should take into account a range of factors including side effect profile and patient preference. The longer the treatment is continued, the more likely a response will be seen. Therefore, clinical guidelines typically recommend that treatment should be continued for at least 6 months with regular review of progress and side effects.

ECT should be considered in patients with severe depression, who either present with significant risk or have not responded to antidepressant treatment.

Figure 8.1 provides a flow chart for the assessment and initial management of older adults with depression.

Chapter summary

We have presented the best available evidence for the identification and initial treatment of depressive episodes in older adults. Depressive disorder is a common condition in older adults and has a significant impact on both functioning and life expectancy.

Although many of the symptoms of a depressive episode are also caused by physical illness, clinicians should have a high index of suspicion that depression may be present in the physically ill, and should not necessarily interpret depressive symptoms as solely caused by physical conditions.

Clinicians should also consider the safety of the patient and involve specialist mental health services in the treatment of patients with severe depression, treatment-resistant depression, or those with suicidal thoughts or suicidal behavior.

Antidepressants and talking therapies (e.g., CBT) are effective in the treatment of older adults with a mild-to-moderately severe depressive episode. The treatment options for more severe episodes of depressive disorder include ECT and antidepressants.

References

1. American Psychiatric Association (ed.) (2000) *Diagnostic and Statistical Manual of Mental Disorders: DSM-IV-TR*, Fourth Edition. Washington: American Psychiatric Association.
2. World Health Organisation (1993) *The ICD-10 Classification of Mental and Behavioural Disorders, Research Criteria*. Geneva: WHO.
3. Ustun TB, et al (2004) Global burden of depressive disorders in the year 2000. *Br J Psychiatry* 184: 386–392.
4. McDougall FA, et al (2007) Prevalence and symptomatology of depression in older people in England and Wales: the MRC CFA Study. *Psychol Med* 37: 1787–1795.
5. McDougall FA, et al (2007) Prevalence and symptomatology of depression in older people living in institutions in England and Wales. *Age Aging* 36: 562–568.
6. Copeland JR, et al (2004) Depression among older people in Europe: the EURODEP studies. *World Psychiatry* 3: 45–49.
7. Mojtabai R, Olfson M (2004) Major depression in community-dwelling middle-aged and older adults: prevalence and 2- and 4-year follow-up symptoms. *Psychol Med* 34: 623–634.
8. Steffens DC, Potter GG (2008) Geriatric depression and cognitive impairment. *Psychol Med* 38: 163–175.
9. Baldwin RC, et al (2006) Prognosis of late life depression: a three-year cohort study of outcome and potential predictors. *Int J Geriatr Psychiatry* 21: 57–63.
10. Alexopoulos GS (2005) Depression in the elderly. *Lancet* 365: 1961–1970.
11. Moussavi S, et al (2007) Depression, chronic diseases, and decrements in health: results from the World Health Surveys. *Lancet* 370: 851–858.
12. Ravaglia G, et al (2008) Prevalent depressive symptoms as a risk factor for conversion to mild cognitive impairment in an elderly cohort. *Am J Geriatr Psychiatry* 16: 834–843.
13. Reynolds SL, Haley WE, Kozlenko N (2008) The impact of depressive symptoms and chronic diseases on active life expectancy in older Americans. *Am J Geriatr Psychiatry* 16: 425–432.
14. Rapp MA, Gerstorf D, Helmchen H, Smith J (2008) Depression predicts mortality in the young old, but not in the oldest old: results from the Berlin Aging Study. *Am J Geriatr Psychiatry* 16: 844–852.
15. Van der Kooy K, et al (2007) Depression and the risk for cardiovascular diseases: systematic review and meta analysis. *Int J Geriatr Psychiatry* 22: 613–626.
16. Cui X, et al (2008) Outcomes and predictors of late-life depression trajectories in older primary care patients. *Am J Geriatr Psychiatry* 16: 406–415.
17. Beekman ATF, et al (2002) The natural history of late-life depression. A 6-year prospective study in the community. *Arch Gen Psychiatry* 59: 605–611.
18. National Institute for Health and Clinical Excellence. (2010) *Depression: the treatment and management in adults.* National Clinical Practice Guideline 90. www.nice.org.uk
19. Gilbody SM, House AD, Sheldon TA (2001) Routinely administered questions for depression and anxiety: a systematic review. *Br Med J* 322: 406–409.
20. O'Connor EA, et al (2009) Screening for depression in adults and older adults in primary care: an updated systematic review. *Ann Intern Med* 151: 784–792.
21. Lowe B, et al (2004) Comparative validity of three screening questionnaires for DSM IV depressive disorders and physicians diagnoses. *J Affect Disord* 78: 131–140.
22. Arroll B, Kim N, Kerse N (2003) Screening for depression in primary care with two verbally asked questions: cross sectional study. *Br Med J* 327: 1144–1146.
23. Whooley MA, Avins AL, Miranda J, Browner WS. (1997) Case-finding instruments for depression two questions are as good as many. *J Gen Intern Med* 12: 439-445.
24. National Institute for Health and Clinical Excellence. (2009) *Depression in adults with a chronic physical health problem: treatment and management.* National Clinical Practice Guideline 91. www.nice.org.uk
25. Kroenke K, Spitzer RL, Williams JB (2001) The PHQ-9: Validity of a brief depression severity measure. *J Gen Intern Med* 16: 606–613.
26. Mallen CD, Peat G (2008) Screening older people with musculoskeletal pain for depressive symptoms in primary care. *Br J Gen Pract* 58: 688–693.
27. Marc LG, Raue PJ, Bruce ML (2008) Screening performance of the 15-item Geriatric Depression Scale in a diverse elderly home care population. *Am J Geriatr Psychiatry* 16: 914–918.
28. Watson LC, Zimmerman S, Cohen LW, et al (2009) Practical depression screening in residential care/assisted living: five methods compared with gold standard diagnoses. *Am J Geriatr Psychiatry* 17: 556–564.
29. Williams JW, et al (2002) Is this patient clinically depressed? *JAMA* 287: 1160–1170.
30. Zimmerman M, Chelminski I, McGlinchey JB, Young D (2006) Diagnosing major depressive disorder X: can the utility of the DSM-IV symptom criteria be improved? *J Nerv Ment Dis* 194: 893–897.
31. Lattanzio F, et al (2009) Improving the diagnostic accuracy of depression in older persons: the depression in the aged female national evaluation cluster randomised trial. *J Am Geriatr Soc* 57: 588–593.
32. Wilson K, Mottram PG, Vassilas C. Psychotherapeutic treatments for older depressed people. Cochrane Database of Systematic Reviews 2008, Issue 1. Art. No.: CD004853.
33. Wilson K, Mottram PG, Sivananthan A, Nightingale A. Antidepressants versus placebo for the depressed elderly. Cochrane Database of Systematic Reviews 2001, Issue 1. Art. No.: CD000561.

34. Nelson JC, Delicchi K, Schneider LS (2008) Efficacy of second generation of antidepressants in late-life depression: a meta-analysis of the evidence. *Am J Geriatr Psychiatry* 16: 558–567.

35. Mottram PG, Wilson K, Strobl JJ. Antidepressants for depressed elderly. Cochrane Database of Systematic Reviews 2006, Issue 1. Art. No.: CD003491.

36. BNF 61 (2011) British National Formulary 61. London: BMJ Publishing and RPS Publishing.

37. Stek ML, Wurff van derFFB, Hoogendijk WJG, Beekman ATF. Electroconvulsive therapy for the depressed elderly. Cochrane Database of Systematic Reviews 2003, Issue 2. Art. No.: CD003593.

CHAPTER 9

A balancing act: preventing and treating falls

Emily Kwan & Sharon Straus
Department of Medicine, Division of Geriatrics, University of Toronto, Toronto, ON, Canada

Introduction

Approximately 30% of community-dwelling individuals aged 65 and older fall and 50% of community dwellers aged 85 and older will fall each year [1]. Of those community-dwelling individuals who fall, 12%–42% will have a fall-related injury, with up to 20% of these requiring medical attention and 10% resulting in fracture secondary to osteoporosis [2]. Falls can also lead to anxiety, depression, social isolation, and immobility. Although vertebral fractures can cause back pain, deformity, disability, and mortality [1, 3], hip fractures have the most devastating prognosis [4]. It is estimated that 1 in 5 people who suffer a hip fracture will die during the first year, and less than one-third will regain their prefracture level of physical function [5]. Recovery from hip fractures is slow, rehabilitation often incomplete, and many patients are permanently institutionalized in nursing homes.

Different definitions of falls have been provided but the one most consistently used is that suggested by the Centers for Disease Control and Prevention, which defines a fall as an "injury received when a person descends abruptly due to force of gravity and strikes a surface at the same or lower level" [6]. Some researchers have modified this definition to include coming to rest on the ground or other lower level than the original position and not due to external forces such as from a motor vehicle accident [6].

The etiology of falls is often multifactorial. Risk factors for falling can be divided into intrinsic and extrinsic factors. Intrinsic factors are normal physical and mental changes related to aging (but not associated with disease) that decrease functional reserve. As a result of these factors, older patients become more susceptible to falls when they are confronted with challenges such as pneumonia, urinary tract infection, or myocardial infarction [1]. Extrinsic factors include environmental factors such as falls due to ice, or tripping on a rug, or due to use of certain medications such as psychotropic medications. Understanding what risk factors for falls are present may help target interventions to prevent falls [1].

Multiple interventions have been studied to prevent falls for older people living in different settings including the community, hospitals, and long-term care. Trials of fall-prevention strategies have shown that approximately one-third of falls can be prevented [7]. Both single and multifactorial interventions for falls prevention have been studied.

In this chapter, we searched the literature for systematic reviews of risk factors for falls and for interventions to prevent falls in patients living in various settings. The focus of this chapter is on falls prevention but we have also included material on recent osteoporosis

Evidence-Based Geriatric Medicine: A Practical Clinical Guide, First Edition. Edited by Jayna M. Holroyd-Leduc and Madhuri Reddy.
© 2012 Blackwell Publishing Ltd. Published 2012 by Blackwell Publishing Ltd.

guidelines since this material should be considered with falls assessments.

Search strategy

For articles on falls risk and prevention, we completed a comprehensive search of the literature including MEDLINE, CINAHL, EMBASE, AGELINE, and COCHRANE from 2005 to May 2011. The search was developed in consultation with an information scientist and used the following terms: "falls", "accidental falls", "aged", "geriatric", "elderly", "senior", "old age", and "older adult". Appropriate wildcards were used in the searching in order to account for plurals and variations in spelling. Additional articles were identified through review of reference lists and discussions with experts.

Inclusion criteria were systematic reviews of studies including those aged 65 years or older, evaluating falls interventions strategies, or of studies assessing risk factors for falls; English language publications; publication date between 2005 and May 2011. The authors of the present chapter independently reviewed each article to identify whether it met inclusion criteria and performed quality assessment.

The systematic reviews were assessed using the Assessment of Multiple Systematic Review (AMSTAR) [8]. If multiple articles were identified on a topic, only those that were rated as high quality (defined as a score of 7 or more out of 11) were included in this review. If a review was unique in its topic, it was included if it scored less than 7 on the AMSTAR.

Osteoporosis management should be considered along with falls prevention. To address this issue, we searched to identify recent guidelines produced in Canada [9], the United States (with the US Preventive Services Task Force (USPSTF) [10], the American College of Preventive Medicine (ACPM) [11]), and the United Kingdom [12]. These guidelines have been appraised using the AGREE (Appraisal of Guidelines for Research and Evaluation) instrument.

What risk factors are associated with falls?

Tools to assess falling were included in three reviews [14–16]. However, no single tool has been found to predict the risk of falls (Table 9.1).

History

Seven articles were identified that described risk factors for falls (Table 9.2). Of the studies that were assessed to be high quality, the most significant risk factors associated with falls included functional limitations/activities of daily living (ADL) disabilities (odds ratio (OR) 2.26), medications (range of OR from 0.96–4.35), visual impairment (OR 1.6–2.0), and balance impairment (OR 1.98).

Medications

Use of various medications and risk of falls has been studied in numerous studies. One of the most frequently studied classes of medications that has been found to be associated with falls is psychotropic medication. Woolcott and colleagues [17] assessed nine classes of medications such as antihypertensives, diuretics, beta-blockers, sedatives and hypnotics, neuroleptics and antipsychotics, benzodiazepines, narcotics, nonsteroidal anti-inflammatory drugs (NSAIDs), and antidepressants. The greatest association with falls was seen with use of sedatives and hypnotics (OR 1.47, 95% confidence interval (CI) 1.35–1.62), neuroleptics and antipsychotics (OR 1.59, 95% CI 1.37–1.83), antidepressants (OR 1.68, 95% CI 1.47–1.91), and benzodiazepines (OR 1.57, 95% CI 1.43–1.72).

Tinetti and colleagues [18] found eight articles that identified an association between use of more than four medications or of psychotropic medications and falls. Ganz and colleagues [13] found two studies that reported likelihood ratios (LR) of 1.7–1.9 (95% CI 1.3–2.5) for use of psychotropic medications and taking four or more medications. In another article in this review, the use of benzodiazepines or antidepressants was associated with falls (LR 27, 95% CI 3.6–207). NSAIDS were found to be associated with falls in a review by Hegeman and colleagues (OR 1.13–4.35, 95% CI 0.57–10.91) [19]. Sterke and colleagues [20] investigated the association between falls and psychoactive medications in patients with dementia and found limited evidence to support this association. However, falls were found to be associated with use of multiple medications.

Functional status

Gait impairment and functional limitations (including limitations in ADL) were associated with falls in one

Table 9.1 Studies evaluating the tools used to assess falls[a]

Review	Study Quality	Studies Included	Population	Tools Studied	Outcome
Gates et al [14]	7	25	5920	• Downton Index • Tinetti Balance scale • Timed Up and Go (TUG) • FRAT (part 1), Mobility Interaction Fall • One leg stance • Tandem stance • Coalition for Community Fall Prevention • Elderly Fall Screen • Falls Risk Assessment • Computerized Dynamic Posturography • Tinetti Mobility Test	• Most tools discriminated poorly between fallers and nonfallers. • Existing studies are methodologically variable and the results are inconsistent. • Insufficient evidence exists that any screening instrument is adequate for predicting falls.
Oliver et al [15]	6	12	3749 Hospital (acute, rehabilitation) setting	• STRATIFY (St Thomas's risk assessment tool in falling elderly inpatients)	Sensitivity 67.2 (95% CI 60.8, 73.6) Specificity 51.2 (95% CI 43.0, 59.3) • May not be optimal for identifying high-risk individuals for fall prevention. • Study demonstrates that population and setting affect STRATIFY performance.
Scott et al [16]	5	34	Unavailable Primarily 65 years and older	38 Tools including: • Berg balance scale • CTSIB • Dynamic gait index • Elderly mobility scale • 5 min walk • Step up test • Tandem stance • TUG • Tinetti balance scale	• Fall-risk assessment tools exist that show moderate to good validity and reliability in most health service delivery areas. • Few tools were tested more than once or in more than one setting. • No single tool can be recommended for implementation in all settings or for all subpopulations within each setting.

[a]All studies were prospective.

high-quality review [13]. In another review, balance impairment was found to be associated with falls (OR 1.98 (1.60, 2.46)) [21].

Bloch and colleagues [22] found an association between impaired ADL (OR 2.26, 95% CI 2.09, 2.45) (disturbance of at least one activity of daily living) and impaired instrumental ADL (IADL) OR 2.10 (95% CI 1.68, 2.64) and falls.

Physical examination

We identified one systematic review that provided details on the accuracy of the clinical exam for assessing

Table 9.2 Studies evaluating the risk factors for falls

Risk Factors	Studies	Study Quality	Number included (Study Design)	OR/RR
Balance impairment	Muir et al [21]	8	60,602 (Prospective studies)	Overall fall risk: rr (Risk Ratio) of 1.42 (1.08, 1.85) and OR of 1.98 (1.60, 2.46)
Visual impairment	Ganz et al [13]	8	19,178 (Prospective cohort studies)	OR 1.6–2.0 range but no other results.
Medications	Hegeman et al [19]	7	209,015 (Observational studies, systematic reviews)	Twelve articles with OR ranges of 1.13–4.35 95% CI 0.57–10.91)—studies on NSAIDS
	Sterke et al [20]	8	61,392 (Prospective cohort design)	Huge range of OR/rr (Risk Ratio) for psychoactive medication for nursing home demented patients.
	168 Woolcott et al [17]	9	79,081 (Cohort, cross-sectional, case-control)	Antihypertensive agents (OR 1.24, 95% CI 1.01–1.50); diuretics (OR 1.07, 95% CI 1.01–1.14); beta-blockers (OR 1.01, 95% CI 0.86–1.17); sedatives and hypnotics (OR 1.47, 95% CI 1.35–1.62); neuroleptics and antipsychotics (OR 1.59, 95% CI 1.37–1.83); antidepressants (OR 1.68, 95% CI 1.47–1.91); benzodiazepines (OR 1.57, 95% CI 1.43–1.72); narcotics (OR 0.96, 95% CI 0.78–1.18); nonsteroidal anti-inflammatory drugs (OR 1.21, 95% CI 1.01–1.44).
				Updated Bayesian adjusted OR estimates for:
				diuretics 0.99 (95% CI 0.78–1.25); neuroleptics and antipsychotics 1.39 (95% CI 0.94–2.00); antidepressants, 1.36 (95% CI 1.13–1.76) benzodiazepines 1.41 (95% CI 1.20–1.71)
Home hazards	Letts et al [23]	7	25,145 (Cross-sectional and cohort studies)	Home hazards (i.e., bathroom, environmental—indoor and outdoor, various list of hazards) are fall risk factors in community dwellers
				Increased risk (OR 1.15, 95% CI 0.997–1.36)
				High quality studies only:
				OR 1.38 (95% CI 1.03–1.87)
				Use of mobility aids significantly increased fall risk in community (OR 2.07, 95% CI 1.59–2.71) and institutional (OR 1.77, 95% CI 1.66–1.89)
Functional limitations, ADL disabilities	Bloch et al [22]	8	19,178 (RCT, observational studies (included cohort, case-control studies, and cross-sectional studies))	OR 2.26 (95% CI 2.09, 2.45) for disturbance in ADL and OR 2.10 (95% CI 1.68, 2.64) for instrumental ADL (IADL)

Continued

Table 9.2 *Continued*

Risk Factors	Studies	Study Quality	Number included (Study Design)	OR/RR
Being married	Bloch et al [22]	8	–	OR 0.68 (95% CI 0.53–0.87)—protective against falling
Low education level	Bloch et al [22]	8	–	OR 0.97 95% CI (0.83–1.13)
Marital status	Bloch et al [22]	8	–	OR 1.04 (95% CI 0.94–1.15)
Confined to bed	Bloch et al [22]	8	–	OR 0.92 (95% CI 0.70–1.20)

RCT, randomized controlled trial.

falls. Ganz et al, 2007 [13] found that history of falls has an LR of 2.3–2.8 and impaired gait has an LR of 1.7–2.4 for predicting falls (Table 9.3) [13].

Home hazards

Letts and colleagues found home hazards to be a risk factor for falls (OR 1.38 (95% CI 1.03–1.87)) [23]. Various home hazards were assessed in these studies including bathroom hazards, unspecified environmental hazards, and various itemized indoor and outdoor environmental hazards.

Clinical bottom line

On assessment for risk of falls, the following should be asked or observed:

1 History of falls
2 Visual impairment
3 Medications
4 Balance impairment
5 Gait impairment and walking difficulty
6 Functional limitations/ADL disability
7 Home hazards
8 Advanced age

What interventions should be considered for fall prevention?

Fifteen systematic reviews of fall-prevention interventions were identified as shown in Table 9.4. Seven of these reviews included participants living in the community, two included those from long-term care settings, one included participants from acute care hospitals, and five included participants from a combination of settings. These reviews assessed interventions including multicomponent strategies (combinations of exercise, balance assessment, home safety assessment, and vitamin D) and single component interventions such as Tai Chi, balance training, group exercise, Otago exercise program, vision correction and home safety assessment and modification.

Zijlstra and colleagues looked at the impact of multifactorial and single interventions on the fear of falling [24]. Single interventions included in this review were Tai Chi, exercise, and hip protector interventions. Home-based exercise, fall-related multifactorial programs, and Tai Chi were found to be effective in the reducing fear of falling. Clemson and colleagues found that environment interventions such as home assessment could reduce risk of falls significantly (relative risk (RR) 0.79; 0.65–0.97) [25].

Michael and colleagues [26] found that multifactorial assessments did not improve quality of life as compared with single intervention. They found that Vitamin D (RR (relative risk) 0.83, 95% CI 0.75–0.91) could decrease risk of falls. Hip protectors showed mixed results in two different trials in the review (one showed significant protective effect but another showed no effect). Vision correction and medication withdrawal did not result in a decreased risk of falls. Exercise and physical therapy did not reduce risk for fall-related fractures but did consistently show a reduced risk of falling.

Exercise training interventions have been assessed. Orr and colleagues [27] showed that progressive resistive training (strength training exercise with progressive overload where muscles exert a force against an external load or contract isometrically) could improve balance, which is an independent intrinsic contributor to falls. The Otago exercise (strength and balance retraining program) was investigated by Thomas and

Table 9.3 Studies evaluating the accuracy of elements of the history and physical exam for diagnosing falls

Risk Factors	Likelihood Ratio (LR)
Previous falls	Four studies reported LR (11 studies found in total)
	Fall in the past year (LR 2.3–2.8)
Gait and impairment of walking difficulty	Four studies reported LR (15 studies found)
	Clinically detected abnormality of gait or balance (LR 1.7–2.4)
Cognitive impairment	Two studied reported LR (8 studies found)
	One study found that five or more errors on the Short Portable Mental Status questionnaire were associated with one or more falls (LR 4.2, 95% CI 1.9–9.6)
	Other study reported that a history of dementia was associated with one or more falls (LR 17, 95% CI 1.9–149) and with two or more falls (LR 13, 95% CI 2.3–79)
Orthostatic hypotension	Four studies found no association when other risk factors were considered
	One study found a weak association between an increased pulse rate of less than 6 per minute, measured 30 seconds after standing up predicts falls (LR 1.4, 95% CI 1.0–1.9)
Functional limitations, ADL disabilities	Two studies reported LR (ten studies found)
	Inability to rise from a chair of knee height without using the chair arms was associated with an increased risk of one or more falls among men (LR 4.3, 95% CI 2.3–7.9)
	Five or more of 11 physical impairments (mostly activities of daily living) was associated with an increased risk of one or more falls (LR 1.9, 95% CI 1.4–2.6)
Age	Three studies reported LR (11 studies found)
	Risk was similar in two studies: for patients aged 65 through 74 years, the fall probability was 31%–32%; for those aged 70 through 74 years, 22%–33%; for those aged 75 through 79 years, 25%–36%; and for those 80 years or older, 34%–37%
	The third study found a statistically increased risk of falling at least once in the next 11 months among older patients (odds ratio per age category, 1.90; $P = .001$): aged 65 through 69 years, the fall probability was 14%; aged 70 through 74 years, 16%; aged 75 through 79 years, 24%; and aged 80 years and older, 34%

All risk factors are from Ganz et al [13] and in general had $N = 19,178$ from prospective cohort studies. (Study quality = 8)

colleagues [28] and was found to reduce the risk of death and falling in community dwellers.

Campbell and colleagues [29] looked to see if multifactorial interventions were superior to single strategies interventions in community dwellers. They found that single interventions (pooled rate ratio (RaR) 0.77, (95% CI 0.67–0.89)) were as effective in reducing falls as interventions with multiple components (RaR 0.78, 0.68–0.89, respectively).

Gillespie and colleagues [30] assessed impact of various multifactorial interventions on falls including a combination of exercise, environment/assistive technology, and knowledge intervention versus medication (drug target). They found exercise intervention reduces risk and rate of falls. Multiple-component group exercise reduced rate of falls and risk of falling (RaR 0.78, (95% CI 0.71–0.86); (RR) 0.83, (95% CI 0.72–0.97)).

Table 9.4 Studies evaluating interventions for preventing falls

Review	Study Quality	Number of Studies Included (Sample Size)	Type of Studies Included	Age	Setting	Intervention	Outcome
Zijlstra et al [24]	8	19 (Unavailable)	RCT	Mean age of 65 and older, special medical conditions were excluded	Community-living older adults	Multifactorial programs and single interventions (i.e., Tai Chi interventions, exercise interventions, and hip protector intervention)	Home-based exercise and fall-related multifactorial programs and community-based Tai Chi delivered in group format have been effective in reducing fear of falling in community-living older people
Agency for Health Care Research and Quality [26]	11	47 (152)	RCT (Questions 1, 2, 4). Question 3 trials and observational studies. Case series and case reports excluded	Older adults	Community-dwelling older adults	Falls interventions (i.e., comprehensive multifactorial assessment and management, exercise/physical therapy interventions, and vitamin D supplementation)	Several types of primary care applicable to falls interventions reduce falls among those selected to be at high risk for falling Risk of falling with multifactorial assessments: Comprehensive assessment (includes multifactorial assessment and provision of medical and social care) Relative risk of risk of falling (RR) 0.75 (95% CI 0.58–0.99) Noncomprehensive assessment (includes a multifactorial assessment but only included referral or limited management) did not reduce risk of falling. Relative risk (RR) 1.04, 95% CI 0.98–1.10

Continued

Table 9.4 *Continued*

Review	Study Quality	Number of Studies Included (Sample Size)	Type of Studies Included	Age	Setting	Intervention	Outcome
Orr et al [27]	8	29 (2174)	RCT	Mean age >60 years (minimum individual age >50)	Community dwellers	Progressive resistive training (PRT) vs. usual daily activity/usual care or activities that enhance the binding of the intervention	PRT does improve balance
Thomas et al [28]	7	7 (1503)	RCT or controlled trials with masked assessment of outcome	65 and older	Community dwellers	Otago exercise program vs. usual care or social visits	Otago exercise program reduces: Risk of death (rr (risk ratio) 0.45, 95% CI 0.25–0.80) Reduced fall rates (incidence rate (RaR) 0.68, 95% CI 0.56–0.79) Injury occurring as the result of a fall (rr (risk ratio) 1.05, 95% CI 0.91–1.22)
Campbell et al [29]	8	14 (5968)	RCT	65 and older	Majority live independently in community	Multifactorial intervention including home assessments, comprehensive geriatric assessment, diagnostic home visits, Stepping On program (group sessions: balance and strengthening exercises, home and community, environmental, and behavioral safety; encouraging regular review of vision and medications, follow-up occupational therapy home visit), physiotherapy and occupational therapy, Tai Chi, balance training Vs. social visits or no intervention or usual care. Also looked at single interventions	For populations at risk, targeted single interventions are as effective as multifactorial interventions; may be more acceptable and cost-effective Reduction of falls using single intervention is similar to multiple components: Single component: pooled RR (rate ratio) 0.77, 95% CI 0.67–0.89 Multicomponent: 0.78, 95% CI 0.68–0.89

| Clemson et al [25] | 8 | 6 (3298) | RCT | Majority of people 65 years and older | Community | Home assessment including hazard reduction, behavioral changes, footwear, ADL, IADL, mobility, home visits, home modifications, vision assessment | Home assessment interventions that are comprehensive, well focused, and incorporate an environmental-fit perspective with adequate follow-up can be successful in reducing falls with significant effects

Home assessments can reduce the fall risk:

RR (relative risk) 0.79 (95% CI 0.65–0.97) |
| Gillespie et al [30] | 10 | 111 (55,303) | RCT and quasi-RCT | 60 years or older | Community | Exercise interventions
This article looks at exercise with 13 other combinations including education, home safety intervention, or with Vitamin D/calcium | Exercise intervention reduces risk and rate of falls

Multiple-component group exercise reduced rate of falls and risk of falling (RaR 0.78, 95% CI 0.71–0.86; rr (risk ratio) 0.83, 95% CI 0.72–0.97)

Tai Chi with reduced rate of falls and risk of falling (RaR 0.63, 95% CI 0.52–0.78; rr (risk ratio) 0.65, 95% CI 0.51–0.82)

Individually prescribed multiple-component home-based exercise with reduced risk of fall and risk of falling (RaR 0.66, 95% CI 0.53–0.82; rr (risk ratio) 0.77, 95% CI 0.61–0.97)

Assessment and multifactorial intervention reduced rate of falls (RaR 0.75, 95% CI 0.65–0.86)

Vitamin D did not reduce falls (RaR 0.95, 95% CI 0.80–1.14; rr (risk ratio) 0.96, 95% CI 0.92–1.01) |

Continued

Table 9.4 *Continued*

Review	Study Quality	Number of Studies Included (Sample Size)	Type of Studies Included	Age	Setting	Intervention	Outcome
Cusimano et al [31]	8	5 (2395)	RCT	60 years of age or older	Residential care including nursing homes	Multifaceted programs (i.e., combinations of education, environment modification, drug regimen review, exercise sessions, vision, hip protectors)	Multifaceted programs show some efficacy
Cameron et al [32]	10	41 (25,422)	RCT	Majority of 65 years and older	Nursing care facilities and hospitals separately	Multifactorial (includes exercise, medication, environment, knowledge, other factors including incontinence, fluid, nutrition, psychological, and vitamin D) and single factor intervention (includes medication, exercise, and knowledge)	Multifactorial interventions reduce falls and fall risks in hospital. Vitamin D is effective in nursing care facilities. Exercise in the subacute hospital setting appears effective

Nursing care (supervised exercise intervention) was inconsistent in multifactorial intervention:

No significant reduction in the rate of falls (RaR 0.82, 95% CI 0.62–1.08) or risk of falling (rr (risk ratio) 0.93, 95% CI 0.86–1.01). But post hoc analysis showed multifactorial intervention reduced the rate of falls (RaR 0.60, 95% CI 0.51–0.72) and risk of falling (rr (risk ratio) 0.85, 95% CI 0.77–0.95).

Vitamin D in nursing homes reduced the rate of falls (RaR 0.72, 95% CI 0.55–0.95), but not risk of falling (rr (risk ratio) 0.98, 95% CI 0.89–1.09) |

Author	No.	Sample (n)	Study type	Population	Setting	Intervention	Results
de Morton et al [33]	10	7 + 2 (4223)	RCT/controlled clinical trial	65 years or older	Hospital	Multidisciplinary interventions, which must include exercise to be compared to "usual hospital care" (vague definition of physiotherapy with discharge planning)	Multifactorial interventions in hospitals reduced rate of falls (RaR 0.69, 95% CI 0.49–0.96 and risk of falling: rr (risk ratio) 0.73, 95% CI 0.56–0.96) Supervised exercise intervention showed significant reduction in risk of falling (rr (risk ratio) 0.44, 95% CI 0.20–0.97) Multidisciplinary interventions indicate small significant increase in discharge to home from hospital Patients discharge to home with multidisciplinary interventions (RR (relative risk) 1.08, 95% CI 1.03–1.14; NNT 16, CI 11–43)
Gates et al [34]	9	19 (6397)	RCT and quasi-RCT, meta-analysis	Older adults	ED, primary care, community	Multifactorial fall-prevention programs (i.e., occupational therapy, home assessment program, comprehensive risk assessment, counseling, motivational video, standardized and individualized fall prevention, nurse home visits) are compared to "usual care" (vague) or no care.	Multifactorial programs can decrease the number of falls Combined to Pooled risk ratio for the number of fallers at follow-up (reduction of number of fallers): 0.91 (95% CI 0.82–1.02) and for fall-related injuries was 0.90 (95% CI 0.68–1.20)
Bischoff-Ferrari et al [35]	7	8 (2) Eight supplements of Vitamin D RCT plus 2 RCT-active forms of Vitamin D (2426)	RCT	Mean age 65 years or older	Community, ambulatory, residential accommodated patients, patients in rehab wards or acute care	Vitamin D of 700–1000 IU	Pooled RR (relative risk) 0.81 (95% CI 0.71–0.92) for seven of the eight articles—reduced fall risk

Continued

Table 9.4 *Continued*

Review	Study Quality	Number of Studies Included (Sample Size)	Type of Studies Included	Age	Setting	Intervention	Outcome
Kalyani et al [36]	10	10 (2932)	RCT	Aged equal or greater than 60 year old	All settings	Vitamin D (200–1000 IU) vs. calcium or placebo	Vitamin D reduces risk of falls: 14% (RR (relative risk) 0.86, 95% (CI 0.79–0.93) Post hoc analysis including seven additional studies (17 total) without explicit fall definitions yielded smaller benefit: RR (relative risk) 0.92(95% CI 0.87–0.98) Significant intergroup differences favoring adjunctive calcium over none
Low et al [37]	7	7 (1972)	RCT	60 years and over	All settings	Single intervention (i.e., Tai Chi)	Tai Chi has the potential to reduce falls or risk of falls among the elderly, provided that they are relatively young and nonfrail
Vaapio et al [38]	8	12 (2357)	RCT	60 years and older	All settings: community, hospitalized and nursing home	Fall-prevention intervention with assessment of quality of life	Only a few fall-prevention studies reported a positive effect on quality of life

Two articles assessed fall interventions for long-term care residents. Cusimano and colleagues [31] showed that multifaceted programs could reduce falls, number of falls, and number of recurrent fallers. In these trials, multifaceted programs consisted of combinations of education, environment modification, drug regiment review, exercise sessions, vision correction, and hip protectors. Cameron and colleagues [32] looked at long-term care residents and hospital populations. Multifactorial interventions (including exercise, medication, environment, knowledge, other factors include incontinence, fluid, nutrition, psychological, and vitamin D) reduced the rate of falls (RaR 0.60, 95% CI 0.51–0.72) and risk of falling (rr "risk ratio" 0.85, 95% CI 0.77–0.95) in nursing home populations.

Cameron and colleagues [32] found that multifactorial interventions reduced the rate of falls (RaR 0.69, 95% CI 0.49–0.96) and risk of falling (rr "risk ratio" 0.73, 95% CI 0.56–0.96) in patients admitted to acute care hospitals. Supervised exercise interventions showed a significant reduction in risk of falling (rr "risk ratio" 0.44, 95% CI 0.20–0.97) in these patients. Among nursing care fallers, multifactorial interventions did not significantly reduce the rate of falls (RaR 0.82, 95% CI 0.62–1.08) or risk of falling (risk ratio (rr) 0.93, 95% CI 0.86–1.01). Morton and colleagues [33] found that multifactorial interventions including exercise led to an increase in discharge from hospital to home (RR "relative risk" 1.08, 95% CI 1.03–1.14).

Five systematic reviews included patients from inpatient and outpatient settings. Gates and colleagues [34] looked at multifactorial fall-prevention programs that included occupational therapy, home assessment, comprehensive risk assessment, counseling, motivational video, standardized and individualized fall prevention, and nurse home visits. They found that these interventions decreased risk of falls and injuries (rr "risk ratio" for falls 0.91 (95% CI 0.82–1.02); for fall-related injuries RR 0.90 (0.68–1.20)).

Bischoff-Ferrari and colleagues [35] and Kalyani and colleagues [36] looked for an association between the use of vitamin D and falls. They found doses of 700–1000-IU supplemental vitamin D reduced fall risk by 19% (RR "relative risk" 0.81, 95% CI 0.71–0.92). They also noted that falls were not reduced by low dose (less than 700 IU) of vitamin D (pooled RR "relative risk" 1.10, 95% CI 0.89–1.35) or by serum

25-hydroxy vitamin D concentrations of less than 60 nmol/L (pooled RR 1.35, 95% CI 0.98–1.84). Kalyani and colleagues [36] also found that vitamin D therapy (200–1,000 IU) decreased falls (RR "relative risk" 0.86, 95% CI 0.79–0.93).

Low and colleagues [37] looked at a single intervention of Tai Chi and found that there may be a benefit to fall reduction, but further studies are needed. Quality of life as an outcome from fall-prevention interventions was assessed by Vaapio and colleagues [38]. They found that fall prevention may also have a positive effect on quality of life, but further studies with larger populations and longer follow-up are needed to determine the association to falls.

Multifaceted versus single Interventions

All of the reviews that assessed multifaceted interventions included different components. And in many of these reviews, it is difficult to understand what the component interventions included. Further studies looking at each component of these multifaceted interventions are needed to further assess if multifaceted interventions are of benefit or whether specific components of that intervention are effective. Exercise seems to be a component in many of the multifaceted interventions and is likely beneficial in all older patients at risk of falls.

Single interventions do seem to work in fall prevention, especially if that specific intervention is targeted to a particular risk factor. For example, in someone with visual impairment due to cataracts, surgery may decrease risk of falls.

Clinical bottom line

Focused single interventions targeted to a particular risk factor or multifactorial interventions (combinations with Vitamin D, exercise, home/environment assessments, and education) should be considered for fall prevention. In mutifactorial interventions, inclusion of an exercise component may be a key element.

How should osteoporosis be addressed among fallers?

Osteoporosis is an important management component when assessing someone at risk for falls and fractures. We identified four national osteoporosis guidelines (one Canadian, two US, and one UK) [9–12, 39] and compared their recommendations in Table 9.5.

Table 9.5 Osteoporosis guidelines for Canada, United Kingdom, and United States

Guideline	Publication Date	Description of Individuals Included	Risk Factors	Diagnostic Assessment Tools Used	Radiological Tests Used	Therapeutic Recommendations						Follow-ups
						Exercise	Calcium	Vitamin D	Bisphosphonates	Reduce Alcohol	Smoking Cessation	
Osteoporosis Canada [9]	October 2010	50 years and older	Age ≥65 years old (male and female) • Clinical risk factors for fracture (menopause women, men age 50–64 years) Fragility fracture after age 40 years • Prolonged use of glucocorticoids (at least 3 months of therapy in the previous year at prednisone equivalent dose ≥7.5 mg daily • Use of other high-risk medication (i.e., aromatase inhibitors) • Parental hip fracture • Vertebral fracture or osteopenia identified on radiography • Current smoking • High alcohol intake • Low body weight (<60 kg) or major weight loss (>10% of body weight at age 25 years)	1 Canadian Association of Radiologists and Osteoporosis Canada (CAROC) (Grade D)[a] 2 Fracture Risk Assessment tool (FRAX) of World Health Organization Canadian Assessment Tool (Grade A)[b]	Bone densitometer Dual-energy X-ray absorptiometry (DXA)	+	+[a]	+	+			Low 10-year fracture risk (defined as calculated score for major osteoporotic fracture is <10%); reassess risk in 5 years. Moderate 10-year fracture risk (defined as 10%–20% risk of osteoporotic fracture); repeat BMD in 1 year and reassess risk

118

Guideline	Date	Indications/Criteria	Risk assessment		
		• Rheumatoid arthritis • Other disorders strongly associated with osteoporosis such as hypogonadism, malabsorption syndromes, chronic inflammatory conditions, and primary hyperparathyroidism			
United Kingdom—National Osteoporosis Guideline Group [12]	July 2010	Female: >65 years and older Men >70 years and older • Age • Sex • History of previous fracture at a site characteristic for osteoporosis (Grade A) • Parental history of hip fracture (Grade A) • Glucocorticoids (any dose, by mouth for 3 months or more) (Grade A) • Current smoking (Grade A) • Alcohol—3 units of more daily (Grade A) • Low body mass index (≤ 10 kg/m^2) (Grade A) • Secondary causes: rheumatoid arthritis (Grade A), untreated hypogonadism in men and women, prolonged immobility, organ transplantation, Type I diabetes, hyperthryoidism, gastrointestinal disease, chronic liver disease, chronic obstructive pulmonary disease	Fracture Risk Assessment tool (FRAX) of World Health Organization	Bone densitometry DXA	+ + + + + + +

Continued

Table 9.5 *Continued*

Guideline	Publication Date	Description of Individuals Included	Risk Factors	Diagnostic Assessment Tools Used	Radiological Tests Used	Therapeutic Recommendations						Follow-ups
						Exercise	Calcium	Vitamin D	Bisphosphonates	Reduce Alcohol	Smoking Cessation	
US Preventive Services Task Force and American College of Preventive Medicine [10, 11]	January/March 2011	Female >65 years and older Men >70 years and older	White women between the ages of 50 and 64 years with equivalent or greater than 10-year fracture risks based on specific risk factors include but are not limited to the following persons: • 50-year-old current smoker with BMI less than 21 kg/m², daily alcohol use, and parental fracture history • 55-year-old woman with parental fracture history • 60-year-old woman with a BMI less than 21 kg/m² and daily alcohol use • 60-year-old current smoker with daily alcohol use	Fracture risk algorithm (FRAX)	Bone densitometer DXA Calcaneal quantitative ultrasound (QUS)	+	+	+	+			DXA not more frequently than every 2 years.

a http://www.osteoporosis.ca/multimedia/tools.html.
b http://www.sheffield.ac.uk/FRAX/tool.jsp?country=19.
c Total daily intake calcium of 1200 mg.

Screening

The Canadian and UK guidelines recommend testing for osteoporosis using dual-energy X-ray absorptiometry (DXA), whereas United States recommends other modalities in addition to DXA including calcaneal ultrasound.

The Canadian guidelines recommend the use of bone mineral density every 1–3 years for those who have risk factors for osteoporosis. The UK guidelines also suggest monitoring but do not give guidance about when it should be done. The US guidelines recommend that bone mineral density not be measured more frequently than every 2 years.

Exercise

The Canadian guidelines recommend that exercises that focus on balance (such as Tai Chi) or on balance and gait training should be considered for those people with osteoporosis who are at risk for falls. In addition, their osteoporosis should be managed with resistance training (in those patients with osteoporosis or increased risk of osteoporosis) or exercises to enhance core stability (for those with vertebral fractures) (Grade B recommendation).

The UK guidelines also recommend exercise but no details are provided on the amount of exercise required. These guidelines suggest weight-bearing exercises and use of exercises that cater to the needs and fitness of the individual patient.

The US (USPSTF) guidelines recommend regular weight-bearing physical activity, but no details are provided on type or duration.

Vitamin D

The Canadian guidelines state that Vitamin D and calcium should be given in the following manner:
- **Calcium:** There is controversy about both the efficacy of calcium supplementation for reducing fractures and the potential adverse effects of high-dose supplementation. Current recommendations suggest that the total daily intake of elemental calcium (dietary and supplements) should be 1200 mg for those 50 years and older (Grade B recommendation).
- **Vitamin D:** If risk of vitamin D deficiency is low, then 400–1000 IU daily is recommended. Low-risk adults are those under age 50, without osteoporosis or conditions affecting vitamin D absorption or action. For moderate risk of vitamin D deficiency, 800–1000 IU is

recommended. Moderate-risk adults include all adults 50 years of age or older. For high-risk and older adults, 800–2000 IU is recommended. Vitamin D levels should be monitored starting 3–4 months after proper supplementation of vitamin D, and when the vitamin D level is optimal ($\geq$75 nmol/L) there is no need for further blood work to monitor the level.

The UK guidelines recommend 800 IU of vitamin D and a calcium dosage of 1.0–1.2 g (for housebound older adults or those living in a nursing home). Community dwellers are recommended 800 IU of Vitamin D but the calcium is lowered to 500–1000 mg/day.

The recommendation from the US (ACPM) guidelines is calcium 1200 mg daily and Vitamin D 800–1000 IU for those aged 50 years and over. The USPSTF guidelines also recommend calcium and vitamin D but no dosage is specified.

Pharmacologic therapy

The Canadian guidelines provide specific recommendations for first-line therapy for osteoporosis according to the type of fracture. For menopausal women with osteoporosis, first-line therapy can include alendronate, risedronate, zoledronic acid, and denosumab for prevention of hip, nonvertebral, and vertebral fractures (Grade A recommendation). Raloxifene is also considered as a first-line agent for fracture prevention but only for vertebral fractures (Grade A recommendation). For those women who are intolerant of first-line therapy, calcitonin or etidronate for vertebral fractures (Grade B recommendation) can be considered. For men with osteoporosis, alendronate, risedronate, and zoledronic acid should be considered as first-line therapy (Grade D recommendation).

The UK guidelines provide similar recommendations for first-line therapy for postmenopausal women. However, etidronate is recommended (Grade A recommendation) for women with vertebral fracture. Ibandronate, calcitonin, calcitriol, raloxifene, strontium ranelate, teriparatide, and recombinant human parathyroid hormone (PTH) are also recommended for vertebral fractures (Grade A recommendation). Men with osteoporosis can be treated with alendronate, risedronate, zoledronate, and teriparatide as first-line therapy.

The USPSTF guidelines recommend bisphosphonates, PTH, raloxifene, estrogen, and calcitonin for fracture prevention.

Clinical bottom line

Based on guideline recommendations, the management of osteoporosis should include exercise, vitamin D, calcium, and an appropriate pharmacologic agent such as a bisphosphonate.

Chapter summary

There are several factors that can increase risk of falls in older people. Clinicians should assess history of falls, visual impairment, medications, balance impairment, gait impairment and walking difficulty, functional limitations and ADL disability, and home hazards.

Falls prevention via single or multifaceted interventions may be beneficial. Further research into multifaceted interventions and whether it is the multifaceted nature of the intervention or a specific component of the interventions (i.e., exercise) that is most effective for preventing falls needs to be investigated. Currently, focused single intervention appears to be as beneficial as multifactorial/multifaceted intervention in preventing risk of falls.

Osteoporosis risk assessment and management should occur alongside falls assessment. Current guidelines recommend exercise, vitamin D, calcium, and bisphosphonates for those who have osteoporosis.

Acknowledgment

Thanks to Laure Perrier who helped with the initial research.

References

1. Akyol AD (2007) Falls in the elderly: what can be done? *Int Nurs Rev* 54: 191–196.
2. Medical Advisory Secretariat, Ministry of Health and Long-Term Care (2008) Prevention of falls and fall-related injuries in community-dwelling seniors. *Ontario Health Technol Assessment Ser* 8.
3. Annweiler C, et al (2010) Fall prevention and vitamin D in the elderly: an overview of the key role of the non-bone effects. *J NeuroEng Rehabil* 7.
4. de Kam D, et al (2009) Exercise interventions to reduce fall-related fractures and their risk factors in individuals in low bone density: a systematic review of randomized controlled trials. *Osteoporos Int* 20: 2111–2125.
5. McGilton K, et al (2009) Outcomes of older adults in an inpatient rehabilitation facility following hip fracture (hf) surgery. *Arch Gerontol Geriatr* 49(1): e23–e31.
6. Huberta-Corazon T, Cesario S (2009) Falls aren't us. *Crit Care Nurs Q* 32: 116–127.
7. Sjosten N, Vaapio S, Kivela SL (2008) The effects of fall prevention trials on depressive symptoms and fear of falling among the aged: a systematic review. *Aging Ment Health* 12: 30–46.
8. Shea B, et al (2007) Development of AMSTAR: a measurement tool to assess the methodological quality of systematic reviews. *BMC Med Res Methodol* 7.
9. Papaioannou A, et al (2010) 2010 clinical practice guidelines for the diagnosis and management of osteoporosis in Canada: summary *CMAJ* 281: 1864–1873.
10. US Preventive Services Task Force (2011) Screening for osteoporosis: US Preventive Services Task Force Recommendation Statement. *Ann Intern Med* 154: 356–364.
11. Lim LS, Hoeksema LJ, Sherin K, ACPM Prevention Practice Committee (2009) Screening for osteoporosis in the adult US population: ACPM position statement on preventive practice. *Am J Prev Med* 36: 366–75.
12. Compston JE, et al (2010) Guideline for the diagnosis and management of osetoporosis in postmenopausal women and men from the age of 50 years in the UK. *Maturitas* 62(2): 105–108.
13. Ganz D, Bao Y, Shekelle P, Rubenstein L (2007) Will my patient fall? *JAMA* 297: 77–86.
14. Gates S, Smith LA, Fisher JD, Lamb SE (2008) Systematic review of accuracy of screening instruments for predicting fall risk among independently living older adults. *J Rehabil Res Dev* 45: 1105–1116.
15. Oliver D, et al (2008) A systematic review and meta-analysis of studies using the STRATIFY tool for prediction of falls in hospital patients: how well it work?. *Age Ageing* 37: 621–627.
16. Scott V, Votova K, Scanlan A, Close J (2007) Multifactorial and functional mobility assessment tools for fall risk among older adults in community, home support, long-term and acute care settings. *Age Ageing* 36: 130–139.
17. Woolcott JC, et al (2009) Meta-analysis of the impact of 9 medication classes on falls in elderly persons. *Arch Intern Med* 169: 1952–1960.
18. Tinetti ME, Kumar C (2010) The patient who falls: "It's always a trade-off ". *JAMA* 303: 258–266.
19. Hegeman J, Van Den Bemt BJ, Duysens J, van Limbeek J (2009) NSAIDs and the risk of accidental falls in the elderly: a systematic review. *Drug Saf* 32: 489–498.
20. Sterke C, et al (2008) The influence of drug use on fall incidents among nursing home residents: a systematic review. *Int Psychogeriatr* 20: 890–910.
21. Muir SW, Berg K, Chesworth B, Klar N, Speechley M (2010) Quantifying the magnitude of risk for balance impairment on falls in community-dwelling older adults: a systematic review and meta-analysis. *J Clin Epidemiol* 63: 389–406.
22. Bloch F, et al (2010) Episodes of falling among elderly people: a systematic review and meta-analysis of social

and demographic pre-disposing characteristics. *Clinics* 65: 895–903.

23. Letts L, et al (2010) The physical environment as a fall risk factor in older adults: systematic review and meta-analysis of cross-sectional and cohort studies. *Aust Occup Ther J* 57: 51–64.

24. Zijlstra GA, et al (2007) Interventions to reduce fear of falling in community-living older people: a systematic review. *J Am Geriatr Soc* 55: 603–615.

25. Clemson L, et al (2008) Environmental interventions to prevent falls in community-dwelling older people: a meta-analysis of randomized trials. *J Aging Health* 20: 954–971.

26. Michael YL, et al (2010) Interventions to prevent falls in older adults: an updated systematic review. *Evidence Synthesis* 80.

27. Orr R, Raymond J, Singh M (2008) Efficacy of progressive resistance training on balance performance in older adults. *Sports Med* 38, 317–343.

28. Thomas S, Mackintosh S, Halbert J (2010) Does the 'Otago exercise programme' reduce mortality and falls in older adults?: a systematic review and meta-analysis. *Age Ageing* 39: 681–687.

29. Campbell AJ & Robertson MC (2007) Rethinking individual and community fall prevention strategies: a meta-regression comparing single and multifactorial interventions. *Age Ageing* 36: 656–662.

30. Gillespie LD, Robertson MC, Gillespie WJ, Lamb SE, Gates S, Cumming RG, Rowe BH. (2009) Interventions for preventing falls in older people living in the community. *Cochrane Database Syst Rev* (2): CD007146.

31. Cusimano MD, Kwok J, Spadafora K (2008) Effectiveness of multifaceted fall-prevention programs for the elderly in residential care. *Inj Prev* 14: 113–122.

32. Cameron ID, Murray GR, Gillespie LD, Robertson MC, Hill KD, Cumming RG, Kerse N (2010) Interventions for preventing falls in older people in nursing care facilities and hospitals. *Cochrane Database Syst Rev* (1): CD005465.

33. de Morton N, Keating JL, Jeffs K. (2007) Exercise for acutely hospitalised older medical patients. *Cochrane Database Syst Rev* (1): CD005955.

34. Gates S, et al (2008) Multifactorial assessment and targeted intervention for preventing falls and injuries among older people in community and emergency care settings: systematic review and meta-analysis. *BMJ* 336: 130–133.

35. Bischoff-Ferrari HA, et al (2009) Fall prevention with supplemental and active forms of vitamin D: a meta-analysis of randomised control trials. *BMJ* 339: 3392–3403.

36. Kalyani RR, et al (2010) Vitamin D treatment for the prevention of falls in older adults: systematic review and meta-analysis. *J Am Geriatr Soc* 58: 1299–1310.

37. Low S, Ang LW, Goh KS, Chew SK (2009) A systematic review of the effectiveness of Tai Chi on fall reduction among the elderly. *Arch Gerontol Geriatr* 48: 325–331.

38. Vaapio SS, Salminen MJ, Ojanlatva A, Kivelä S (2009) Quality of life as an outcome of fall prevention interventions among the aged: a systematic review. *Cent Eur J Public Health* 19: 7–15.

39. Hanley D, et al (2010) Vitamin D in adult health and disease: a review and guideline statement from Osteoporosis Canada. *CMAJ* 182: E610–E618.

CHAPTER 10

Keeping dry: managing urinary incontinence

Cara Tannenbaum[1,2]

[1]*Faculties of Medicine and Pharmacy, Université de Montréal, Montréal, QC, Canada*
[2]*Geriatric Incontinence Clinic, Institut Universitaire de Gériatrie,Université de Montréal, Montréal, QC, Canada*

Introduction

In community-dwelling adults aged 65 years and older, urinary incontinence (UI) affects up to 55% of women and 20% of men [1]. In long-term care (LTC), the prevalence of incontinence can exceed 70% [2, 3]. Incontinence is not an innocuous condition. In seniors, UI is associated with poor quality of life [4], poor self-rated health [5], social isolation [6], depression [7], and a decline in instrumental activities of daily living [8]. Among debilitated LTC residents, UI also contributes to falls [9] and pressure ulcers [10].

Effective evidence-based evaluation and treatment strategies for the management of UI exist. In well-functioning, healthy older people, treatment can be relatively straightforward [11, 12]. For the frail elderly who experience cognitive or mobility impairments, the management approach may require more complex multimodal interventions [13]. Regardless of functional status, important improvements and cures for UI are obtainable at all ages [14].

Managing UI requires a systematic approach aimed at identifying the type or types, and ascertaining the underlying cause or causes of UI experienced by each patient. A precise diagnosis of the types and causes of UI begins with a thorough understanding of the lower urinary tract system and its neural control. In the geriatric patient, the contribution of other factors outside the urinary tract and the existence of comorbid pathologies that affect continence or the ability to toilet successfully may also play a part in precipitating or maintaining UI.

The aging lower urinary tract

The healthy bladder spends about 99% of its time storing urine, and only 1% of its time expelling urine, or voiding. Storage of urine is mediated by sympathetically mediated relaxation of the bladder detrusor muscle and a concomitant increase in tone of the internal urethral sphincter to prevent urine leakage during filling (Figure 10.1). Somatic input via pudendal nerves activates the external urethral sphincter, an integral part of the pelvic floor musculature. When the bladder is full, parasympathetic (S2–S4) sacral nerve roots mediate detrusor muscle contraction, and coordinated sympathetically mediated sphincter relaxation occurs, which results in voiding. Central nervous system control of voiding acts via a tonic inhibitory influence from the frontal lobes and pontine micturition center down through the spinal cord onto the sacral nerve roots. The inhibitory influence is removed when voiding is deemed physiologically and socially acceptable.

With age, changes occur in the lower urinary tract that predispose an individual to incontinence [13]. These include a decline in detrusor contraction strength, decreased bladder capacity, and increased nighttime urine production. Women experience a reduction in urethral closure pressures and men have an

Evidence-Based Geriatric Medicine: A Practical Clinical Guide, First Edition. Edited by Jayna M. Holroyd-Leduc and Madhuri Reddy.
© 2012 Blackwell Publishing Ltd. Published 2012 by Blackwell Publishing Ltd.

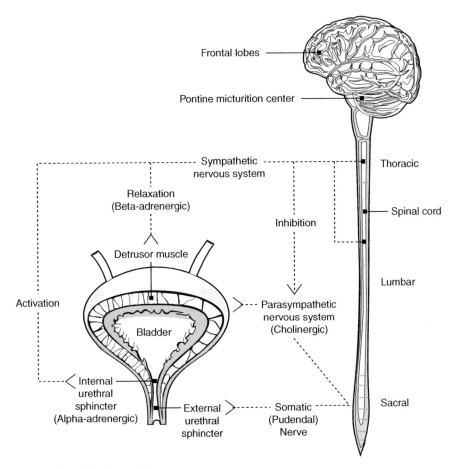

Figure 10.1 Innervation of the lower urinary tract.

increased incidence of prostatic enlargement. While these changes increase the likelihood of UI, they are rarely the sole explanation for new onset UI and other causes must be sought. Other causes include disease-related pathology, functional impairments, or the effect of medications on the lower urinary tract.

Any pathologic disturbance of the urinary storage mechanism can result in involuntary urine loss. The dysfunction may involve complete incompetence at the level of the urinary sphincters, or may be due to an overactive or underactive detrusor muscle. Many factors outside the lower urinary tract can also cause or contribute to UI. Central or spinal cord pathologies (stroke, neurodegenerative diseases, normal pressure hydrocephalus, tumors) that interrupt normal inhibition of the sacral voiding reflex may lead to uninhibited detrusor contractions and unwanted voiding.

Comorbidity affects continence through a variety of mechanisms. For example, in diabetes mellitus, diabetic neuropathy (causing detrusor dysfunction) and hyperglycemia (causing osmotic diuresis and polyuria) may contribute. In Parkinson's disease, continence may be affected by medications, constipation, or cognitive or mobility impairment. Patients with pedal edema will likely suffer from nocturia (voiding at night) and possible nocturnal incontinence due to redistribution of fluid from their lower extremities.

Several medication classes have a deleterious effect on the lower urinary tract by increasing urine production, or contributing to pedal edema, or by affecting the neural mechanisms controlling bladder and sphincter function [13]. Medications may also interfere with the ability to toilet successfully through independent effects on the central nervous system [15]. For

Table 10.1 Commonly used medications that can affect the lower urinary tract and the ability to toilet successfully

Type of Medication	Mechanism
Diuretics Lithium	Polyuria
Nonsteroidal anti-inflammatory drugs Certain calcium channel blockers (i.e., nifedipine XL) Certain oral hypoglycemics (glitazones)	Pedal edema/fluid retention that redistributes and causes nocturnal diuresis
Alpha adrenergic agonists (nasal decongestants)	Increased urethral sphincter tone/obstruction/ retention (especially in men with prostate disease)
Alpha adrenergic antagonists (antihypertensive agents)	Decreased urethral sphincter tone
Anticholinergics: tricyclic antidepressants, antihistamines, antiparkinsonian agents opioid analgesics	Impaired bladder emptying, retention, overflow, incontinence
Cholinesterase inhibitors	Increased bladder contractility
Benzodiazepines and other hypnotics Narcotics and some other pain medications Antipsychotics	Altered sensorium, psychomotor slowing, mobility impairment
Angiotensin converting enzyme inhibitors	Cough
Estrogens	Unknown

instance, benzodiazepines and narcotics affect arousal and induce psychomotor slowing, which may result in delayed toileting. Antipsychotic medications can cause rigidity or mobility impairments, which also impact the ability to get to the toilet in a timely fashion. Table 10.1 lists medications that increase the risk of UI.

Types of UI

Different types of UI are categorized according to distinguishing characteristics. The types include stress, urge, mixed, overflow, functional, and nocturnal UI [16]. In geriatric patients, several types of UI may co-exist due to the presence of multifactorial etiologies.

Stress UI is characterized by the involuntary leakage of small amounts of urine on effort or exertion, or on sneezing or coughing. The predominant symptom of urge UI is involuntary leakage accompanied or immediately followed by urgency (a sudden strong need to void). Mixed UI is the combination of stress and urge UI episodes in the same individual.

Overflow UI is characterized by continuous or discrete UI episodes without the hallmark features of stress and urge UI. Overflow UI generally occurs as a sequelae to urinary retention (most commonly in men with prostatic obstruction).

Functional UI is incontinence resulting from cognitive, functional, or mobility difficulties in a person who may or may not have lower urinary tract deficits. Nighttime episodes of UI may occur with any of the aforementioned UI types. However, if UI occurs exclusively at night, the term "nocturnal UI" is generally used. Finally, multifactorial or geriatric UI indicates the presence of a classic geriatric syndrome characterized by a constellation of contributing etiologic factors, which, when they occur concomitantly, leads to a failure of the continence mechanism.

Each UI type has an underlying differential diagnosis (Table 10.2). Investigating and treating the disorder(s) responsible for the UI symptoms is an essential component of optimal management and minimization of treatment failure. This chapter on the evidence-based management of UI addresses three clinical topics: (1) the best way to assess UI in the office setting; (2) the best options for treating UI once the incontinence type and underlying cause(s) has (have) been established; (3) the best treatment approach for LTC residents and patients with dementia.

Search strategy

The search strategy sought all systematic reviews on the evaluation of UI, and all meta-analyses and Cochrane reviews of randomized controlled trials (RCTs) examining pharmacologic and nonpharmacologic treatment of UI in the Cochrane Library and MEDLINE. The search of MEDLINE using Ovid (1966–February 2011) employed the terms "urinary incontinence," "diagnostic tests," "management," "treatment," "aged,"

Table 10.2 Incontinence types and their underlying causes

Type of UI	Potential Causes
Stress	Bladder neck (internal sphincter) hypermobility Poor intrinsic sphincter function Weak pelvic floor muscles Vesico-vaginal fistula post surgery or pelvic radiation in women Postprostatectomy in men Chronic cough (due to chronic pulmonary disease) may contribute Medications
Urge	Polyuria due to hyperglycemia, hypercalcemia, diabetes insipidus, potomania, excessive alcohol, or caffeine consumption Urinary tract infection Medications Bladder polyp, tumor, or calculus Interstitial cystitis Idiopathic detrusor overactivity Neurological disorders: Parkinson's disease, multisystem atrophy, multiple sclerosis, cerebrovascular disease and stroke, normal pressure hydrocephalus, paraplegia, spinal stenosis, spinal cord injury
Mixed	Any combination of the causes of stress and urge UI
Overflow	Medications Sacral peripheral neuropathy Cauda equine syndrome Idiopathic detrusor underactivity Prostatic obstruction in men Urethral obstruction due to prolapse in women Urethral stricture
Functional	Delirium Neurodegenerative disorders Arthritis/degenerative joint disease Medications
Nocturnal	Nocturnal polyuria from lower extremity edema due to: • Chronic venous insufficiency • Congestive heart failure • Nephrotic syndrome and chronic kidney disease • Certain neurologic disorders (autonomic neuropathy) • Medications Obstructive sleep apnea and related sleep disorders Idiopathic detrusor overactivity Medications
Geriatric	Any combination of the above Medications Cognitive impairment Mobility impairment Depression Caffeine consumption Sarcopenia (and weak pelvic floor muscles) Environmental factors (e.g., inaccessible toilets or unavailable caregivers for toileting assistance)

"elderly," and "geriatrics," and was restricted to the English language. Additional material was sought from published recommendations of the International Consultation on Incontinence.

For this chapter, we graded relevant clinical studies using the Oxford Centre for Evidence-based Medicine Levels of Evidence.

What is the best way to assess urinary incontinence in the office setting?

Evidence to answer this question was derived from four systematic reviews [11, 13, 17, 18] (Level 1 evidence), one cross-sectional study in the LTC setting [19] (Level 2 evidence), and one geriatric expert opinion on UI [20] (Level 5 evidence). Two of the systematic reviews are published recommendations from the 4th International Consultation on Incontinence [13, 17].

History

Clinicians should screen for UI during the review of systems for all older men and women during their routine annual checkup. If a patient initiates discussion about urine leakage, the symptoms should not be ignored. As with dementia, the initial evaluation for incontinence may be time consuming, especially in frail older adults, and a separate office visit may need to be scheduled for a comprehensive workup and physical exam.

The history should identify whether the onset of UI is acute or of long-standing duration. The nature of the UI symptoms should be elicited as well as the presence of other concomitant neurological symptoms (e.g., lower extremity weakness), relevant coexisting diseases (e.g., diabetes, stroke, dementia, Parkinsonism, and arthritis), previous pelvic surgeries, current medications, functional status including mobility and cognitive impairment, review of environmental factors that could impact the ability to toilet successfully, and lifestyle factors such as the amount and type of fluid intake. Risk factors for UI such as the consumption of caffeinated beverages (coffee, tea, and colas), obesity, constipation, and smoking should be established [11]. UI associated with potentially treatable and reversible factors such as restricted mobility has commonly been called "transient" [11, 19, 20].

Establishing the type of incontinence will depend on the answers to several questions [18]. If a patient responds "yes" to the question, "Do you lose urine during physical exertion, lifting, coughing, laughing, or sneezing?" the patient is twice as likely to experience stress UI compared to a patient who responds "no" to this question (positive likelihood ratio (LR) 2.2; 95% confidence interval (CI), 1.6–3.2; negative LR 0.39; 95% CI 0.25–0.61). Even more telling is the patient who responds "yes" when asked "Do you ever experience such a strong and sudden urge to void that you leak before reaching the toilet?" This patient is four-times as likely to have urge UI than a patient who does not experience feelings of urgency associated with urine leakage (positive LR 4.2; 95% CI 2.3–7.6; negative LR 0.48; 95% CI 0.36–0.62). Positive answers to both these questions strongly suggest mixed UI. A patient who experiences urine leakage at night will have nocturnal UI. If the onset of UI corresponds to or is exacerbated by the onset or worsening of mobility or cognitive impairments, then there is likely a functional component. Geriatric UI often originates from multifactorial etiologies [11, 20].

Although positive answers to the questions listed above increase the likelihood that a patient will have a certain type of UI, history alone is insufficient to establish diagnostic certainty (sufficient diagnostic evidence is defined as a positive likelihood ratio >5 to confirm the diagnosis, and a negative likelihood ratio <0.2 to exclude the diagnosis) [18]. As such, diagnostic interviews need to be complemented by a targeted physical exam and sound clinical judgment to establish a probable diagnosis. Comprehensive assessment, including the history, physical exam, and targeted investigation, still holds the most value for diagnosing stress UI (positive LR 3.7; 95% CI 2.6–5.2; negative LR 0.20; 95% CI 0.08–0.51) and urge UI (positive LR 4.6; 95% CI 1.7–12.6; negative LR 0.11; 95% CI 0.04–0.33) in older women.

Physical examination

The physical examination should include an abdominal exam to detect an overdistended bladder, and a gynecological exam for women to rule out prolapse and fistulas. A digital vaginal exam should be used to assess pelvic floor muscle strength, determined by asking the patient to contract their pelvic floor muscles while the examiner inserts a finger into the vaginal introitus. This will also help determine if the woman knows how to correctly identify her pelvic floor muscles for contraction, which may be important when targeting management strategies. In both men and women, a rectal exam is needed to evaluate rectal tone and the presence of stool impaction, and in men the prostate size should be determined. At a minimum, the neurological exam should test perineal sensation, anal wink, and bulbocavernosus reflexes to ensure the integrity of the sacral nerves S2–S4 that mediate bladder contraction. Signs of Parkinsonism and gait disturbances should also be sought. A cognitive screen and detailed exam of the lower extremities is also recommended in all frail older patients, who may potentially have occult neurological disease. In patients with nocturnal UI, a targeted search for pedal edema is recommended to determine whether patients could benefit from compression stockings or daytime leg elevation to diminish nocturnal polyuria [17].

Special maneuvers that can be performed at the office assessment include the stress test, the Q-tip test, and the pad test. The stress test involves direct observation for urine loss with coughing in the upright or decubitus position. This test is best preformed with a full bladder. Instantaneous leakage is a positive test and suggests a threefold greater likelihood of stress UI [18]. A negative test is nondiagnostic. The Q-tip test involves placement of a lubricated cotton swab in the urethra to enable observation of urethral hypermobility if the Q-tip moves above the horizontal axis during coughing or straining. There is insufficient evidence to support the use of the Q-tip test to diagnose stress UI in women [18]. The pad test involves the continuous wearing of continence pads for a set period of time. The pads are weighed on their removal and checked for abnormal increases (>15 g) in pad weight gain. The pad test is used for research purposes and has no utility in the office setting for distinguishing the type of UI.

Investigations

Measurement of the postvoid residual urine volume by a portable bladder ultrasound scanner is helpful for determining detrusor underactivity and overflow UI, especially if a distended bladder is palpated on abdominal exam or if sacral nerve deficits are detected. If a portable bladder ultrasound is not available in the office setting and overflow incontinence is suspected, the patient should be sent for outpatient imaging studies. In-and-out bladder catheterization is an alternate modality. We did not identify any studies of postvoid urine volume measurement as a test for determining UI type in the literature. Measurement of the postvoid urine volume is commonly used in clinical practice and is also an important test for older women with urge UI because of the risk of detrusor hyperactivity with impaired contractility (DHIC). DHIC is associated with a heightened risk of urinary retention if treated with anticholinergic medication [21].

A urinalysis screening for hematuria, glucosuria, pyuria, and bacteriuria should also be performed to help rule out bladder neoplasia, diabetic polyuria, and urinary tract infection respectively, along with other tests as indicated from the history and physical examination (e.g., calcium levels) [17].

The bladder diary is a tool that is used by the patient to document the frequency and volume of urine output, as well as the amount and type of fluid intake. There is no evidence to support its accuracy in diagnosing the type of UI [18]. A bladder diary can often be useful to the clinician in the initial assessment of UI and is effective for monitoring changes in the patient's condition during follow-up.

Clinical bottom line

A comprehensive assessment including a focused history, a targeted physical exam of the genitourinary tract and related neurological conditions, a stress test, urinalysis, and measurement of the postvoid residual urine volume are required to posit a probable diagnosis of the type of UI and its underlying cause(s).

Use of a bladder diary is helpful initially, as well as during follow-up to evaluate the effects of treatment.

Evidence supports the use of a systematic evaluation to help diagnose stress and urge incontinence [18].

What are the best options for treating urinary incontinence?

Thirteen systematic reviews [11, 13, 22–32] (Level 1 evidence), 13 RCTs [33–45] (Level 2 evidence), two nonrandomized intervention studies [46, 47] (Level 3 evidence), four case series [14, 48–50] (Level 4 evidence), and two expert opinion papers [12, 51] (Level 5 evidence) provided evidence to answer this question.

Models of care

Many different models of UI management exist. An individual with incontinence may attempt to self-manage or choose to engage in a doctor–patient dyad with their primary care physician. Nurse continence advisors may become involved by working alone, in tandem with specialty clinics, or by overseeing community triage. Urology or urogynecology specialist clinics usually offer second-line surgical interventions. Comprehensive geriatric assessment units will integrate a multidisciplinary approach using a geriatrician, nurse specialist, physiotherapist, and sometimes a pharmacist or social worker.

Nurse-led continence advisor programs achieve important improvements and at least 25% cure rates through conservative management of UI, with urology and urogynecology specialty practices offering minimal advantages (Level 1 evidence) [40–42]. Outpatient geriatric assessment units also report obtainable dryness rates up to 25% and improvement in an additional 45% of frail older patients who consult their services (Level 3 evidence) [14, 49, 50].

After identifying and treating all underlying causes and contributing factors, the management of UI is divided into conservative (including behavioral), pharmacologic, and surgical measures. Table 10.3 summarizes the level of evidence for each type of intervention according to the underlying UI type for women and men.

Conservative and behavioral interventions

Behavioral treatment includes lifestyle interventions, pelvic floor muscle training, and bladder training. Other conservative measures include the use of different bulking agents and various other medical devices for women and men for stress UI.

There is Level 1 evidence from randomized controlled clinical trials that behavioral interventions are warranted as first-line treatment for all types of UI in women [22–24]. Data for men are sparser, although a trial of behavioral therapy is recommended for all men with urge UI (Level 4 evidence) [12] and persistent postprostatectomy stress UI (Level 2 evidence) [33].

Lifestyle interventions

Lifestyle changes include appropriate fluid management, reducing caffeine intake, weight control, and bowel management. Weight loss has achieved Level 1 evidence for reducing stress and urge UI [34, 35]. Intensive lifestyle therapy to maintain loss of at least 7% of initial body weight and engagement in regular physical activity reduced stress UI by 15% after 2.9 years of follow-up in the Diabetes Prevention Program RCT among 2191 overweight prediabetic women with a mean body mass index of 24 kg/m^2 or greater (relative risk (RR) 0.85; 95% CI 0.73–0.99) [34]. A similar weight loss program in overweight women yielded a 47% reduction in UI (vs. 28% in the nonintervention group, $p = 0.01$) with a mean of 8% weight loss [35]. No data on weight loss programs are available for men. Caffeine reduction, fluid management, and treatment of constipation empirically reduce UI in men and women, and are used routinely as adjuvant measures in clinical practice, despite the lack of large RCTs investigating their effectiveness (Level 2–4 evidence) [23, 43, 44, 46].

Pelvic floor muscle training

The goal of pelvic floor muscle training is to teach cognitively intact and motivated individuals how to control and strengthen the periurethral muscles of the external urethral sphincter in order to reduce or prevent urine leakage, either during exertion, coughing or sneezing, or on the way to the bathroom during episodes of urinary urgency. The first step is proper identification of the pelvic floor muscles and to be able to contract and relax them selectively (without increasing intra-abdominal pressure on the bladder or pelvic floor). The second step is performance of a daily exercise program aimed at improving the strength, coordination, and endurance of the muscles. A typical strength-training exercise is to ask the patient to perform three sets of ten series of sustained pelvic floor muscle contractions, (each contraction lasting 8–10 seconds, with a 1:1 or 2:1 relaxation period in between), daily over a 12-week period. It should be reinforced that the pelvic floor muscles will take time to strengthen and therefore, improvement in UI will generally not be seen until the exercises have been preformed consistently over several weeks. The strength-training exercise may be performed in the lying, sitting, or standing position. A well-known coordination exercise, the "knack," requires the patient to remain in the standing position and contract their pelvic floor muscles prior to initiating a cough.

Table 10.3 Evidence-based interventions for different UI types in women and men

Type of UI	Interventions	
	Women	Men
Stress	Weight loss programs (7%–8% loss of initial body weight) are effective (Level 1) Pelvic floor muscle training is effective (Level 1) Injectable bulking agents may be effective (Level 2) Pessaries may be effective (Level 3 evidence)	Pelvic floor muscle training is *not* effective for acute postprostatectomy stress UI (Level 1), yielding the same resolution rates as watchful waiting. Pelvic floor muscle training and bladder control strategies may be effective for persistent (>1 year) postprostatectomy stress symptoms (Level 2) External penile compression devices (clamps) are effective, but there are safety problems that need to be resolved (Level 2)
Urge	Pelvic floor muscle training is effective (Level 1) Bladder training is effective (Level 1) Weight loss programs are effective (Level 1) Other lifestyle interventions (fluid management, caffeine consumption, bowel management) may be effective (Levels 2–4) A combination of behavioral management strategies is *most* effective (Level 1) Pharmacologic therapy with antimuscarinic agents is effective (Level 1)	Lifestyle interventions may be effective (Level 4) Bladder training and pelvic floor muscle training are probably effective (Level 4) A combination of behavioral management strategies is probably *most* effective (Level 4) Pharmacologic therapy with antimuscarinic agents is effective (Level 1) Combination pharmacologic therapy with antimuscarinic and alpha-adrenergic blocking agents is effective for symptoms of overactive bladder (Level 2)
Mixed	Same as for stress and urge	Not studied in men
Overflow	In-and-out catheterization and indwelling catheters can effectively manage urinary retention (Level 2)	In-and-out catheterization and indwelling catheters can effectively manage urinary retention (Level 2)
Nocturnal	Combination therapy with behavioral strategies is effective (Level 2) The use of desmopressin for the treatment of nocturia is not recommended in the elderly because of the high risk of hyponatremia (Level 4)	Combination therapy with behavioral strategies and treatment of medical and sleep disorders is effective (Level 2) The use of desmopressin for the treatment of nocturia is not recommended in the elderly because of the high risk of hyponatremia (Level 4)
Geriatric	All of the above Comprehensive geriatric assessment is probably effective (Levels 3, 4)	All of the above Comprehensive geriatric assessment is probably effective (Levels 3, 4)

RCT, randomized controlled trials.
Levels of evidence: Level 1 = systematic reviews, meta-analyses, good quality RCTs; Level 2 = RCTs, good quality prospective cohort studies; Level 3 = case-control studies, case series; Level 4 = expert opinion.

The use of pelvic floor muscle training alone resolves or improves UI in women compared with usual care, although the effect size is inconsistent across RCTs (Level 1 evidence) [11, 22, 26]. The benefits of pelvic floor muscle training are augmented when combined with bladder training for stress, mixed, and urge UI (Level 1 evidence) [22], with a pooled risk difference of 13% (0.13; 95% CI 0.10–0.61) across studies. Supervised training programs with a skilled physiotherapist or nurse practitioner are decidedly more effective than self-administered programs using a self-help booklet (risk difference 0.24; 95% CI 0.08–0.39). Many pelvic floor muscle-training programs use biofeedback-assisted technologies to help women correctly identify their pelvic floor muscles, and this appears helpful for women who are unable to perform a pelvic floor muscle contraction during vaginal palpation. Electrical stimulation and active magnetic stimulation of the pelvic floor muscles yields no additional benefit over placebo in women (Level 1 evidence) [22, 23]. Pelvic floor muscle training is not more effective than watchful waiting for reducing symptoms of stress UI, immediately postprostatectomy in men (Level 1 evidence) [25]. However, in men with persistent (<1 year) symptoms of stress UI, pelvic floor muscle exercises combined with bladder control strategies may provide benefit (Level 2 evidence) [33].

Bladder training

Bladder training is used for cognitively intact and motivated individuals to regain or improve continence, by increasing the time interval between voids and to diminish the sensation of urgency. Urge suppression and urge control techniques are the two main components of bladder training. Urge suppression involves teaching the patient to pause, sit down if possible, relax, and contract the pelvic floor muscles repeatedly to diminish urgency, inhibit detrusor contractions, and prevent urine loss. After the urge to urinate has subsided, the patient is encouraged to walk slowly at a normal pace to the toilet. Urge control techniques require the patient to distract themselves from focusing on the urge to void during this waiting interval. Mental arithmetic or consciously concentrating on another problem-solving challenge are commonly used distraction techniques employed to help the patient control the urge to void while waiting for the voiding interval to pass. A bladder drill procedure imposes a progressively lengthened 5–15 minute interval between voids over days-to-weeks based on individual tolerance, to a maximum of every 3–4 hours. In RCTs using bladder training, mean reductions in urge incontinence range from 60%–80%, often yielding better results than drug treatment alone (Level 1 evidence) [22, 23, 27, 36]. Bladder training, in combination with other behavioral strategies and treatment of sleep and related medical disorders (including the use of compression stockings when warranted), also improves nocturia in older men and women (Level 3 evidence) [45, 47]. There have been no studies of bladder training alone in men with urge UI.

Bulking agents and medical devices

A limited number of RCTs have shown improved rates of continence and improvement in stress UI in women using various injectable bulking agents such as collagen (Level 2 evidence) [22]. There is limited evidence to recommend the use of vaginal cones, pessaries, or disposable intravaginal devices in women with stress UI (Level 3 evidence) [22]. External penile compression devices (clamps) are effective for containing incontinence postprostatectomy in men, but there are safety problems that need to be resolved before recommending their use (Level 2 evidence) [25].

Pharmacologic management

Level 1 evidence supports the use of antimuscarinic agents for the treatment of urge UI in men and women [22, 28–31]. Oxybutynin, tolterodine, propiverine, fesoterodine, solifenacin, darifenacin, and trospium chloride all have similar proven efficacy in overactive bladder, reducing incontinence episodes by up to 70%, and resulting in cure in 50% of the individuals included in the trials. One study suggests that antimuscarinic agents may be less effective in persons aged 60 years and older [37], although this observation is not consistent across trials [38]. Tolerability of the antimuscarinic drugs is limited by a high incidence of dry mouth and gastrointestinal side effects, including constipation [28–30]. In older adults, anticholinergic safety concerns have been raised around cognitive impairment and tachycardia [28, 51]. Table 10.4 lists the available antimuscarinic agents with their theoretical propensity for crossing the blood–brain barrier, as well as other implications for causing drug–drug interactions in the older adults [28].

Combination therapy with antimuscarinic agents and alpha-adrenergic antagonists may be more effective than either drug alone for the treatment of symptoms of overactive bladder in men with prostatic enlargement (Level 2 evidence), although this combination has not been extensively studied for urge UI (Level 4 evidence) [12, 39].

Botulinum toxin in an intravesical injectable form has also been used in small trials for the treatment of urge UI in patients with neurologic and refractory idiopathic cases of detrusor overactivity (Level 2 evidence), but cannot as yet be recommended as part of the routine treatment armamentarium for urge UI in

Table 10.4 Characteristics of the different antimuscarinic agents used in the treatment of overactive bladder

Characteristic	Trospium Chloride IR	Trospium LA	Oxybutynin IR/LA	Oxybutynin Transdermal	Tolterodine IR/LA	Fesoterodine	Darifenacin	Solifenacin	Propiverine
Chemical structure	Quaternary amine	Quaternary amine	Tertiary amine	Tertiary amine	Tertiary amine	Tertiary amine	Tertiary amine	Tertiary amine	Tertiary amine
Muscarinic receptor selectivity	Nonselective	Nonselective	Nonselective	Nonselective	More selective for M2 receptors	More selective for M2 receptors	More selective for M3 receptors	More selective for M3 receptors	Nonselective
Oral bioavailability	<10%; take on an empty stomach	<10%; take on an empty stomach	2%–15%	None	75%	52%	15%–20%	90%	40%–50%
Metabolism	Ester hydrolysis by non-CYP450	Ester hydrolysis by non-CYP450	CYP2D6 and CYP3A4	CYP2D6 and CYP3A4	CYP2D6 and CYP3A4	Ester hydrolysis by non-CYP450; levels may be affected by CYP2D6 and 3A4 inhibition	CYP2D6 and CYP3A4	CYP3A4	CYP3A4
Metabolites contributing to clinical effect	None	None	Des-ethyl-oxybutynin	Des-ethyl-oxybutynin	5-hydroxy-methyl-tolterodine	5-hydroxy-methyl-tolterodine	None	None	N-oxide
Excretion	Tubular secretion, ~80% of parent compound unchanged in urine	Tubular secretion, ~60% of parent compound unchanged in urine	<5% of active compound in urine	<5% of active compound in urine	<5% of active compound in urine	~70% is excreted in the urine	3% of active compound in urine	<15% of active compound in urine	<10% of active compound in urine

Continued

Table 10.4 *Continued*

Characteristic	Trospium Chloride IR	Trospium LA	Oxybutynin IR/LA	Oxybutynin Transdermal	Tolterodine IR/LA	Fesoterodine	Darifenacin	Solifenacin	Propiverine
Half-life (h)	20	35	2/13	7–8	2/8.5	7–8	12	45–68	20
Adverse effects	Dry mouth constipation, headache, blurred vision, urinary retention	Dry mouth constipation, headache, blurred vision, urinary retention	Highest incidence of dry mouth in the IR form (>60%), constipation, somnolence, blurred vision	Lowest incidence of dry mouth (<10%), constipation, somnolence, blurred vision, application site pruritus & erythema (~15%)	Dry mouth, headache, constipation, abdominal pain[a]	Dry mouth, dry eyes, dyspepsia, constipation, dizziness	Dry mouth constipation, dry eyes, upper abdominal pain	Dry mouth constipation, headache, blurred vision, urinary retention[b]	Dry mouth, constipation, dry eyes
Propensity for crossing the blood–brain barrier	*Low:* Hydrophilic, positive charge, large molecular size	*Low:* Hydrophilic, positive charge, large molecular size	*High:* Lipophilic, neutral charge, small molecular size	*High:* Lipophilic, neutral charge, small molecular size	*Medium:* Low lipophilicity, partially charged, relatively "larger" molecular size	*Medium:* Low lipophilicity, neutral charge, small molecular size	*Medium:* Low lipophilicity, partially charged, relatively "larger" molecular size	*Medium:* Low lipophilicity, partially charged, relatively "larger" molecular size	*Medium:* Low lipophilicity, partially charged, small molecular size
Dosing	20 mg twice daily, 20 mg once daily for renal impairment creatinine clearance <30 mL/min	60 mg once daily in the morning on an empty stomach; contraindicated in patients with creatinine clearance <30 mL/min	*IR:* 2.5 mg tid up to 15 mg max per day *LA:* 5–30 mg once daily	3.9 mg twice weekly applied to hips, buttocks, or abdomen	*IR:* 1–2 mg twice daily *LA:* 2–4 mg once daily; max 2 mg per day in severe renal impairment	*IR:* 4–8 mg once daily; maximum 4 mg daily in severe renal impairment	7.5–15 mg once daily	5–10 mg daily; maximum 5 mg daily in severe renal impairment	15 mg one to three times daily

IR, immediate release; LA, long-acting.

[a]Tachycardia, warning re: long-QT syndrome.

[b]Warning: long QT syndrome.

the older adult because of an increased risk of urinary retention [28, 32].

The 2008 International Consultation on Incontinence found insufficient evidence to recommend the use of duloxetine or any other adrenergic agent for treatment of stress UI, and similarly declared that good evidence was lacking to justify the use of tricyclic antidepressants or flavoxate for urge UI. Although desmopressin may reduce nocturia (Level 2 evidence), its use has been contraindicated in frail older adults because of a high risk of hyponatremia (Level 4 evidence) [13, 28].

Surgical management

There are a number of minimally invasive surgical treatment options available for stress UI in women who fail conservative therapy. Limited evidence suggests that older women who are appropriate candidates may significantly benefit from surgery, with only slightly higher treatment failure rates for stress UI than younger women (20% vs. 11%, $p = 0.03$) (Level 3 evidence) [48].

Clinical bottom line

Weight loss and pelvic floor muscle strengthening provide a Level 1 evidence base for the treatment of stress UI in women. Level 1 evidence therapeutic options for urge UI in women include weight loss, pelvic floor muscle exercises, bladder retraining, and antimuscarinic drug therapy. In men, antimuscarinic therapy provides the highest level of evidence for the treatment of urge UI. Several other therapies such as caffeine restriction are used empirically, but future research is needed to provide a stronger evidence base for these types of interventions. There appears to be no single best model of care, with all models resulting in UI cures for up to 25% of patients.

What is the best treatment approach for LTC residents and people with dementia?

The answer to this question was informed by three systematic reviews [52–54] (Level 1 evidence), one RCT [56] (Level 2 evidence), two cohort studies [57, 58] (Level 3 evidence), six case series [19, 55, 59–63] (Level 4 evidence), and three expert opinion papers [64–66] (Level 5 evidence).

UI affects up to 77% of all LTC residents. In many of these residents, dementia and incontinence coexist [52, 64]. In some instances, incontinence may be a direct result of neurodegenerative changes in central nervous system pathways controlling normal urine voiding and storage functions. However, incontinence may also occur due to difficulties with dressing and undressing, mobility, or motivation and executive function [52, 65]. A urodynamic case study of 94 institutionalized incontinent persons with incontinence revealed urge UI in 61%, with concomitant impaired detrusor contractility present in half these patients [59]. Other causes among women were stress UI (21%), underactive detrusor (8%), and outlet obstruction (4%). Among the relatively few men in this sample, outlet obstruction accounted for 29% of the cases. In 35% of the patients, at least two coexisting probable causes of UI were identified. Moreover, urodynamic abnormalities frequently coexisted with functional impairments and other contributing causes [59]. Contributing factors and multiple potentially reversible causes frequently occur in LTC residents, and should be aggressively sought and corrected [19, 66].

A number of effective continence interventions are available for LTC residents (Level 1 evidence) [53]. However, continence care programs in the LTC setting are more difficult to implement and sustain, requiring continued efforts and implication by the LTC administration and staff [60].

A recent systematic review of randomized trials of treatment interventions in LTC residents with UI revealed that prompted voiding alone or prompted voiding plus exercise are two effective techniques to reduce daytime incontinence (Level 1 evidence) [53]. A 7-step prompted voiding strategy is illustrated in Figure 10.2 [60]. The response to treatment can be monitored with wet checks by care-providers and recorded in bladder diaries. Eligible residents are those with intact self-care skills, ability to ambulate independently, baseline UI frequency of fewer than four episodes per 12-hour period, and who are able to say their name or reliably point to one of two named objects [60]. All incontinent residents who fit these criteria should be given a 3-day trial of prompted voiding every 2–3 hours. Targeting the intervention to those who are most likely to respond promotes cost-effectiveness and best use of staff time. In general, nighttime prompted voiding disrupts sleep, is not effective, and should not be carried

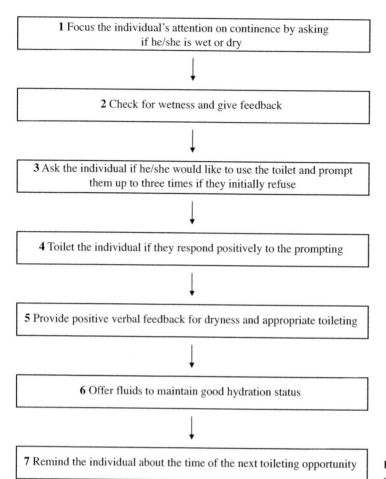

1 Focus the individual's attention on continence by asking
if he/she is wet or dry

2 Check for wetness and give feedback

3 Ask the individual if he/she would like to use the toilet and prompt
them up to three times if they initially refuse

4 Toilet the individual if they respond positively to the prompting

5 Provide positive verbal feedback for dryness and appropriate toileting

6 Offer fluids to maintain good hydration status

7 Remind the individual about the time of the next toileting opportunity

Figure 10.2 Seven-step-prompted voiding strategy.

out except for residents who express a preference and willingness to toilet at night [55].

There appears to be no benefit of habit retraining in the management of UI in frail older adults with cognitive impairment (Level 1 evidence) [54]. Habit retraining involves identifying an incontinent person's toileting pattern and developing an individualized toileting schedule to preempt involuntary bladder emptying.

Pharmacologic therapy may provide a small additional benefit in reducing UI in LTC residents when used with prompted voiding (Level 2 evidence) [53]. However, there is some concern about the anticholinergic side effects of antimuscarinic agents in residents with dementia [61]. One small randomized, 4-week trial of extended-release oxybutynin 5 mg per day in 50 female LTC residents (mean age 89) with dementia and urge incontinence showed no decline in cognitive function or increased rates of delirium or falls with oxybutynin treatment compared to placebo [56]. No participant in this study was taking a concomitant cholinesterase inhibitor therapy for the treatment of dementia.

Concomitant use of cholinesterase inhibitors and anticholinergics in patients with dementia and urge incontinence remains controversial, because of their opposing mechanisms of action. Three studies have examined the effects of this regimen (Level 3 evidence) [58, 62, 63]. A Japanese study examined the addition of a 3-month trial of propiverine 20 mg per day to donepezil in 26 cognitively impaired older adults, and found improved dryness rates with no deleterious effect on cognition [62]. The second study, a 6-month trial compared the effects of trospium, galantamine, or trospium plus galantamine in 178 older adults with urge incontinence ($n = 99$), dementia ($n = 43$), or dementia and incontinence ($n = 36$), respectively [63]. Treatment with 45–60 mg per day of trospium chloride and combined use of trospium with galantamine 24 mg per day was found to have no adverse effect on cognitive or physical function scores in this group of patients. A larger observational study of 3563 LTC residents with dementia also failed to document an increased rate of cognitive decline with combined use of a cholinesterase inhibitor and anticholinergic therapy (oxybutynin or tolterodine) compared to cholinesterase therapy alone [58]. However, a 50% faster rate of physical function decline was observed in higher functioning participants on dual therapy compared to cholinesterase inhibitor therapy alone. As the cognitive measures used in these studies (MDS-Cog and MMSE) probably do not have sufficient sensitivity to detect early evidence of worsening cognitive function, evidence for worsening cognitive effects during combination therapy remains inconclusive. The extent to which specific antimuscarinic agents cross the blood–brain barrier or selectively block subtypes of antimuscarinic receptors may be counterbalanced by neuropharmacologic and blood–brain barrier permeability changes that occur in vascular or neurodegenerative dementia [51], so larger randomized controlled studies are required.

Clinical bottom line

Incontinence is highly prevalent in the LTC setting, where cognitive and mobility impairments frequently coexist.

Transient and reversible causes of UI should be sought and treated.

Prompted voiding is effective for daytime UI in patients with mild dementia (Level 1 evidence), with exercise and drug therapy offering minimal additional benefit (Level 1 evidence).

Concomitant use of anticholinergic drugs and acetylcholinesterase inhibitors may worsen functional status (Level 3 evidence), so this treatment strategy is generally not recommended at the present time (Level 4 evidence).

Summary

UI affects one in two women, and up to 20% of men aged 65 years and older. Unfortunately, incontinence often remains undertreated despite the availability of successful evidence-based evaluation and management strategies that can be easily implemented in the office and LTC setting. A comprehensive assessment including a targeted history, physical exam, and specific investigations, such as a stress test, urinalysis, and measurement of the postvoid residual urine volume, yields the highest rate of diagnostic certainty for establishing the type(s) and underlying cause(s) of UI. A wide range of evidence-based treatment options exists for both men and women suffering from different types of UI. Nonpharmacological strategies such as lifestyle modifications, pelvic floor muscle exercises, and bladder training should be considered as first-line therapy. In the LTC setting, reversible causes of UI should be sought and treated. Prompted voiding should be introduced for patients with mild dementia. Management of UI in the LTC setting may be difficult to implement unless the support staff is sensitized to the importance of reducing both the incidence and prevalence of this often neglected condition.

References

1. Thom D (1998) Variation in estimates of urinary incontinence prevalence in the community: effects of differences in definition, population characteristics, and study type. *J Am Geriatr Soc* 46: 473–480.
2. Ouslander JG, Schnelle JF (1995) Incontinence in the LTC. *Ann Intern Med* 122: 438–449.
3. Ouslander JG, Palmer MH, Rovner BW, German PS (1993) Urinary incontinence in LTCs: incidence, remission and associated factors. *J Am Geriatr Soc* 41: 1083–1089.
4. Temml C, Haidinger G, Schmidbauer J, Schatzl G, Madersbacher S (2000) Urinary incontinence in both sexes: prevalence rates and impact on quality of life and sexual life. *Neurourol Urodyn* 19: 259–271.
5. Johnson TM, 2nd, Kincade JE, Bernard SL, Busby-Whitehead J, Hertz-Picciotto I, DeFriese GH (1998) The association of urinary incontinence with poor self-rated health. *J Am Geriatr Soc* 46: 693–699.
6. Wyman JF, Harkins SW, Fantl JA (1990) Psychosocial impact of urinary incontinence in the community-dwelling population. *J Am Geriatr Soc* 38: 282–288.
7. Dugan E, et al (2000) The association of depressive symptoms and urinary incontinence among older adults. *J Am Geriatr Soc* 48: 413–416.
8. Holroyd-Leduc JM, Mehta KM, Covinsky KE (2004) Urinary incontinence and its association with death, LTC admission, and functional decline. *J Am Geriatr Soc* 52: 712–728.
9. Kron M, Loy S, Sturm E, Nikolaus T, Becker C (2003) Risk indicators for falls in institutionalized frail elderly. *Am J Epidemiol* 158: 645–653.

10. Berlowitz DR, Brandeis GH, Anderson J, Brand HK (1997) Predictors of pressure ulcer healing among LTC residents. *J Am Geriatr Soc* 45: 30–34.

11. Holroyd-Leduc JM, Straus SE (2004) Management of urinary incontinence in women: scientific review. *JAMA* 291: 986–995.

12. Abrams P, Chapple C, Khoury S, Roehrborn C, de la Rosette J (2009) Evaluation and treatment of lower urinary tract symptoms in older men. *J Urol* 181: 1779–1787.

13. DuBeau CE, Kuchel GA, Johnson T, Palmer MH, Wagg A (2010) Incontinence in the frail elderly: report from the 4th International Consultation on Incontinence. *Neurourol Urodyn* 29: 165–178.

14. Tannenbaum C, Bachand, G, DuBeau CE, Kuchel GA (2001) Experience of an incontinence clinic for older women: no apparent age limit for potential physical and psychological benefits. *J Women Health & Gend Based Med* 10: 751–756.

15. Ruby CM, Hanlon JT, Fillenbaum GG, Pieper CF, Branch LG, Bump RC (2005) Medication use and control of urination among community-dwelling older adults. *J Aging Health* 17: 661–674.

16. Abrams P, et al (2002) The standardization of terminology in lower urinary tract function: report from the Standardization Sub-committee of the International Continence Society. *Neurourol Urodyn* 21: 167–178.

17. Staskin D, et al (2009) Chapter 5: Initial assessment of urinary and faecal incontinence in adult male and female patients. In: P Abrams, L Cardozo, S Khoury, A Wein (eds) *Incontinence.* Plymouth, MA: Health Publications Ltd.

18. Holroyd-Leduc JM, Tannenbaum C, Thorpe KE, Strauss SE (2008) What type of urinary incontinence does this woman have? *JAMA* 299: 1446–1456.

19. Brandeis GH, Baumann MM, Hossain M, Morris JN, Resnick NM (1997) The prevalence of potentially remediable urinary incontinence in frail older people: a study using the minimum data set. *J Am Geriatr Soc* 45(2): 179–184.

20. Resnick NM (1995) Urinary incontinence. *Lancet* 346: 94–99.

21. Taylor JA, Kuchel GA (2006) Detrusor underactivity: clinical features and pathogenesis of an underdiagnosed geriatric condition. *J Am Geriatr Soc* 54: 1920–1932.

22. Shamliyan TA, Kane RL, Wyman J, Wilt TJ (2008) Systematic review: randomized, controlled trials of nonsurgical treatments for urinary incontinence in women. *Ann Inter Med* 148: 459–773.

23. Burgio KL (2009) Behavioral treatment of urinary incontinence, voiding dysfunction, and overactive bladder. *Obstet Gynecol Clin N Am* 36: 475–491.

24. Teunissen TAM, de Jonge A, van Weel C, Lagro-Janssen ALM (2004) Treating urinary incontinence in the elderly – conservative measures that work: a systematic review. *J Fam Practice* 53: 25–32.

25. Hunter KE, Moore KN, Glazener CMA (2007) Conservative management for post-prostatectomy urinary incontinence. *Cochrane Database Syst Rev* (2) Art. No. CD001843.

26. Dumoulin C, Hay-Smith J (2010) Pelvic floor muscle training versus no treatment, or inactive control treatments, for urinary incontinence in women. *Cochrane Database Syst Rev* (1) Art. No. CD005654.

27. Roe B, Ostaszkiewicz J, Milne J, Wallace S (2007) Systematic reviews of bladder training and voiding programmes in adults: a synopsis of findings from data analysis and outcomes using metastudy techniques. *J Advanced Nurs* 57: 15–31.

28. Andersson KE, et al (2009) Pharmacological treatment of overactive bladder: report from the International Consultation on Incontinence. *Curr Opin Urol* 19: 380–394.

29. Chapple CR, Khullar V, Gabriel Z, Muston D, Bitoun CE, Weinstein D (2008) The effects of antimuscarinic treatments in overactive bladder: an update of a systematic review and meta-analysis. *Eur Urol* 54: 543–562.

30. Novara G, et al (2008) A systematic review and meta-analysis of randomized controlled trials with antimuscarinic drugs for overactive bladder. *Eur Urol* 54: 740–764.

31. Nabi G, Cody JD, Ellis G, Hay-Smith J, Herbison GP (2006) Anticholinergic drugs versus placebo for overactive bladder syndrome in adults. *Cochrane Database Syst Rev* (4) Art. No. CD003781.

32. Duthie JB, Herbison GP, Wilson DI, Wilson D (2007) Botulinum toxin injections for adults with overactive bladder syndrome. *Cochrane Database Syst Rev* (3) Art. No. CD005493.

33. Goode PS, et al (2011) Behavioral therapy with or without biofeedback and pelvic floor electrical stimulation for persistent postprostatectomy incontinence: a randomized controlled trial. *JAMA* 305: 151–9.

34. Brown JS, et al (2006) Diabetes Prevention Program Research Group. Lifestyle intervention is associated with lower prevalence of urinary incontinence: the Diabetes Prevention Program. *Diabetes Care* 29: 385–390.

35. Subak LL, et al (2009) Weight loss to treat urinary incontinence in overweight and obese women. *N Engl J Med* 360: 481–490.

36. Burgio KL, et al (1998) Behavioral versus drug treatment for urge incontinence in older women: a randomized clinical trial. *JAMA* 23: 1995–2000.

37. Malone-Lee JG, et al (2001) Tolterodine: a safe and effective treatment for older persons with overactive bladder. *J Am Geriatr Soc* 49: 700–705.

38. Zinner NR, Mattiasson A, Stanton SL (2002) Efficacy, safety and tolerability of extended-release once-daily tolterodine treatment for overactive bladder in older versus younger patients. *J Am Geriatr Soc* 50: 799–807.

39. Kaplan SA, et al (2006) Tolterodine and tamsulosin for treatment of men with lower urinary tract symptoms and overactive bladder: a randomized controlled study. *JAMA* 296: 2319–2328.

40. Borrie MJ, Bawden M, Speechley M, Kloseck M (2002) Interventions led by nurse continence advisers in the management of urinary incontinence: a randomized controlled trial. *CMAJ* 166: 1267–1273.

41. Moore KH, O'Sullivan RJ, Simons A, Prashar S, Anderson P, Louey M (2003) Randomised controlled trial of nurse continence advisor therapy compared with standard

urogynaecology regimen for conservative incontinence treatment: efficacy, costs and two year follow up. *BJOG* 110: 649–657.

42. Williams KS, Assassa RP, Cooper NJ (2005) Clinical and cost-effectiveness of a new nurse-led continence service: a randomized controlled trial. *Br J Gen Practice* 55: 696–703.

43. Swithinbank L, Hashim H, Abrams P (2005) The effect of fluid intake on urinary symptoms in women. *J Urol* 174: 187–189.

44. Bryant CM, Dowell CJ, Fairbrother G (2002) Caffeine reduction education to improve urinary symptoms. *Br J Nurs* 11: 560–565.

45. Johnson TM II, et al (2005) Effects of behavioral and drug therapy on nocturia in older incontinent women. *J Am Geriatr Soc* 53: 846–850.

46. Tomlinson BU, et al (1999) Dietary caffeine, fluid intake and urinary incontinence in older rural women. *Int Urogynecol J Pelvic Floor Dysfunct* 10: 22–28.

47. Vaughan C, et al (2009) A multicomponent behavioral and drug intervention for nocturia in elderly men: rationale and pilot results. *BJU INt* 104: 9–74.

48. Sung VW, Joo K, Marques F, Myers DL (2009) Patient-reported outcomes after combined surgery for pelvic floor disorders in older compared to younger women. *Am J Obstet Gynecol* 201: 534.e1–534.e5.

49. Harari D, Igbedioh C (2009) Restoring continence in frail older people living in the community: what factors influence successful treatment outcomes? *Age Ageing* 38: 228–233.

50. Padros J, Peris T, Salva A, Denkinger MD, Coll-Planas L (2008) Evaluation of a urinary incontinence unit for community-dwelling older adults in Barcelona: implementation and improvement of the perceived impact on daily life, frequency and severity of urinary incontinence. *Z Gerontol Geriatr* 41: 291–297.

51. Kay GG, Abou-Donia MB, Messer WS, Murphy DG, Tsao JW, Ouslander JG 2005 Antimuscarinic drugs for overactive bladder and their potential effects on cognitive function in older patients. *J Am Geriatr Soc* 53: 2195–2201.

52. Offermans MPW, Du Moulin MFMT, Hamers JPH, Dassen T, Halfens RJG (2009) Prevalence of urinary incontinence and associated risk factors in LTC residents: a systematic review. *Neurourol Urodyn* 28: 288–294.

53. Fink HA, Taylor BC, Tacklind JW, Rutks IR, Wilt TJ (2008) Treatment interventions in LTC residents with urinary incontinence: a systematic review of randomized trials. *Mayo Clin Proc* 83: 1332–1343.

54. Ostaszkiewicz J, Chestney T, Roe B. (2004) Habit retraining for the management of urinary incontinence in adults. *Cochrane Database Syst Rev* (2) Art. No. CD002801.

55. Ouslander JG, Al-Samarrai N, Schnelle JF (2001) Prompted voiding for nighttime incontinence in LTCs: is it effective? *J Am Geriatr Soc* 49: 706–709.

56. Lackner TE, Wyman JF, McCarthy TC, Monigold M, Davey C (2008) Randomized, placebo-controlled trial of the cognitive effect, safety, and tolerability of oral extended-release oxybutynin in cognitively impaired LTC residents with urge urinary incontinence. *J Am Geriatr Soc* 56: 862–870.

57. Ouslander JG, et al (1995) Predictors of successful prompted voiding among incontinent LTC residents. *JAMA* 273: 1366–1370.

58. Sink KM, Thomas J, Xu H, Craig B, Kritchebsky S, Sands LP (2008) Dual use of bladder anticholinergics and cholinesterase inhibitors: long-term functional and cognitive outcomes. *J Am Geriatr Soc* 56: 847–853.

59. Resnick NM, Yalla SV, Laurino E (1989) The pathophysiology of urinary incontinence among institutionalized elderly persons. *N Engl J Med* 320: 1–7.

60. Etheridge F, Tannenbaum C, Couturier Y (2008) A systemwide formula for continence care: overcoming barriers, clarifying solutions and defining team members' roles. *J Am Med Dir Assoc* 9: 178–189.

61. Jewart RD, Green J, Lu CJ, Cellar J, Tune L (2005) Cognitive, behavioral and physiological changes in Alzheimer disease patients as a function of incontinence medications. *Am J Geriatr Psychiatry* 13: 324–328.

62. Sakadkibara R, et al (2009) How to manage overactive bladder in elderly individuals with dementia? Combined use of donepezil, a central acetylcholinesterase inhibitor, and propiverine, a peripheral muscarine receptor antagonist. *J Am Geriatr Soc* 57: 1515–1517.

63. Isik AT, Celik T, Bozoglu E, Doruk H (2009) Trospium and cognition in patients with late onset Alzheimer disease. *J Nutr Health Aging* 13: 672–676.

64. Ouslander JG, Schnelle JF (1995) Incontinence in the LTC. *Ann Intern Med* 122: 438–449.

65. DuBeau CE, Resnick NM (1995) Urinary incontinence and dementia: the perils of guilt by association. *J Am Geriatr Soc* 43: 310–311.

66. Tannenbaum C, DuBeau CE (2004) Urinary incontinence in the LTC: practical approach to evaluation and management. *Clin Geriatr Med* 20: 437–452.

CHAPTER 11

Keeping things moving: preventing and managing constipation

Dov Gandell[2,4] *& Shabbir M.H. Alibhai*[1,2,3]

[1]*Departments of Medicine and Health Policy, Management, and Evaluation, University of Toronto, Toronto, ON, Canada*
[2]*Toronto Rehabilitation Institute, Toronto, ON, Canada*
[3]*Internal Medicine and Geriatrics, University Health Network, Toronto, ON, Canada*
[4]*University of Toronto, ON, Canada*

Introduction

Chronic constipation is a common issue among older adults [1]. Complaints about constipation and its prevalence increase with age, particularly over the age of 65 [2, 3]. Prevalence rates vary depending on the setting, with approximately 40% of community-dwelling seniors and 60% in long-term care suffering from constipation [4–6]. Female gender, regular medication use, lower socioeconomic class, nonwhite race, as well as symptoms of anxiety and depression, have all been associated with the increased prevalence of constipation in the older adult [7–10]. Patients with constipation rate their quality of life significantly lower than nonconstipated healthy individuals [11]. Costs associated with treating the problem in the elderly are high, estimated at US$2253 per year per long-term care resident for labor and supplies [12].

Over 50% of long-term care residents use laxatives [13]. Although there is little overall objective evidence on the efficacy of most commonly used laxatives [14], there are randomized trials of several laxatives and systematic reviews to help guide clinical decisions, even in the older patient.

Clinicians, whether practicing in clinic, hospital, or long-term care, need an evidence-based skill set to understand and manage constipation when caring for the older adult.

Search strategies

We sought to identify treatment trials that specifically recruited older patients (defined as age 65 or over) or trials with at least 50% of the population over the age of 65. MEDLINE was searched from 1966 to July 2010 for randomized controlled trials on constipation treatment. Key search terms included: "laxatives," "stimulant," "osmotic," 'bulk,' and "irritant laxatives," "fecal softener," "sorbitol," "lactulose," "magnesium," "milk of magnesia," "magnesium sulfate," "bisacodyl," "calcium polycarbophil," "polyethylene glycol," "danthron," "cascara," "ispaghula," "psyllium," "bran," "celandin," "docusate," "poloxalkol," "mineral oil," "glycerine," "methylcellulose," "senna," "tegaserod," "prucalopride," and "lubiprostone." Limits above and below the age of 65 were added to isolate trials that specifically focused on the geriatric population. All randomized trials on the treatment of chronic constipation, excluding irritable bowel syndrome (IBS), were reviewed. Finally, reference lists from the identified articles and from previously published systematic reviews and review articles were scanned for relevant articles.

To determine the prevalence and etiology of chronic constipation, two MEDLINE searches from 1966 to July 2010 were conducted using constipation as the subject heading and prevalence or etiology as the subheading. Limits to exclude pediatric and adolescent

Evidence-Based Geriatric Medicine: A Practical Clinical Guide, First Edition. Edited by Jayna M. Holroyd-Leduc and Madhuri Reddy.
© 2012 Blackwell Publishing Ltd. Published 2012 by Blackwell Publishing Ltd.

populations were applied. Previous systematic reviews and review articles on chronic constipation were scanned for relevant references.

For this chapter, we graded relevant clinical studies using the Oxford Centre for Evidence-based Medicine Levels of Evidence.

How do you define and diagnose chronic constipation?

Due to the subjective nature of the condition, no single clinical definition of constipation exists [15, 16]. Standardized criteria used in the research setting come from the Rome Foundation Committee (a nonprofit group that promotes recognition, scientific understanding, and treatment of functional gastrointestinal disorders) on functional constipation (Table 11.1) [17].

Bowel movement frequency is just one of the six cardinal symptoms of constipation. In the clinical setting, strict adherence to the Rome Criteria is difficult and constipation is usually diagnosed on the basis of patient's complaint of difficulty with defecation, incomplete defecation [17], or infrequent stools [18]. The older adult and physicians tend to differ on their viewpoint, with the older adult identifying straining as the predominant symptom [19]; whereas physicians tend to focus on stool frequency despite patients often

Table 11.1 Rome III Criteria for the diagnosis of functional constipation

---

Must include two or more of following six symptoms:

Straining during at least 25% of defecations

Lumpy or hard stools in at least 25% of defecations

Sensation of incomplete evacuation for at least 25% of defecations

Sensation of anorectal obstruction/blockage for at least 25% of defecations

Manual maneuvers (digital evacuation/support of pelvic floor) to facilitate at least 25% of defecations

Fewer than three defecations per week

Loose stools are rarely present without the use of laxatives

Insufficient criteria for irritable bowel syndrome

Criteria fulfilled for the last 3 months with symptom onset at least 6 months prior to diagnosis

---

underestimating their number of movements [20–22]. The range of normal stool frequency can vary between three bowel movements per day to three per week [23]. Frequency of movements outside that range may also be normal in the absence of a change from baseline and without other symptoms. For individuals with moderate-to-severe cognitive impairment, clinicians usually rely on caregiver observation for diagnosis.

What are the common causes of constipation in the older adult?

As with most geriatric syndromes, the cause of constipation is usually multifactorial [24]. Age-related changes in colonic anatomy and physiology have been described but are not considered to be a major cause of constipation in the elderly. Collagen fibers become smaller and more tightly packed in the left colon with aging and myenteric plexus neurons are reduced in number and decreased in function [3]. Impaired rectal sensitivity and compliance as well as decrease in anal sphincter pressures have also been described [25, 26]. Studies in healthy older adults have shown either similar [27, 28] or delayed colonic transit time and motility relative to younger adults [29].

Dietary and lifestyle factors have also been implicated as causes of constipation but decreased mobility, low fiber intake, and limited fluid intake in nondehydrated persons do not have strong evidence from cohort or randomized trials to support those claims (Level 1b evidence) [9, 27, 30–32].

Constipation in the older adult is classified as either primary or secondary. Medications (Table 11.2) and disease states (Table 11.3) account for the majority of secondary causes, although the relative frequency of each cause is not well described. It is unclear which pathophysiologic process is most prevalent in community-dwelling older adult with constipation [3].

Constipation is labeled primary when secondary causes have been excluded. Primary constipation can be further subdivided into three groups: (1) normal transit constipation, (2) slow transit constipation, and (3) disordered or dyssynergic defecation. There is overlap among the subtypes of primary constipation, a patient may have more than one underlying mechanism, and history alone is insufficient to discriminate

Table 11.2 Drugs commonly associated with constipation

Over-the-Counter Preparations	Prescription Drugs
Antacids (calcium containing)	Anticholinergic drugs
Calcium supplements	Anti-Parkinsonian drugs
Oral iron	Antipsychotics
Antidiarrheal agents	Antihistamines
Anti-inflammatory agents	Calcium channel blockers
	Diuretics
	Opiates
	Tricyclic antidepressants
	Sympathomimetics

between subtypes [33]. In primary care settings, the value of distinguishing between the primary subtypes is not known and does not influence the initial therapeutic options.

Normal transit constipation, the most frequent cause in one surgical series [34], is characterized by 72 hours or less for colonic transit time, and is interchangeable with the term "functional" constipation. Bowel movement frequency is typically normal and complaints of hard stool, pain, bloating, and psychological symptoms are often present.

Slow transit constipation usually starts in adolescence and is more prevalent in women. Infrequent urges to defecate, abdominal pain, and bloating are common symptoms. Changes to myenteric nerve cell expression and neurotransmitter levels are thought to play a role. Postprandial colonic high-amplitude contractions may be reduced [16, 35].

Dyssynergic defecation refers to the inability to adequately empty the rectum with the passage of stool. It results from a paradoxical increase in the anal sphincter pressure and/or difficulty with the pelvic floor. Patients often complain of excessive straining and use of manual maneuvers (e.g., digital disimpaction) to assist in evacuating the rectum.

Clinical bottom line

Neither low fiber, low fluid intake nor immobility has been conclusively shown to cause constipation in older adults. Primary constipation is subdivided into normal transit, slow transit, and dyssynergic defecation. Medications and disease states account for the majority of secondary causes of constipation.

What is the suggested diagnostic workup of constipation?

Although not strictly evidence-based, a thorough history and physical exam should be performed to reveal potential contributing factors and to exclude secondary causes of chronic constipation. On history, the most

Table 11.3 Disease states associated with constipation

Metabolic	Gastrointestinal	Neurologic	Psychiatric	Connective Tissue
Diabetes mellitus	Colorectal carcinoma	Stroke	Depression	Primary systemic sclerosis
Hypothyroidism	Diverticular disease	Parkinson's disease	Anxiety	Amyloidosis
Hypercalcemia	Colonic stricture	Dementia	Somatization	
Hypokalemia	Rectal prolapse	Autonomic neuropathy		
	Rectocele	Spinal cord lesion		
	Megacolon	Multiple sclerosis		
	Hemorrhoids/fissure			

Source: Adapted from Gallager et al [35].

Box 11.1 Bristol stool chart

Type 1 Separate hard lumps, like nuts (hard to pass)
Type 2 Sausage-shaped but lumpy
Type 3 Like a sausage but with cracks on its surface
Type 4 Like a sausage or snake, smooth and soft
Type 5 Soft blobs with clear cut edges (passed easily)
Type 6 Fluffy pieces with ragged edges, a mushy stool
Type 7 Watery, no solid pieces, entirely liquid

Box 11.2 Alarm symptoms

Family history of colon cancer or inflammatory bowel
 disease
Hematochezia
Anemia
Weight loss ≥ 10 lbs
Positive fecal occult blood test
Severe or persistent constipation that is unresponsive
 to treatment
New onset constipation in elderly patient without any
 evidence of a likely underlying cause of constipation

Source: Data from [4].

troubling symptom(s) to the patient, date of onset, frequency of motions, size and consistency of stool, pain (abdominal and rectal), bleeding, weight loss, straining, and need for manual maneuvers or unusual postures to expel stool should be elicited. Mobility, fluid intake, dietary habits, medications, and cognitive and psychiatric history should also be reviewed. In constipated adults, an assessment of stool form, particularly with a score of <3 as measured by the Bristol Stool Scale (Box 11.1), correlates with both delayed whole gut and colonic transit time [36, 37].

An abdominal examination, including the perineum and digital rectal exam, should be performed. The perineum should be inspected for fistulas, fissures, and hemorrhoids. A more detailed examination, such as that done by a gastroenterologist, can also include an assessment of perineal descent. Perineal descent, normally between 1 and 3.5 cm, can be observed with the patient at rest and while bearing down in order to detect features of disordered defecation. Reduced descent may indicate failure of the pelvic floor musculature to relax during defecation [16]. Excessive descent indicates laxity of the perineum and may lead to incomplete evacuation [16]. The digital exam can further assess sphincter tone and for fecal impaction, anal strictures, and rectal masses. However, the reliability and validity of these physical exam maneuvers have not been reported.

In older patients with alarming symptoms (Box 11.2), it is recommended to exclude secondary causes of constipation with the appropriate tests. Systematic reviews have not revealed an evidence base for the routine use of diagnostic investigations such as blood tests (electrolytes, calcium, thyroid indices), plain radiographs, barium enema, flexible sigmoidoscopy, or colonoscopy in all patients presenting with chronic constipation [38]. This does not discount the

need for colon cancer screening in elder candidates according to evidence-based cancer screening guidelines.

More sophisticated physiologic testing may be done to investigate the mechanisms of chronic constipation in patients who fail to respond to conventional treatment. Anorectal manometry, balloon expulsion, and defecography assist in evaluation of disordered defecation, whereas colonic transit study distinguishes normal from delayed transit time. The utility of physiologic testing has not been formally evaluated in large-scale prospective studies.

Clinical bottom line

Although the evidence is limited, it is reasonable to perform a thorough history, physical exam, and a few simple laboratory tests, such as calcium and thyroid indices, in the diagnostic workup of chronic constipation. Older adults should be screened for colon cancer according to local or national evidence-based guidelines.

What are the potential complications of constipation?

In susceptible frail older adults, excessive straining can lead to cardiovascular compromise, including syncope and coronary or cerebral ischemia. The most serious local complications of chronic constipation are fecal impaction and incontinence. Fecal impaction refers to stool, of any consistency, that is stuck from further passage. Putative risk factors for fecal impaction in the older patient include immobility, cognitive impairment, colonic disorders, neurologic disorders, and medications. Fecal impaction can present as a change in bowel habit or with abdominal symptoms of anorexia, nausea, vomiting, or pain. Paradoxical overflow diarrhea can occur where liquid contents of the colon bypass the impacted mass or the outer layer of the impacted mass. More severe cases can be associated with delirium, urinary retention or incontinence, bowel obstruction, or stercoral ulceration. Most impactions occur in the rectal vault and can be diagnosed on rectal examination. Patients with fecal incontinence and a normal rectal exam should be imaged for obstructive impaction; usually a plain abdominal radiograph is sufficient. Treatment may require manual evacuation although laxatives, particularly polyethylene glycol (PEG) [39], and enemas are sometimes successful. Future prevention of repeated impaction with both nonpharmacologic and pharmacologic treatments of chronic constipation is suggested [40].

Clinical bottom line

The possibility of fecal impaction should be considered in patients with chronic constipation and can be diagnosed by rectal examination and/or plain abdominal radiograph.

What are the methods of preventing constipation?

Two prospective randomized trials that refer to prevention of constipation in older hospitalized patients were found [41, 42]. In a nonblinded trial of 16 postoperative orthopedic patients with unknown prior status of constipation, 20 g of wheat bran mixed into the diet did not prevent constipation relative to controls [41]. The second trial of 200 general medical inpatients given 20 g of bran twice daily also failed to detect a decrease in the number of days requiring laxatives, irrespective of baseline constipation status (Level 2b evidence) [42].

Clinical bottom line

Increasing fiber intake does not clearly prevent constipation. Firm evidence-based recommendations on preventing constipation cannot be made at this time. However, it is reasonable to proactively address potentially related dietary and lifestyle factors, along with minimizing unnecessary medications that can contribute to constipation.

What are the nonpharmacological treatments of constipation?

Nonpharmacologic treatments of constipation include general recommendations on bowel habits, dietary fiber and fluid intake, exercise, and lifestyle techniques. Although there is a paucity of high-quality studies evaluating any of these approaches, these strategies should be attempted prior to initiating pharmacological treatments (Level 5 evidence).

Patients should attempt defecation, and cognitively impaired individuals should be prompted to toilet with adequate time on the toilet, 30 minutes after the morning meal to take advantage of the gastrocolic reflex. If laxatives are eventually prescribed, dosing the evening prior may assist the gastrocolic reflex shortly following the morning meal (Level 5 evidence).

Dietary fiber intake of at least 20–30 grams per day promotes greater stool bulk [43]. Dietary sources of fiber include bran, whole grains, fruits, vegetables, nuts, and legumes. A review of the evidence concluded that increasing fluid intake in nondehydrated patients has not been shown to help treat chronic constipation (Level 4 evidence) [31]. Ambulation and mobility are also thought to promote forward flow of contents through the gastrointestinal tract, given the increased prevalence of constipation seen in settings with higher proportions of immobile older adults [5]. A trial in eight ambulatory patients, three of them 65 years or older, involving increased exercise did not show any benefit in a constipation index ($p = 0.68$) (Level 2b evidence) [44]. In long-term care residents, exercise combined with increased fiber and fluid intake has been found to decrease laxative use (Level 2b evidence) [45]. The seated position during defecation is favored to optimize abdominal and pelvic dynamics. In young healthy volunteers, the lying position relative to the seated position was associated with increased pattern of dyssynergic defecation [46].

On a program level, in poststroke patients recruited from rehabilitation facilities, a single systematized nursing evaluation leading to targeted patient and caregiver education, provision of a booklet, and a diagnostic summary and treatment recommendations sent to the patient's general practitioner revealed more bowel movements per week at 1 ($p = 0.011$) and 6 months ($p = 0.05$) compared to controls but not at 12 months. No difference in fecal incontinence was seen (Level 2b evidence) [47]. A nonblinded trial of light abdominal and hand massage (15 minutes per massage, 5 days per week) in 50 patients revealed beneficial effects on a nonvalidated gastrointestinal symptoms rating scale (Level 2b evidence) [48].

Clinical bottom line

Modifying bowel habits, increasing fiber and fluid intake, as well as exercise and positioning may all help alleviate symptoms of constipation. Given their relative safety, these strategies should be considered prior to pharmacologic treatment.

What are the pharmacological treatments of constipation?

When nonpharmacological measures fail to provide adequate relief from constipation, pharmacotherapy is often required (Table 11.4).

Overall, there is lack of objective evidence of efficacy for many of the laxatives used to treat chronic constipation (Level 1a evidence) [14]. Two widely cited systematic reviews on chronic constipation reported data on trials primarily conducted with younger adults [4, 50]. In this chapter, therapeutic trials on the older patient are preferentially reviewed despite the potential pitfalls in the interpretation of clinical studies involving older persons [51]. Where few, if any, trials were available in the older population, a broader perspective on a given treatment's effect is summarized from studies in the broader adult population.

Bulking agents

Seven randomized trials of bulking agents versus placebo or controls in older adults were found (Level 2b evidence) [52–58]. Five more trials evaluated bulking agents or mixtures of agents, compared to other active agents [59–63]. A number of fibers, including psyllium, bran, prune, linseed, galacto-oligosaccharides, calcium polycarbophil, and plantain rind, were studied. Overall, the results are mixed. When compared to controls or placebo, three studies of bulking agents revealed improvement in stool frequency. No study demonstrated benefit in stool consistency. A ten-patient study, most with disordered defecation, comparing psyllium to placebo revealed decreased total gut transit time with treatment but no effect on stool frequency [52]. Psyllium was compared to calcium polycarbophil and no

difference in stool frequency, consistency, or straining was found, although more people (26 vs. 6, $p<0.01$) favored calcium polycarbophil [60]. Semisynthetic and synthetic fibers may be better tolerated since they do not undergo bacterial breakdown and fermentation in the colon, yielding less bloating and gas.

These findings are consistent with previous systematic reviews evaluating the efficacy of bulking agents in chronic constipation in the broader adult population (Level 2a evidence) [4, 50]. However, both systematic reviews gave a stronger recommendation for psyllium compared to other bulking agents on the basis of an additional four studies that recruited predominantly younger adults (Level 2a evidence) [18, 64–66]. The other bulking agents, including methylcellulose, did not have sufficient evidence for or against their use (Level 2a evidence) [67]. An earlier review that pooled results of six trials evaluating bulking agents or dietary fiber in the adult population arrived at a point estimate of 1.4 more bowel movements per week with fiber (95% confidence interval (CI) 0.6–2.2) [50].

Stool softeners

Three randomized trials of stool softeners in the elderly were found (Level 2b evidence) [68–70]. Dioctyl sodium sulfosuccinate (DSS or docusate sodium) and dioctyl calcium sulfosuccinate (DCS or docusate calcium) were trialed versus placebo. Conflicting results on improvements in stool frequency were found with both agents, and DCS revealed mixed results on impressions of stool consistency.

These findings are consistent with previously published systematic reviews evaluating the efficacy of stool softeners on chronic constipation in the broader adult patient population (level 2b evidence) [67]. One additional trial in adults compared docusate sodium 100 mg BID to psyllium 5.1g BID and found stool frequency to be better with psyllium (3.5 BM/week vs. 2.6 BM/week, $p = 0.021$) [71].

Osmotic laxatives

Polyethylene glycol

PEG was primarily evaluated in older patients in two randomized studies [72, 73] and two other studies with a relatively high proportion of older patients enrolled [74, 75].

Hypotonic PEG was shown to be noninferior to isotonic PEG in a 4-week, double-blind trial of

Table 11.4 Pharmacological treatment of constipation

Category	Dose	Mechanism	Adverse Effects [49]	Contraindications
Bulk forming agents		Increase fecal mass, stimulating peristalsis	Bloating, flatulence, gastrointestinal obstruction, or impaction	Dysphagia, gastrointestinal obstruction, impaction, colonic atony
Psyllium (Metamucil, Fybogel)	Up to 20 g/day			
Methylcellulose (Citrucel)	Up to 20 g/day	Natural fibers undergo bacterial degradation	Rare reports of anaphylaxis and asthma with psyllium; better tolerated if slowly titrated over 1–2 weeks	
Polycarbophil (FiberCon)	Up to 20 g/day			
Stimulants		Increase intestinal motility	Cramps, hypokalemia, melanosis coli (benign condition, usually reversible 12 months after cessation), no definite relation to myenteric nerve damage or carcinoma has been established	Intestinal obstruction
Senna (Senokot, Ex-Lax)	Up to 68.8 g/day			Castor oil may cause severe diarrhea and cramping
Bisacodyl (Dulcolax)	5–10 mg/day			
Cascara	5 mL/day			
Sodium picosulfate	5–15 mg/day			
Castor oil	15–30 mL daily			
Stool softeners		Decrease stool surface tension leading to increased water penetration	Diarrhea, abdominal cramping	
Docusate sodium (Colace)	100 mg twice daily			
Docusate calcium (Surfak)	240 mg twice daily			
Osmotic agents		Increase water content in large bowel	Bloating, flatulence, colic, diarrhea	Gastrointestinal obstruction, paralytic ileus, inflammatory conditions of the gastrointestinal tract (Crohn's, ulcerative colitis (UC))
Polyethylene Glycol (Miralax, Colyte)	17–36 mg/day—twice/day			
Lactulose (Duphalac, Chronulac)	15–30 mL/day—twice/day	Fermentation of lactulose decreases stool pH	Hypermagnesemia, case reports of fatalities even with normal renal function	
Sorbitol (Cystosol)	15–30 mL/day—twice/day		Hyperphosphatemia, hypocalcemia, hypernatremia, hypokalemia	
Magnesium hydroxide (Phillips' Milk of Magnesia)	15–30 mg/day—twice/day			Magnesium is partially absorbed and can lead to hypermagnesemia in patients, particularly those with impaired renal function
Magnesium citrate	150–300 mL			
Sodium phosphate (Fleet phospho-soda, fleet enema)	10–25 mL with 350 mL water			
Lubricants	No more than once daily		Anal seepage of oily material	Generally not recommended in elderly patients
Mineral oil (Fleet mineral oil)			Lipoid pneumonia if taken orally and aspirated	
			May interfere with absorption of fat-soluble vitamins	
Chloride channel stimulators		Stimulates type 2 chloride channel on intestinal epithelial cells promoting a net secretion of fluid into the intestinal lumen	Nausea, headache, diarrhea	Not studied in patients with renal or hepatic impairment
Lubiprostone (Amitiza)	24 μg PO BID			Postmarketing reports of dyspnea following first dose

Table 11.4 *Continued*

Category	Dose	Mechanism	Adverse Effects [49]	Contraindications
Prokinetics Prucalopride	2 mg daily	Stimulates specific 5-HT4 intestinal receptors stimulating peristalsis	Nausea, vomiting, flatulence, headache	Potential cardiac rhythm and vascular abnormalities as seen with two previous drugs of the same class (cisapride and tegaserod)
Rectal enema or suppository Phosphate enema (Fleet enema) Tap water enema Soapsuds enema Glycerin bisacodyl suppository Mineral oil retention enema	120 mL daily 500 mL daily 1500 mL daily 10 mg daily 100 mL daily	Enemas distend the rectum and initiate the reflex to defecate, soften stool, and topically stimulate colonic muscle to contract	Phosphate enema can cause hyperphosphatemia and other electrolyte abnormalities if the enema is retained Soapsuds enema may carry more risk to rectal mucosa than tap water enema	Bowel obstruction

Source: Adapted from Lembo [16].

59 patients, mean age 86, who were chronically constipated and living in long-term care (Level 1b evidence) [72]. Stool frequency was similar at 8.5 and 8.4 bowel movements per week, respectively. PEG was also evaluated in 71 constipated Parkinson's patients and found to be superior to placebo on a composite endpoint of overall subjective relief from symptoms and reduction in Rome Criteria (Level 1b evidence) [73]. Overall, 78.3% of patients on PEG responded versus 25% on placebo, $p = 0.0012$. Stool frequency ($p = 0.002$) and consistency ($p = 0.001$) were also shown to be better with PEG.

PEG was favored (improved stool frequency, straining, overall subjective improvement, and less flatulence) over lactulose in a study with 37% of 115 outpatient participants described as geriatric (mean age 55) (Level 2b evidence) [74]. Another study, with approximately 30% of 100 trial participants over the age of 65, revealed PEG to give more effective relief from constipation secondary to medications than placebo (Level 2b evidence) [75]. Overall, 78% of PEG-treated versus 39% of placebo participants showed improved Rome Criteria ($p < 0.001$). Stool frequency was also statistically higher with PEG ($p < 0.01$). No subgroup analysis by age group was reported in either study.

Lastly, a single-arm trial, with 117 of 311 patients over the age of 65 (mean age of older subgroup = 73.9), evaluated the effects and safety of 17 g of PEG daily over 12 months (Level 2b evidence) [76]. Mean exposure to PEG was 3.7 kg over the 12 months. Subjective reports of improvement were reported by the vast majority, including in the older subgroup. The Rome Criteria revealed that 91%–95% of the older subgroup no longer met diagnostic criteria for constipation. Only 4% dropped out for lack of efficacy. No significant differences in adverse events were noted based on age. Overall, 12.8% of elderly reported diarrhea, 8.5% flatulence, 6.8% nusea, 4.3% loose stool, and 2.6% abdominal pain. No significant laboratory parameter changes were seen in the elderly subgroup [76].

In the broader adult population, PEG has been shown to increase both stool frequency and consistency compared to placebo in several trials (Level 1a evidence) [77–80] and carries a Grade A recommendation from the American College of Gastroenterology [4]. A recent Cochrane review that included both adult and pediatric populations concluded that PEG should be used in preference to lactulose in the treatment of chronic constipation [81]. The study noted PEG to be superior in measures of stool frequency, form of stool, relief of abdominal pain, and the need for additional products. Only four of the ten trials included were conducted in adults. They also noted that findings were consistent in subgroup analyses restricted to adults, but few of the adult trials reported all of the above outcomes.

Lactulose

Three randomized trials evaluate lactulose in the older population (Level 2b evidence) [82–84]. Two were placebo-controlled [82, 83], while the third compared lactulose to sorbitol [84]. Lactulose was favored over placebo in 86% versus 60% of trial participants, respectively ($p < 0.02$), and did not require more than one additional laxative in 21 days [82]. Mean age was not reported but trial participants were described as older. Lactulose also improved stool frequency (0.63 bowel movements per day compared to 0.58 with placebo; $p < 0.02$) in another trial of older volunteers at a 400-bed Home and Medical Care center [83]. Further, episodes of fecal impaction were fewer with lactulose relative to placebo (6 vs. 66; $p < 0.015$).

In the broader adult population, lactulose was studied in a double blind, randomized controlled trial that demonstrated improved stool frequency and consistency [85]. A previous systematic review also rated lactulose as a Grade A recommendation [4].

Sorbitol

One randomized trial found sorbitol to be equivalent to lactulose in stool frequency, consistency, use of additional laxatives, and in a subjective visual analog scale in 30 older patients (Level 2b evidence) [84].

Magnesium

One randomized trial of magnesium hydroxide compared to laxamucil (a mixture of plantain rind and sorbitol) was carried out in 64 older patients (Level 2b evidence) [86]. In nonblinded fashion, magnesium hydroxide was shown to produce a mean of 2.8 more bowel movements over 4 weeks ($p < 0.001$) [86]. Stool consistency ($p < 0.01$) and use of additional laxatives ($p < 0.01$) were also significantly better with magnesium. Adverse events were not reported, but serum magnesium levels averaged 1.46 mmol/L and 1.37 mmol/L in patients with elevated and normal creatinine values, respectively. Magnesium toxicity has in-

frequently been reported in older adults with normal renal function [49].

Stimulants

Four randomized trials evaluating the effects of stimulants in older adults with chronic constipation were found (Level 2b evidence) [59, 87–89]. Bisacodyl, sodium picosulfate, dihydroxyanthraquinone, and senna were all studied compared to other active treatments. The methodology of two trials made the results difficult to interpret [87, 88]. In a comparison of two mixtures of differing proportions of fiber and senna, the preparation with higher senna content revealed superior stool frequency but no test of statistical inference was reported [59]. Lastly, a senna and fiber combination revealed improved stool frequency (0.8 bowel movements per day) versus lactulose (0.6 bowel movements per day; $p < 0.001$) [89]. Stool consistency ($p < 0.005$) and straining ($p = 0.02$) were also improved with the senna/fiber combination.

In the broader adult patient population, previous reviews establish similar levels of evidence [4, 67]. In one placebo-controlled trial conducted over 3 days in patients with acute on chronic constipation, bisacodyl was found to be more effective at improving stool frequency ($p = 0.006$) and consistency ($p < 0.001$) than placebo [90]. Another trial revealed bisacodyl not to be superior to bisoxatin acetate among 61 male prisoners with constipation [91]. A variety of stimulant laxatives were inferior to lactulose in the proportion of patients subjectively experiencing normal stool consistency at 7 days (42.1% vs. 57.8%, respectively; $p < 0.001$) [92].

Prokinetics

One randomized, phase II, safety study of prucalopride (a newer specific 5-HT4 receptor agonist) conducted in older adults was found. Eighty-nine constipated long-term care residents (88% of whom had a cardiovascular disease history) did not show an increase in adverse events with up to 2 mg daily of prucalopride over placebo [93].

In the adult population, there are several trials demonstrating the efficacy of prucalopride in the treatment of chronic constipation (Level 1b evidence) [94–96]. Despite these trials, concerns over prucalopride's electrophysiologic effects, overall safety, and significant delays in data publication have been noted [97]. Previous generation compounds affecting the gastrointestinal serotonergic system, cisapride and tegaserod, were both removed from the market due to safety concerns. Cisapride was associated with a prolonged QT interval and sudden cardiac death, whereas tegaserod increased cardiovascular events.

Lubiprostone

No randomized trials of lubiprostone in the older population were found. In a study that primarily enrolled adult women, 24 μg of lubiprostone twice daily outperformed placebo in improving stool frequency and associated symptoms of constipation (Level 1b evidence) [98]. Nausea was more frequently seen with treatment (31.7% vs. 3.3%; $p < 0.001$). Pooled data from approximately 1000 patients (10%–18% aged 65 years or older) showed no changes in serum electrolytes (Level 2c evidence) [99]. Dyspnea within 1 hour of the first dose has been seen in postmarketing data and the drug has not been studied in patients with renal or hepatic impairment [99].

Enemas and suppositories

In one randomized trial, frail, long-term care residents with a history of fecal impaction and incontinence were treated with oral lactulose or oral lactulose with a daily glycerine suppository and weekly tap water enema [100]. Over 5 weeks, the suppositories and enemas did not affect the primary outcome of episodes of incontinence and soiled laundry. A subgroup of responders, defined as three consecutive rectal examinations yielding an empty vault, did show a significant difference in the primary outcome in favor of the combined treatment arm ($p < 0.02$).

Clinical bottom line

Studies of bulking agents have not shown consistent improvement in constipated elders. In younger adults, psyllium demonstrates more consistent improvement in stool frequency compared to placebo than other bulking agents.

Studies of stool softeners have not shown consistent results in constipated elders.

Studies of PEG in older adults with chronic constipation have consistently shown improvement, similar to findings in younger adults. In one study involving older adults, PEG 17 g daily for a year was shown to be safe. Studies of lactulose in older adults with chronic constipation have consistently shown benefit.

Stimulant agents have not been trialed versus placebo in older patients with chronic constipation.

Safety concerns have LED TO removal OF previous generation prokinetic agents from the market and relatively few older adults have been exposed to the newest agent, prucalopride, in published trials. As such, we do not recommend prucalopride in older adults with chronic constipation AT THIS TIME.

Due to the limited experience with lubiprostone, the significantly increased incidence of nausea, and potential for adverse pulmonary events, a recommendation for its use in the older adult population cannot be made at this time.

Enemas and suppositories have not been well studied in the management of chronic constipation, though there may be a role for them when used in combination with other laxatives.

How should constipation be managed among patients on opioid analgesics?

Conventional thought claims that stimulants are generally required in patients who suffer constipation secondary to opioids. No randomized trials were found to confirm or refute that claim. A trial of methylnaltrexone compared to placebo in 133 terminally ill older adults (mean age = 72) on high doses of narcotics (median morphine equivalent = 100 − 150 mg) revealed improved rescue-free laxation within 4 hours after each dose without increased pain ($p < 0.001$) (Level 1b evidence) [101].

In adults, one randomized trial evaluating PEG in relieving constipation secondary to medications (any medication with a 3% or higher incidence of constipation according to a reference manual) found PEG superior to placebo (78% relief vs. 39%; $p < 0.001$) (Level 1b evidence) [75]. Thirty-two of the 100 study patients were using opioids. Subgroup analysis in older patients revealed a trend toward improvement with PEG but was limited by sample size [75]. Finally, a three-arm randomized trial of 57 younger adults (mean age unknown) in a methadone maintenance program who complained of constipation revealed similar beneficial effects of both PEG and lactulose over placebo at improving stool consistency but not frequency (Level 2b evidence) [102].

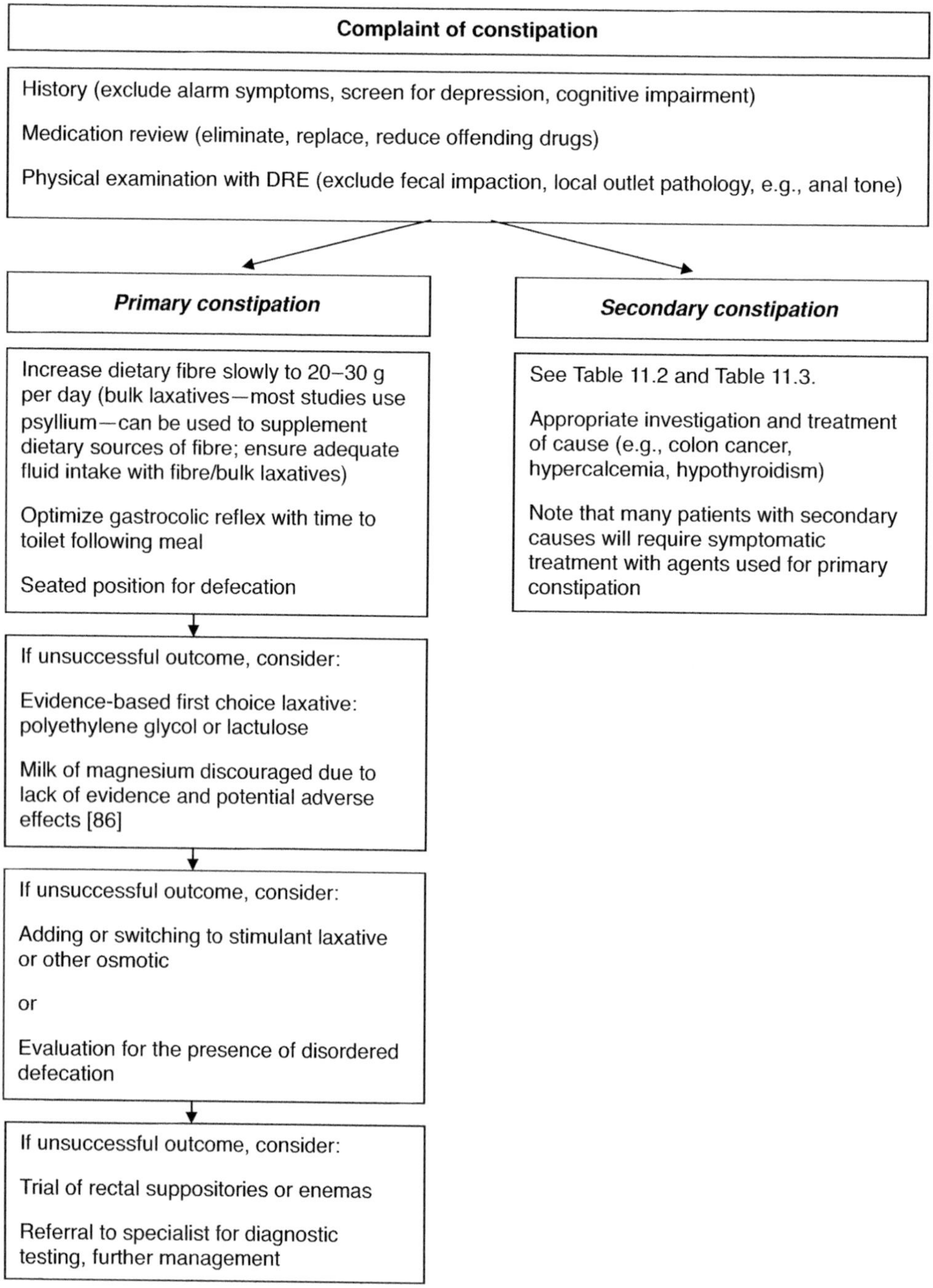

Complaint of constipation

History (exclude alarm symptoms, screen for depression, cognitive impairment) Medication review (eliminate, replace, reduce offending drugs) Physical examination with DRE (exclude fecal impaction, local outlet pathology, e.g., anal tone)

Primary constipation	Secondary constipation
Increase dietary fibre slowly to 20–30 g per day (bulk laxatives—most studies use psyllium—can be used to supplement dietary sources of fibre; ensure adequate fluid intake with fibre/bulk laxatives) Optimize gastrocolic reflex with time to toilet following meal Seated position for defecation	See Table 11.2 and Table 11.3. Appropriate investigation and treatment of cause (e.g., colon cancer, hypercalcemia, hypothyroidism) Note that many patients with secondary causes will require symptomatic treatment with agents used for primary constipation

If unsuccessful outcome, consider: Evidence-based first choice laxative: polyethylene glycol or lactulose Milk of magnesium discouraged due to lack of evidence and potential adverse effects [86]

If unsuccessful outcome, consider: Adding or switching to stimulant laxative or other osmotic or Evaluation for the presence of disordered defecation

If unsuccessful outcome, consider: Trial of rectal suppositories or enemas Referral to specialist for diagnostic testing, further management

Figure 11.1 Management algorithm for constipation.

Clinical bottom line

PEG appears to help relieve constipation secondary to opioids.

Should my patient with severe constipation have colonic surgery?

No randomized trials where found of surgical versus medical treatment for severe constipation in older adults. Surgery, including subtotal colectomy, for chronic constipation is rarely required. The evaluation of the risks and benefits should be made in consultation with an expert only after conventional therapies have failed.

Is there evidence to treat constipation with biofeedback?

In the adult population, multiple trials have shown biofeedback to be effective in the treatment of chronic constipation secondary to dyssynergic defecation [103–105]. Older adults with cognitive impairment, depending on severity, are not likely candidates for biofeedback therapy.

Chapter summary

A diagnosis of chronic constipation can be made more rigorously by using the Rome Criteria and a suggested management algorithm is provided in Figure 11.1. A careful history and physical exam should be performed in older patients who present with chronic constipation with particular attention to medications, alarm symptoms, signs of fecal impaction, and candidacy for local colon cancer screening guidelines. Thereafter, nonpharmacologic measures are recommended to facilitate satisfactory bowel movements. Bulking agents can be considered, particularly if it is difficult to increase dietary fiber to 20–30 g per day; psyllium is the most studied of the bulking agents. Often, pharmacologic treatment will be necessary and evidence suggests either PEG or lactulose to be the preferred options. Stimulant laxatives may be substituted or added if treatment with PEG or lactulose is insufficient, although there is little formal evidence to confirm their usefulness.

If symptoms persist, based on history and physical examination, dyssynergic defecation should be considered (either by the primary care physician or with the assistance of a specialist) and use of enemas or suppositories may help relieve the problem. For willing and able older patients, a referral to a specialist for more definitive testing and treatment can also be made.

References

1. Sonnenberg A, Koch TR (1989) Physician visits in the united states for constipation: 1958 to 1986. *Dig Dis Sci* 34(4): 606–611.
2. Wald A (1994) Constipation and fecal incontinence in the elderly. *Semin Gastrointest Dis* 5(4): 179–188.
3. Camilleri M, Lee JS, Viramontes B, Bharucha AE, Tangalos EG (2000) Insights into the pathophysiology and mechanisms of constipation, irritable bowel syndrome, and diverticulosis in older people. *J Am Geriatr Soc* 48(9): 1142–1150.
4. Brandt LJ, Prather CM, Quigley EM, Schiller LR, Schoenfeld P, Talley NJ. (2005) Systematic review on the management of chronic constipation in North America. *Am J Gastroenterol* 100(Suppl. 1): S5–S21.
5. Kinnunen O (1991) Study of constipation in a geriatric hospital, day hospital, old people's home and at home. *Aging Clin Exp Res* 3(2): 161–170.
6. Campbell AJ, Busby WJ, Horwath CC (1993) Factors associated with constipation in a community based sample of people aged 70 years and over. *J Epidemiol Community Health* 47(1): 23–26.
7. Tariq SH (2007) Constipation in long-term care. *J Am Med Dir Assoc* 8(4): 209–218.
8. Stewart RB, Moore MT, Marks RG, Hale WE (1992) Correlates of constipation in an ambulatory elderly population. *Am J Gastroenterol* 87(7): 859–864.
9. Towers AL, Burgio KL, Locher JL, Merkel IS, Safaeian M, Wald A (1994) Constipation in the elderly: influence of dietary, psychological, and physiological factors. *J Am Geriatr Soc* 42(7): 701–706.
10. Choung RS, Locke GR, 3rd, Schleck CD, Zinsmeister AR, Talley NJ (2007) Cumulative incidence of chronic constipation: a population-based study 1988–2003. *Aliment Pharmacol Ther* 26(11-12): 1521–1528.
11. Glia A, Lindberg G (1997) Quality of life in patients with different types of functional constipation. *Scand J Gastroenterol* 32(11): 1083–1089.
12. Frank L, et al (2002) Time and economic cost of constipation care in nursing homes. *J Am Med Dir Assoc* 3: 215–223.
13. Hosia-Randell H, Suominen M, Muurinen S, Pitkala KH (2007) Use of laxatives among older nursing home residents in Helsinki, Finland. *Drugs Aging* 24(2): 147–154.
14. Jones MP, Talley NJ, Nuyts G, Dubois D (2002) Lack of objective evidence of efficacy of laxatives in chronic constipation. *Dig Dis Sci* 47(10): 2222–2230.
15. McCrea GL, Miaskowski C, Stotts NA, Macera L, Varma MG (2008) Pathophysiology of constipation in the older adult. *World J Gastroenterol* 14(17): 2631–2638.
16. Lembo A, Camilleri M (2003) Chronic constipation. *N Engl J Med* 349(14): 1360–1368.

17. Longstreth GF, Thompson WG, Chey WD, Houghton LA, Mearin F, Spiller RC (2006) Functional bowel disorders. *Gastroenterology* 130(5): 1480–1491.

18. Ashraf W, Park F, Lof J, Quigley EM (1995) Effects of psyllium therapy on stool characteristics, colon transit and anorectal function in chronic idiopathic constipation. *Aliment Pharmacol Ther* 9(6): 639–647.

19. Whitehead WE, Drinkwater D, Cheskin LJ, Heller BR, Schuster MM (1989) Constipation in the elderly living at home. Definition, prevalence, and relationship to lifestyle and health status. *J Am Geriatr Soc* 37(5): 423–429.

20. Harari D, Gurwitz JH, Avorn J, Bohn R, Minaker KL (1996) Bowel habit in relation to age and gender. Findings from the national health interview survey and clinical implications. *Arch Intern Med* 156(3): 315–320.

21. Harari D, Gurwitz JH, Avorn J, Bohn R, Minaker KL (1997) How do older persons define constipation? Implications for therapeutic management. *J Gen Intern Med* 12(1): 63–66.

22. Ashraf W, Park F, Lof J, Quigley EM (1996) An examination of the reliability of reported stool frequency in the diagnosis of idiopathic constipation. *Am J Gastroenterol* 91(1): 26–32.

23. Schaefer DC, Cheskin LJ (1998) Constipation in the elderly. *Am Fam Physician* 58(4): 907–914.

24. McCrea GL, Miaskowski C, Stotts NA, Macera L, Varma MG (2008) Pathophysiology of constipation in the older adult. *World J Gastroenterol* 14(17): 2631–2638.

25. Merkel IS, Locher J, Burgio K, Towers A, Wald A (1993) Physiologic and psychologic characteristics of an elderly population with chronic constipation. *Am J Gastroenterol* 88(11): 1854–1859.

26. Bannister JJ, Abouzekry L, Read NW (1987) Effect of aging on anorectal function. *Gut* 28(3): 353–357.

27. Evans JM, Fleming KC, Talley NJ, Schleck CD, Zinsmeister AR, Melton LJ, 3rd (1998) Relation of colonic transit to functional bowel disease in older people: a population-based study. *J Am Geriatr Soc* 46(1): 83–87.

28. Loening-Baucke V, Anuras S (1984) Sigmoidal and rectal motility in healthy elderly. *J Am Geriatr Soc* 32(12): 887–891.

29. Madsen JL (1992) Effects of gender, age, and body mass index on gastrointestinal transit times. *Dig Dis Sci* 37(10): 1548–1553.

30. Leung FW (2007) Etiologic factors of chronic constipation: review of the scientific evidence. *Dig Dis Sci* 52(2): 313–316.

31. Muller-Lissner SA, Kamm MA, Scarpignato C, Wald A (2005) Myths and misconceptions about chronic constipation. *Am J Gastroenterol* 100(1): 232–242.

32. Lindeman RD, Romero LJ, Liang HC, Baumgartner RN, Koehler KM, Garry PJ (2000) Do elderly persons need to be encouraged to drink more fluids? *J Gerontol A Biol Sci Med Sci* 55(7): M361–M365.

33. Mertz H, Naliboff B, Mayer EA (1999) Symptoms and physiology in severe chronic constipation. *Am J Gastroenterol* 94(1): 131–138.

34. Nyam DC, Pemberton JH, Ilstrup DM, Rath DM (1997) Long-term results of surgery for chronic constipation. *Dis Colon Rectum* 40(3): 273–279.

35. Gallagher P, O'Mahony D (2009) Constipation in old age. *Best Pract Res Clin Gastroenterol* 23(6): 875–887.

36. Lewis SJ, Heaton KW (1997) Stool form scale as a useful guide to intestinal transit time. *Scand J Gastroenterol* 32(9): 920–924.

37. Saad RJ, et al (2010) Do stool form and frequency correlate with whole-gut and colonic transit? Results from a multicenter study in constipated individuals and healthy controls. *Am J Gastroenterol* 105(2): 403–411.

38. Rao SS, Ozturk R, Laine L (2005) Clinical utility of diagnostic tests for constipation in adults: a systematic review. *Am J Gastroenterol* 100(7): 1605–1615.

39. Culbert P, Gillett H, Ferguson A (1998) Highly effective new oral therapy for faecal impaction. *Br J Gen Pract* 48(434): 1599–1600.

40. Wrenn K (1989) Fecal impaction. *N Engl J Med* 321(10): 658–662.

41. Schmelzer M (1990) Effectiveness of wheat bran in preventing constipation of hospitalized orthopaedic surgery patients. *Orthop Nurs* 9(6): 55–59.

42. Kochen MM, Wegscheider K, Abholz HH (1985) Prophylaxis of constipation by wheat bran: a randomized study in hospitalized patients. *Digestion* 31(4): 220–224.

43. Graham DY, Moser SE, Estes MK (1982) The effect of bran on bowel function in constipation. *Am J Gastroenterol* 77(9): 599–603.

44. Meshkinpour H, Selod S, Movahedi H, Nami N, James N, Wilson A (1998) Effects of regular exercise in management of chronic idiopathic constipation. *Dig Dis Sci* 43(11): 2379–2383.

45. Karam SE, Nies DM (1994) Student/staff collaboration: a pilot bowel management program. *J Gerontol Nurs* 20(3): 32–40.

46. Rao SS, Kavlock R, Rao S (2006) Influence of body position and stool characteristics on defecation in humans. *Am J Gastroenterol* 101(12): 2790–2796.

47. Harari D, Norton C, Lockwood L, Swift C (2004) Treatment of constipation and fecal incontinence in stroke patients: randomized controlled trial. *Stroke* 35(11): 2549–2555.

48. Lamas K, Lindholm L, Stenlund H, Engstrom B, Jacobsson C (2009) Effects of abdominal massage in management of constipation–a randomized controlled trial. *Int J Nurs Stud* 46(6): 759–767.

49. Xing JH, Soffer EE (2001) Adverse effects of laxatives. *Dis Colon Rectum* 44(8): 1201–1209.

50. Tramonte SM, Brand MB, Mulrow CD, Amato MG, O'Keefe ME, Ramirez G (1997) The treatment of chronic constipation in adults. A systematic review. *J Gen Intern Med* 12(1): 15–24.

51. Scott IA, Guyatt GH (2010) Cautionary tales in the interpretation of clinical studies involving older persons. *Arch Intern Med* 170(7): 587–595.

52. Cheskin LJ, Kamal N, Crowell MD, Schuster MM, Whitehead WE (1995) Mechanisms of constipation in older

persons and effects of fiber compared with placebo. *J Am Geriatr Soc* 43(6): 666–669.

53. Rajala SA, Salminen SJ, Seppanen JH, Vapaatalo H (1988) Treatment of chronic constipation with lactitol sweetened yoghurt supplemented with guar gum and wheat bran in elderly hospital in-patients. *Compr Gerontol [A]* 2(2): 83–86.

54. Teuri U, Korpela R (1998) Galacto-oligosaccharides relieve constipation in elderly people. *Ann Nutr Metab* 42(6): 319–327.

55. Howard LV, West D, Ossip-Klein DJ (2000) Chronic constipation management for institutionalized older adults. *Geriatr Nurs* quiz 82-3; 21(2): 78–82.

56. Snustad D, Lee V, Abraham I, Alexander C, Bella D, Cumming C (1991) Dietary fiber in hospitalized geriatric patients: too soft a solution for too hard a problem?. *J Nutr Elder* 10(2): 49–63.

57. Sairanen U, Piirainen L, Nevala R, Korpela R (2007) Yoghurt containing galacto-oligosaccharides, prunes and linseed reduces the severity of mild constipation in elderly subjects. *Eur J Clin Nutr* 61(12): 1423–1428.

58. Finlay M (1988) The use of dietary fibre in a long-stay geriatric ward. *J Nutr Elder* 8(1): 19–30.

59. Pers M, Pers B. (1983) A crossover comparative study with two bulk laxatives. *J Int Med Res* 11(1): 51–53.

60. Mamtani R, Cimino JA, Kugel R, Cooperman JM (1989) A calcium salt of an insoluble synthetic bulking laxative in elderly bedridden nursing home residents. *J Am Coll Nutr* 8(6): 554–556.

61. Passmore AP, Wilson-Davies K, Stoker C, Scott ME (1993) Chronic constipation in long stay elderly patients: a comparison of lactulose and a senna-fibre combination. *BMJ* 307(6907): 769–771.

62. Kinnunen O, Winblad I, Koistinen P, Salokannel J (1993) Safety and efficacy of a bulk laxative containing senna versus lactulose in the treatment of chronic constipation in geriatric patients. *Pharmacology* 47(Suppl. 1): 253–255.

63. Stern FH (1966) Constipation—an omnipresent symptom: effect of a preparation containing prune concentrate and cascarin. *J Am Geriatr Soc* 14(11): 1153–1155.

64. Fenn GC, Wilkinson PD, Lee CE, Akbar FA (1986) A general practice study of the efficacy of regulan in functional constipation. *Br J Clin Pract* 40(5): 192–197.

65. Rouse M, Mahapatra M, Atkinson SN, Prescott P (1991) An open, randomised, parallel group study of lactulose versus ispaghula in the treatment of chronic constipation in adults. *BJCP* 45(1): 28–30.

66. Dettmar PW, Sykes J (1998) A multi-centre, general practice comparison of ispaghula husk with lactulose and other laxatives in the treatment of simple constipation. *Curr Med Res Opin* 14(4): 227–233.

67. Ramkumar D, Rao SS (2005) Efficacy and safety of traditional medical therapies for chronic constipation: systematic review. *Am J Gastroenterol* 100(4): 936–971.

68. Hyland CM, Foran JD (1968) Dioctyl sodium sulphosuccinate as a laxative in the elderly. *Practitioner* 200(199): 698–699.

69. Fain AM, Susat R, Herring M, Dorton K (1978) Treatment of constipation in geriatric and chronically ill patients: a comparison. *South Med J* 71(6): 677–680.

70. Castle SC, Cantrell M, Israel DS, Samuelson MJ (1991) Constipation prevention: empiric use of stool softeners questioned. *Geriatrics* 46(11): 84–86.

71. McRorie JW, Daggy BP, Morel JG, Diersing PS, Miner PB, Robinson M (1998) Psyllium is superior to docusate sodium for treatment of chronic constipation. *Aliment Pharmacol Ther* 12(5): 491–497.

72. Seinela L, Sairanen U, Laine T, Kurl S, Pettersson T, Happonen P (2009) Comparison of polyethylene glycol with and without electrolytes in the treatment of constipation in elderly institutionalized patients: a randomized, double-blind, parallel-group study. *Drugs Aging* 26(8): 703–713.

73. Zangaglia R, et al (2007) Macrogol for the treatment of constipation in Parkinson's disease. A randomized placebo-controlled study. *Mov Disord* 22(9): 1239–1244.

74. Attar A, et al (1999) Comparison of a low dose polyethylene glycol electrolyte solution with lactulose for treatment of chronic constipation. *Gut* 44(2): 226–230.

75. DiPalma JA, Cleveland MB, McGowan J, Herrera JL (2007) A comparison of polyethylene glycol laxative and placebo for relief of constipation from constipating medications. *South Med J* 100(11): 1085–1090.

76. Di Palma JA, Cleveland MV, McGowan J, Herrera JL (2007) An open-label study of chronic polyethylene glycol laxative use in chronic constipation. *Aliment Pharmacol Ther* 25(6): 703–708.

77. Andorsky RI, Goldner F (1990) Colonic lavage solution (polyethylene glycol electrolyte lavage solution) as a treatment for chronic constipation: a double-blind, placebo-controlled study. *Am J Gastroenterol* 85(3): 261–265.

78. Corazziari E, et al (1996) Small volume isosmotic polyethylene glycol electrolyte balanced solution (PMF-100) in treatment of chronic nonorganic constipation. *Dig Dis Sci* 41(8): 1636–1642.

79. Corazziari E, et al (2000) Long term efficacy, safety, and tolerability of low daily doses of isosmotic polyethylene glycol electrolyte balanced solution (PMF-100) in the treatment of functional chronic constipation. *Gut* 46(4): 522–526.

80. Cleveland MB, Flavin DP, Ruben RA, Epstein RM, Clark GE (2001) New polyethylene glycol laxative for treatment of constipation in adults: a randomized, double-blind, placebo-controlled study. *South Med J* 94(5): 478–481.

81. Lee-Robichaud H, Thomas K, Morgan J, Nelson RL (2010) Lactulose versus polyethylene glycol for chronic constipation. *Cochrane Database of Systematic Reviews* (7): CD007570.

82. Wesselius-De Casparis A, Braadbaart S, Bergh-Bohlken GE, Mimica M (1968) Treatment of chronic constipation with lactulose syrup: results of a double-blind study. *Gut* 9(1): 84–86.

83. Sanders JF (1978) Lactulose syrup assessed in a double-blind study of elderly constipated patients. *J Am Geriatr Soc* 26(5): 236–239.

84. Lederle FA, Busch DL, Mattox KM, West MJ, Aske DM (1990) Cost-effective treatment of constipation in the elderly: a randomized double-blind comparison of sorbitol and lactulose. *Am J Med* 89(5): 597–601.

85. Bass P, Dennis S (1981) The Laxative effects of lactulose in normal and constipated subjects. *J Clin Gastroenterol* 3(Suppl. 1): 23–28.

86. Kinnunen O, Salokannel J (1987) Constipation in elderly long-stay patients: its treatment by magnesium hydroxide and bulk-laxative. *Ann Clin Res* 19(5): 321–323.

87. Christopher LJ (1969) A controlled trial of laxatives in geriatric patients. *Practitioner* 202(212): 821–825.

88. Williamson J, Coll M, Connolly M (1975) A comparative trial of a new laxative. *Nursing Times* 23: 1705–1707.

89. Passmore AP, Davies KW, Flanagan PG, Stoker C, Scott MG (1993) A comparison of agiolax and lactulose in elderly patients with chronic constipation. *Pharmacology* 47(Suppl. 1): 249–252.

90. Kienzle-Horn S, Vix JM, Schuijt C, Peil H, Jordan CC, Kamm MA (2006) Efficacy and safety of bisacodyl in the acute treatment of constipation: a double-blind, randomized, placebo-controlled study. *Aliment Pharmacol Ther* 23(10): 1479–1488.

91. Rider JA (1971) Treatment of acute and chronic constipation with bisoxatin acetate and bisacodyl. Double-blind crossover study. *Curr Ther Res Clin Exp* 13(6): 386–392.

92. Connolly P, Hughes IW, Ryan G (1974-1975) Comparison of "duphalac" and "irritant" laxatives during and after treatment of chronic constipation: a preliminary study. *Curr Med Res Opin* 2(10): 620–625.

93. Camilleri M, Beyens G, Kerstens R, Robinson P, Vandeplassche L (2009) Safety assessment of prucalopride in elderly patients with constipation: a double-blind, placebo-controlled study. *Neurogastroenterol Motil* 21(12): 1256-e117.

94. Camilleri M, Kerstens R, Rykx A, Vandeplassche L (2008) A placebo-controlled trial of prucalopride for severe chronic constipation. *N Engl J Med* 358(22): 2344–2354.

95. Coremans G, Kerstens R, De Pauw M, Stevens M (2003) Prucalopride is effective in patients with severe chronic constipation in whom laxatives fail to provide adequate relief. Results of a double-blind, placebo-controlled clinical trial. *Digestion* 67(1-2): 82–89.

96. Emmanuel AV, Roy AJ, Nicholls TJ, Kamm MA (2002) Prucalopride, a systemic enterokinetic, for the treatment of constipation. *Aliment Pharmacol Ther* 16(7): 1347–1356.

97. Moss AJ (2008) The long and short of a constipation-reducing medication. *N Engl J Med* 358(22): 2402–2403.

98. Johanson JF, Morton D, Geenen J, Ueno R. (2008) Multicenter, 4-week, double-blind, randomized, placebo-controlled trial of lubiprostone, a locally-acting type-2 chloride channel activator, in patients with chronic constipation. *Am J Gastroenterol* 103: 170–177.

99. Lacy BE, Chey WD (2009) Lubiprostone: chronic constipation and irritable bowel syndrome with constipation. *Expert Opin Pharmacother* 10(1): 143–152.

100. Chassagne P, et al (2000) Does treatment of constipation improve faecal incontinence in institutionalized elderly patients?. *Age Ageing* 29(2): 159–164.

101. Thomas J, et al (2008) Methylnaltrexone for opioid-induced constipation in advanced illness. *N Engl J Med* 358(22): 2332–2343.

102. Freedman MD, Schwartz HJ, Roby R, Fleisher S. (1997) Tolerance and efficacy of polyethylene glycol 3350/electrolyte solution versus lactulose in relieving opiate induced constipation: a double-blinded placebo-controlled trial. *J Clin Pharmacol* 37: 904–907.

103. Rao SS, et al (2007) Randomized controlled trial of biofeedback, sham feedback, and standard therapy for dyssynergic defecation. *Clin Gastroenterol Hepatol* 5(3): 331–338.

104. Rao SS, Valestin J, Brown CK, Zimmerman B, Schulze K (2010) Long-term efficacy of biofeedback therapy for dyssynergic defecation: randomized controlled trial. *Am J Gastroenterol* 105(4): 890–896.

105. Heymen S, Jones KR, Scarlett Y, Whitehead WE (2003) Biofeedback treatment of constipation: a critical review. *Dis Colon Rectum* 46(9): 1208–1217.

CHAPTER 12

Preventing and treating pressure ulcers

*Madhuri Reddy[1], Sudeep S. Gill[2], Sunila R. Kalkar[3], Wei Wu[3], &
Paula A. Rochon[3,4,5]*

[1]*Hebrew Senior Life, Boston, MA, USA*
[2]*Department of Medicine, Division of Geriatric Medicine Queen's University, Kingston, ON, Canada*
[3]*Women's College Research Institute, Women's College Hospital, Toronto, ON, Canada*
[4]*Institute for Clinical Evaluative Sciences, Toronto, ON, Canada*
[5]*Department of Medicine, University of Toronto, Toronto, ON, Canada*

Introduction

Pressure ulcers are a common but potentially preventable condition seen most often in high-risk populations, such as the older adult [1]. These wounds most often develop over bony prominences such as the coccyx or heels [1–3]. The incidence rates of pressure ulcers vary by clinical setting, and range from 0.4%–38% in acute care, 2.2%–23.9% in long-term care (LTC), and 0%–17% in home care [2].

Pressure ulcers can contribute to pain and infection, and result in longer lengths of hospital stays [4]. Pressure ulcers are a marker of poor overall prognosis, and may contribute to premature mortality [5, 6]. Treatment is costly, and is estimated at $11 billion per year in the United States [8, 9].

While it is possible to prevent most pressure ulcers, many patients continue to develop them [2, 4]. Hundreds of wound care products are currently available [4], but only a few have been evaluated in randomized controlled trials (RCTs) [5–9].

Diagnosing infection in pressure ulcers and wounds resulting from other causes (e.g., venous insufficiency) is a common challenge faced by clinicians. In older adults, infected pressure ulcers can lead to sepsis and be a precursor to death [10]. Infected pressure ulcers are one of the leading causes of infections in LTC facilities [11]. The classic signs of infection (such as purulent exudate and erythema) may be absent in chronic wounds [12].

This chapter is based on three of our previous publications [4, 9, 13] and is written for physicians, nurses, and other healthcare professionals working in LTC or acute care, who are not specialists in wound care. We have updated our previous findings and have also included information from more recent systematic reviews. In this chapter, we review interventions for the prevention and treatment of pressure ulcers. We also review important issues related to the diagnosis of infection in chronic wounds.

The methodological quality of RCTs evaluating interventions to prevent and treat pressure ulcers is relatively poor. Consequently, in addition to providing guidance on evidence-based interventions, we have also included in this chapter a compilation of the major guidelines for the prevention and treatment of pressure ulcers (Tables 12.1 and 12.2). Some of these recommendations are based on little evidence or expert opinion.

Search strategy

We employed a systematic literature search and selection process in order to identify the available articles investigating pressure ulcers and also the diagnosis of infection in chronic wounds. Because of the paucity of

Evidence-Based Geriatric Medicine: A Practical Clinical Guide, First Edition. Edited by Jayna M. Holroyd-Leduc and Madhuri Reddy.
© 2012 Blackwell Publishing Ltd. Published 2012 by Blackwell Publishing Ltd.

Table 12.1 Prevention of pressure ulcers

Topic	Guideline
Risk assessment	Establish a risk assessment policy in all healthcare settings All patients admitted to a healthcare setting should have a risk assessment (e.g., Braden scale) performed and documented within the time frame specified by regulations Risk assessment should be repeated regularly as required by patient acuity Patients should be rescreened when there is a significant change in their condition Risk assessment should include a complete skin assessment
Skin assessment	Skin assessment should be performed regularly and more frequently if the patient's condition deteriorates Skin assessment should include assessment for signs of redness, localized heat, edema, or induration; and for pressure damage caused by medical devices (e.g., catheters)
Skin care	Use moisturizers for dry skin Use a topical barrier product to reduce excessive skin moisture
Positioning	Frequency of repositioning varies depending on such variables as the patient's level of activity, overall treatment objectives, and the support surface used Document repositioning regimens (including frequency and positions) Use transfer aids to reduce friction and shear. Lift (don't drag) the patient during repositioning Avoid positions that increase pressure, such as the 90° side lying position or the semirecumbent position. Reposition using, for example, the 30° tilted side lying position For patients in chairs, place the feet on a footrest when the feet do not reach the floor
Support surfaces	Continue to reposition patients at risk of pressure ulcer development, regardless of the type of mattress used Use high-specification foam mattresses rather than standard hospital foam mattresses for those at risk of pressure ulcer development Keep heels off the surface of the bed (e.g., use a pillow under the calf muscles to "float" heels) For those seated and at risk of pressure ulcer development, use a pressure-redistributing seat cushion Avoid donut-shaped devices and synthetic sheepskin pads Natural sheepskin may help to prevent pressure ulcers Use a pressure-redistributing mattress on the operating table, as well as prior to and after surgery, for all patients at risk of pressure ulcer development
Nutrition	Screen all patients at risk of pressure ulcers in each healthcare setting Refer patients at risk of poor nutrition and pressure ulcer development to a registered dietitian Offer adequate protein and total caloric intake for patients at risk of poor nutrition and pressure ulcer development

Source: Data from Prevention and Treatment of Pressure Ulcers: Clinical Practice Guideline (developed by the National Pressure Ulcer Advisory Panel and European Pressure Ulcer Advisory Panel) and Guidelines for the Prevention of Pressure Ulcers (Wound Healing Society)[a,b]

[a]National Pressure Ulcer Advisory Panel and European Pressure Ulcer Advisory Panel (2009) Prevention and treatment of pressure ulcers: clinical practice guideline. Washington DC: National Pressure Ulcer Advisory Panel.

[b]Stechmiller JK, Cown L, Whitney J, et al (2008) Guidelines for the prevention of pressure ulcers. *Wound Rep Reg* 16: 151–168.

well-designed wound trials, we did not limit our search to older adults.

For the first question, "What are the best ways to prevent pressure ulcers?," we had performed a previous systematic review, published in 2006 [4]. For that sys-tematic review, we searched MEDLINE, EMBASE, and CINAHL from inception through June 2006, and the Cochrane Database (Issue 1, 2006), to identify relevant RCTs and systematic reviews. We also searched UMI Proquest Digital Dissertations, ISI Web of Science,

Table 12.2 Medical management of pressure ulcers

Topic	Guideline
Positioning	Reposition regardless of the support surface being used Establish a repositioning schedule and do not position patients on a pressure ulcer Maintain the head of the bed ≤30° unless contraindicated (higher elevation, plus a slouched position, places pressure and shear on the sacrum and coccyx) 30°–40° side lying position or flat in bed (rather than 90° side lying) position is recommended for sleeping Use transfer aids and lift (rather than drag) while repositioning, in order to reduce friction and shear Limit time on a bedpan to the minimum necessary
Support surfaces	Support surfaces alone do not heal pressure ulcers A nonpowered support surface may be appropriate for Stage I & II pressure ulcers: • High-specification foam • Pressure-redistribution cushion in a chair • Minimize seating time and consult a seating specialist if pressure ulcers continue to deteriorate • Relieve heel pressure by placing pillows under the calf muscles to elevate heels off the bed, or by using pressure-reducing devices with heel suspension A powered support surface may be appropriate for patients with a pressure ulcer: • who cannot be repositioned, • has pressure ulcers on two or more turning surfaces, or • who fails to heal or deteriorates despite comprehensive care In patients who have a large stage III or stage IV pressure ulcer, or multiple pressure ulcers involving several turning surfaces, a low-air loss or air-fluidized bed may be indicated. For pressure ulcers secondary to sitting: • Minimize seating time • Use a seat cushion based on the needs of the individual. • Consult a seating specialist if pressure ulcers continue to deteriorate. Avoid donut-shaped devices
Nutrition	Nutritional assessment should be performed on entry to a new healthcare setting and whenever there is a change in an individual's condition that may increase the risk of under nutrition Encourage dietary intake or supplementation if an individual who is undernourished is at risk of developing a pressure ulcer Ensure adequate dietary intake to prevent undernutrition to the extent that this is compatible with the individual's wishes If dietary intake continues to be inadequate, impractical, or impossible, nutritional support (usually tube feeding) should be considered Give vitamin and mineral supplements if deficiencies are confirmed or suspected
Debridement	Initial and maintenance debridement is required if consistent with overall goals of care No one debridement method is consistently superior to another. One of a number of debridement methods (including sharp surgical, autolytic, mechanical, or enzymatic) can be selected Perform a thorough vascular assessment before debriding lower extremity pressure ulcers Use sharp debridement with caution in the presence of compromised vascular supply to the limb Tunneling wounds, sinuses, or cavities must be deroofed and treated
Wound bed preparation	Examine the patient's systemic diseases and medications Examine the patient's tissue perfusion and oxygenation Wounds should be cleansed initially and at each dressing change using a neutral, nonirritating, nontoxic solution Infection control should be achieved by reducing wound bacterial burden and achieving wound bacterial balance

continued

Table 12.2 *Continued*

Topic	Guideline
	Achieve local moisture balance by management of exudate
	There should be an ongoing and consistent documentation of wound history, recurrence, and characteristics (location, staging, size, base, exudates, infection, condition of surrounding skin, and pain)
	The rate of wound healing should be evaluated to determine whether treatment is optimal
Dressings	Choose a dressing that will keep the wound bed moist
	Select a dressing that will manage the wound exudate and protect the periulcer skin
	Select a dressing that is cost-effective
	Consider hydrocolloid dressing for clean Stage II and noninfected, shallow Stage III pressure ulcers
	Consider a hydrogel dressing for shallow, minimally exudating pressure ulcers
	Consider an alginate dressing for moderately and heavily exudating pressure ulcers
	Consider a foam dressing on exudative Stage II and shallow Stage III pressure ulcers
	Consider silver dressings for pressure ulcers at high risk of infection
	Consider silver dressing FOR PRESSURE ULCERS that are infected or heavily colonized
	Consider use of cadexomer iodine dressings in moderately to highly exudating pressure ulcers
	Avoid use of gauze dressings for clean pressure ulcers
	Consider silicone dressings for atraumatic dressings changes (e.g., when the periwound tissue is fragile)

Source: Data from Prevention and Treatment of Pressure Ulcers: Clinical Practice Guideline (developed by the National Pressure Ulcer Advisory Panel and European Pressure Ulcer Advisory Panel) and Guidelines for the Treatment of Pressure Ulcers (by the Wound Healing Society)[a,b]

[a]National Pressure Ulcer Advisory Panel and European Pressure Ulcer Advisory Panel (2009) Prevention and treatment of pressure ulcers: clinical practice guideline. Washington DC: National Pressure Ulcer Advisory Panel.

[b]Whitney J, Phillips L, Aslam R, et al (2006) Guidelines for the treatment of pressure ulcers. *Wound Repair Regen* 14(6): 663–679.

and Cambridge Scientific Abstracts. We used the following search terms: "pressure ulcer," "pressure sore," "decubitus," "bedsore," "prevention," "prophylactic," "reduction," "randomized," and "clinical trials." The bibliographies of identified articles were also searched. Criteria for selection of studies included RCTs that reported objective, clinically relevant outcome measures (such as incidence and severity of pressure ulcers). There were no restrictions on language, publication date, or setting. The search strategy identified 763 citations, from which 59 relevant RCTs were selected. The 59 studies we selected enrolled a total of 13,845 patients in mixed settings. For this chapter, we searched MEDLINE through 2010 to identify any new systematic reviews and update our previous systematic review. One new systematic review was selected from this updated search [14].

For the second question, "What are the best ways to treat pressure ulcers?," we had performed a previous systematic review, published in 2008 [9]. For that systematic review, we searched MEDLINE, EM-BASE, and CINAHL from inception through August 23, 2008, to identify relevant RCTs. We used the following search terms: "pressure ulcer," "pressure sore," "decubitus," "bedsore," "chronic wound," "treatment," "therapy," "management," "randomized," and "clinical trials." We also performed a hand search to identify any other articles. Inclusion criteria were English-language RCTs that reported objective, clinically relevant outcome measures such as healing rates or wound size. The search identified 872 abstracts, from which 103 relevant RCTs were selected. The 103 RCTs included 5889 participants. For this chapter, we searched MEDLINE through 2010 to update our previous systematic review. Four new RCTs [15–18] and three new systematic reviews [19–21] were identified from this search.

For the third question, "What are the best noninvasive ways to diagnose infection in chronic wounds?," we performed a previous systematic review, for publication in 2012 [13]. We searched MEDLINE, EM-BASE, and CINAHL databases through November 18, 2011 using nine exploded Medical Subject Headings (physical examination, medical history taking, professional competence, "sensitivity and specificity," reproducibility of results, observer variation, "diagnostic tests, routine," decision support techniques, and Bayes theorem). We added the search terms: "chronic wound" and "infection." The search was restricted to English language and humans. Studies of acute wounds (including traumatic wounds, acute postoperative surgical wounds, and burns) and osteomyelitis were excluded. The search strategy identified 305 abstracts from which 15 relevant studies were selected [22–36].

For this chapter, we graded relevant clinical studies using the Oxford Centre for Evidence-based Medicine Levels of Evidence [37].

What are the best ways to prevent pressure ulcers?

In this section, we describe the evidence related to interventions for preventing pressure ulcer formation (i.e., support surfaces, repositioning, exercise, treatment of incontinence, nutritional supplementation, and skin care).

Support surfaces

Specialized support surfaces (such as mattresses and cushions) reduce or relieve the pressure that the patient's body weight exerts on skin and subcutaneous tissues as it presses against the surface of a bed or chair. If a patient's mobility is compromised and this pressure is not relieved, pressure ulcer formation can result.

The National Pressure Ulcer Advisory Panel (NPUAP) categorizes support surfaces as "nonpowered" (support surfaces such as foam, which do not need electricity, previously known as "static") and "powered" (support surfaces such as rotating beds, which require electricity, previously known as "dynamic") [38]. Powered support surfaces include alternating pressure mattresses, low-air loss beds, and air-fluidized mattresses. Alternating pressure mattresses produce alternating high and low pressures between the patient and mattress, thus diminishing the period of high pressure. Low-air loss mattresses consist of air sacs through which warmed air passes. Air-fluidized mattresses contain silicone-coated beads that liquefy when air is pumped through them. Powered support surfaces are typically more costly than nonpowered surfaces, with air-fluidized mattresses being

the most costly type of powered support surface [39]. Standard hospital mattresses (i.e., not a specialized support surface) usually incur a one-time cost in the hundreds of dollars, but specialized support surfaces are usually rented and can cost thousands of dollars a month [40]. Specialized foams (e.g., convoluted foam, cubed foam) and specialized sheepskin (denser than regular sheepskin) are the only surfaces that are consistently superior to standard hospital mattresses in reducing the incidence of pressure ulcers (Level 1a-evidence) [4]. Specialized foam mattress overlays on operating tables reduce the incidence of postoperative pressure ulcers in patients undergoing elective major surgery (Level 1b evidence) [41]. An overlay is a support surface designed to be placed on top of another support surface. Rotating beds do not reduce the incidence of pressure ulcers when compared to either standard hospital beds or ICU beds (Level 1a-evidence) [4]. One well-designed RCT compared powered and nonpowered support surfaces in 447 patients and found no difference in pressure ulcer incidence between the two types of surfaces (Level 1b evidence) [42]. In another well designed RCT, no difference was found in the incidence of pressure ulcers when powered support surface mattress overlays were used instead of powered support surface mattresses in acute care (Level 1b evidence) [43]. The mattresses were more expensive than the overlays, but an economic evaluation has suggested that the mattresses may be more cost effective and are more acceptable to patients than the overlays [44]. There is insufficient evidence regarding the optimal surface to prevent heel pressure ulcers (Level 2a-evidence) [14].

Repositioning

Repositioning, like support surfaces, is meant to reduce or eliminate interface pressure and reduce the risk for pressure ulcer development. There is insufficient evidence regarding how often to turn and which patient position is optimal in terms of risk reduction (Level 1a-evidence) [4]. Repositioning of patients is usually recommended to be performed every 2 hours in most pressure ulcer prevention protocols.

Exercise and treatment of incontinence

One RCT examined the effects of providing both exercise and care for incontinence (both urinary and fecal) in the nursing home. This care was provided to residents for 2 hours per day for 32 weeks, but did not reduce pressure ulcer incidence relative to usual care (Level 1b evidence) [45].

Nutritional supplementation
Nutritional intake is frequently assumed to affect the risk for developing pressure ulcers. The best designed study we found was an RCT that studied 672 critically ill inpatients over age 65 years, and compared standard diet alone to standard diet plus two oral nutritional supplements per day [46]. Patients in the control group had a relative risk of pressure ulcer development of 1.57 (95% confidence interval (CI) 1.30–2.38) when compared to those in the intervention group (Level 1b evidence). Other RCTs studying nutrition did not find a reduction in pressure ulcer risk when patients were supplemented nutritionally, but this may be because these studies were underpowered (Level 1a-evidence) [4].

Skin care
Dry sacral skin is a risk factor for developing pressure ulcers [12]. However, we were unable to find evidence that any specific topical agent has a beneficial effect on the prevention of pressure ulcers [4].

Clinical bottom line
The nonpowered support surfaces of specialized foam and specialized sheepskin, both reduce pressure ulcer incidence when compared with standard hospital mattresses (Level 1b-evidence) [4]. On operating tables, mattress overlays may decrease the incidence of postoperative pressure ulcers (Level 1b-evidence) [41]. It is unclear whether powered support surfaces are superior to nonpowered support surfaces, so costs are important to consider when deciding between these two types of surfaces [4]. In acute care hospitals, although alternating pressure mattresses are initially more expensive than alternating pressure overlays, inpatients prefer the mattresses and in the long-term they may be more cost-effective than overlays (Level 1b-evidence) [44].

Nutritional supplementation may help to reduce the risk of pressure ulcers, but it is not clear which nutrients are best. We outline some additional guidelines for the prevention of pressure ulcers in Table 12.1.

What are the best ways to treat pressure ulcers?

In this section, we describe the evidence related to interventions for treating pressure ulcers (i.e., support surfaces, repositioning, exercise, nutritional supplementation, wound cleansing, wound dressings, biological agents, and adjunctive therapies).

Support surfaces
We found inconsistent results regarding the benefits of powered (e.g., alternating pressure) versus nonpowered (e.g., foam) support surfaces [47–52]. It is unclear whether one type of powered mattress is superior to any other type. Evans et al [53] and Nixon et al [54] found no differences in ulcer healing between the two powered support surfaces they compared (Level 1b evidence). Allman et al [55] found that ulcer surface area decreased with an air fluidized powered mattress but increased on an alternating pressure mattress (median changes -1.2 cm^2 vs. $+0.5$ cm^2; 95% CI for the difference, -9.2 to -0.6 cm^2) (Level 1b evidence).

For people in wheelchairs, use of an individually adjusted automated wheelchair seat that provides cyclic pressure relief may improve healing as compared with the combination of a standard wheelchair and performing arm push-ups every 20–30 minutes for pressure relief (Level 1b evidence) [15].

Repositioning
No trials have examined the effects of repositioning alone, so there is insufficient evidence regarding the optimal frequency or type of repositioning for the treatment of pressure ulcers [19].

Nutritional supplementation
In one RCT, LTC residents were randomized to either a collagen protein supplement or placebo combined with standard care [56]. Healing was measured over 8 weeks with the PUSH (Pressure Ulcer Scale for Healing) tool (0 = healed, 17 = worst possible score) [57]. Residents randomized to the supplement had better healing than those randomized to placebo (mean improvement in PUSH scores 3.55 +/− 4.66 vs. 3.22 +/− 4.11 respectively; $P < 0.05$) (Level 1b-evidence).

In another RCT, high- and low-dose vitamin C (500 mg twice daily and 10 mg twice daily, respectively) were given for either 12 weeks or until pressure ulcer healing (whichever came first) [58]. No differences were found in either wound closure rates or mean change in ulcer surface area per week (Level 1b evidence) [58]. Another RCT found that 500 mg of vitamin C twice daily significantly decreased the size of pressure ulcers as compared with placebo (Level 1b-evidence) [59]. The inconsistent results of these two RCTs make it difficult to draw firm conclusions about the efficacy of vitamin C in pressure ulcer treatment. Although there may be benefit of vitamin C supplementation for pressure ulcer healing, the dose to use is unclear.

A small RCT of 28 older LTC residents demonstrated that healing was faster in those who received a disease-specific nutrition treatment consisting of a standard diet plus a supplement of protein (20% of the total calories), arginine, zinc, and vitamin C ($P < 0.001$ for all nutrients vs. control), than in LTC residents who received the standard diet alone (Level 1b-evidence) [18].

An RCT of 160 undernourished older adults with heel ulcers examined the effects of supplementation with ornithine alpha-ketoglutarate [17]. Participants with small pressure ulcers and treated with ornithine alpha-ketoglutarate in addition to standard care showed some benefit in healing as compared to participants treated with standard care alone (Level 1b-evidence).

Wound cleansing

No particular wound cleansing solution or technique is superior to another in terms of increasing healing rate of pressure ulcers (Level 1a-evidence) [20].

Wound dressings

Most high quality RCTs have found no difference in wound healing with the specific products studied: collagenase versus fibrinolysin/deoxyribonuclease (both are enzymatic debriding agents), collagenase versus hydrocolloid (an occlusive dressing containing gel-forming agents), radiant heat dressing versus hydrocolloid +/− alginate (alginates are absorbant dressings extracted from seaweed), and topical phenytoin solution versus normal saline [60–64]. No debriding agent was found to be consistently superior to other debriding agents [60, 61, 65–67].

The RCTs that did find an advantage to a specific dressing found that calcium alginate was superior to

dextranomer paste (mean wound surface area reduction per week was 2.39 cm^2 (SD = 3.54) vs. 0.27 cm^2 (SD = 3.21); $P = 0.0001$) [68] and oxyquinolone was superior to lanolin/petrolatum (Level 1b evidence) [69].

Biological agents

The highest quality RCT of biological agents compared three doses of recombinant human platelet derived growth factor (rPDGF-BB isoform) with placebo [70]. The incidence of complete healing was greater in all three rPDGF-BB groups ($P < 0.025$ in all groups), compared with placebo (Level 1b-evidence).

Adjunctive therapies

No good quality RCT has shown benefits of laser [71] (compared to moist saline gauze) or of ultrasound [72] (compared to sham ultrasound). One single-blind RCT of electrostimulation demonstrated that it may improve healing in people with spinal cord injury, but the control group was not subjected to sham electrostimulation therapy so definitive conclusions cannot be drawn from this study [16].

Vacuum therapy has not been shown to be more effective than various control interventions in the treatment of pressure ulcers (Level 1a-evidence) [21]. There are a large number of prematurely terminated and unpublished trials of vacuum therapy [73]. No RCTs of hyperbaric oxygen therapy (HBOT) met our inclusion criteria. Two previous systematic reviews were not able to confirm any benefit of HBOT for the healing of pressure ulcers (Level 1a-evidence) [74, 75].

Clinical bottom line

Powered support surfaces have not been found to be consistently superior to nonpowered mattresses for healing pressure ulcers. It is not known whether repositioning is comparable or superior to specific support surfaces [76].

Nutritional supplementation has not been shown to improve pressure ulcer healing in patients without specific nutritional deficiencies, although there may be some benefit to vitamin C administration. Pressure ulcer healing may be improved in LTC residents who are supplemented with protein.

It is unknown whether the often costly biological agents are cost-effective as compared to standard wound care (Level 1b-evidence) [70, 77].

We did not find any one specific dressing that was consistently superior to any other dressing. Similar conclusions have been reached for arterial ulcers [78], venous stasis ulcers [6], and surgical wounds healing by secondary intention [79].

There is no good evidence that adjunctive therapies improve pressure ulcer healing.

Overall, there have been few significant outcome differences in RCTs of specific pressure ulcer treatment strategies. Pressure ulcers may require multifactorial wound care interventions (e.g., a combination of repositioning and local wound care) rather than a single treatment. We outline some of the guidelines for the medical management of pressure ulcers in Table 12.2.

What are the best noninvasive ways to diagnose infection in chronic wounds?

In terms of clinical symptoms of chronic wound infection, we found that the likelihood of infection is greatly increased when an ulcer is causing increasing pain, although the absence of increasing pain has only a modest effect on lowering the likelihood of infection (Level 2a-evidence) [13]. Items in the history and physical examination, in isolation or in combination, do not appear to adequately rule in or rule out infection in chronic wounds. This is true of both the classical signs and symptoms of wound infection (purulent exudate, heat, edema, and erythema) and the atypical signs and symptoms said by experts to be more characteristic of chronic wound infection [13].

Diagnostic tests that help to diagnose chronic wound infection include wound fluid cultures, which are highly accurate in determining infection in a chronic wound when compared to the reference standard of deep tissue biopsy culture [29]. An infection of chronic wounds is more likely (positive LR (likelihood ratio) 6.3) when a quantitative swab culture using Levine's technique (i.e., a swab is rotated over a 1 cm × 1 cm area for 5 seconds with sufficient pressure to extract fluid from within the wound tissue) is positive, while a negative swab culture decreases the likelihood (negative LR 0.47). This same study also demonstrated that wound swabs performed using the Z-technique (applying in a zigzag manner covering the entire wound surface while simultaneously rotating the swab between the thumb and forefinger) neither predicted nor excluded wound infection [28].

Clinical bottom line

The clinical symptom that may be most helpful in diagnosing infection in a chronic wound is an increase in the level of pain. However, the absence of an increase in the level of pain does not necessarily rule out infection (Level 2a-evidence). A quantitative swab culture might help physicians estimate the probability of infection when they do not have results from deep tissue biopsy culture. Further evidence is required to determine which, if any, type of swab is most diagnostic. In some clinical situations, both clinical features and diagnostic tests will aid in diagnosis, and in other situations only the latter is helpful.

Summary

The methodological quality of some older RCTs evaluating interventions to prevent and treat pressure ulcers has been relatively poor but new good quality RCTs are emerging and further high quality studies are needed to better establish the efficacy and safety of many commonly used treatments. Appropriate support surfaces (mattress overlays on operating tables, specialized foam, and specialized sheepskin), optimizing nutritional status, and moisturizing sacral skin are probably beneficial in terms of preventing pressure ulcers. For treating existing pressure ulcers, there is little evidence to justify a specific support surface or dressing, or the routine use of nutritional supplements, biological agents, and adjunctive therapies as compared to standard care.

The clinical symptom that may be most helpful in diagnosing infection in a chronic wound is an increase in the level of pain, which essentially rules in infection. However, the absence of an increase in the level of pain does not necessarily rule out infection. Further evidence is required to determine which, if any, type of quantitative swab culture is most diagnostic.

References

1. European Guidelines for Pressure Ulcer Treatment (2004) http://www.epuap.org/gltreatment.html (accessed October 29, 2007).

2. Cuddigan J, Frantz RA (1998) Pressure ulcer research: pressure ulcer treatment. A monograph from the National Pressure Ulcer Advisory Panel. *Adv Wound Care* 11(6): 294–300.

3. Whitney J, et al (2006) Guidelines for the treatment of pressure ulcers. *Wound Repair Regen* 14(6): 663–679.

4. Reddy M, Gill SS, Rochon PA (2006) Prevention of pressure ulcers: a systematic review. *JAMA* 296(8): 974–984.

5. Nelson E, Bradley M (2003) Dressings and topical agents for arterial leg ulcers. *Cochrane Database Syst Rev* 1: CD001836.

6. Palfreyman SJ, Nelson EA, Lochiel R, Michaels JA (2006) Dressings for healing venous leg ulcers. *Cochrane Database Syst Rev* 3: CD001103.

7. Adderley U, Smith R (2007) Topical agents and dressings for fungating wounds. *Cochrane Database Syst Rev* 2: CD003948.

8. Vermeulen H, Ubbink D, Goossens A, de Vos R, Legemate D (2004) Dressings and topical agents for surgical wounds healing by secondary intention. *Cochrane Database Syst Rev* 2: CD003554.

9. Reddy M, et al (2008) Treatment of pressure ulcers: a systematic review. *JAMA* 300(22): 2647–2662.

10. Redelings MD, Lee NE, Sorvillo F (2005) Pressure ulcers: more lethal than we thought? *Adv Skin Wound Care* 18(7): 367–372.

11. Smith PW, Black JM, Black SB (1999) Infected pressure ulcers in the long-term-care facility. *Infect Control Hosp Epidemiol* 20(5): 358–361.

12. Gardner SE, et al (2001) A tool to assess clinical signs and symptoms of localized infection in chronic wounds: development and reliability. *Ostomy Wound Manage* 47(1): 40–47.

13. Reddy M, Gill SS, Wu W, *et al.* Does my patient have an infected chronic wound? Pending publication.

14. Junkin J, Gray M (2009) Are pressure redistribution surfaces or heel protection devices effective for preventing heel pressure ulcers? *J Wound Ostomy Continence Nurs* 36: 602–608.

15. Makhsous M, et al (2009) Promote pressure ulcer healing in individuals with spinal cord injury using an individualized cyclic pressure-relief protocol. *Adv Skin Wound Care* 22(11): 514–521.

16. Houghton PE, et al (2010) Electrical stimulation therapy increases rate of healing of pressure ulcers in community-dwelling people with spinal cord injury. *Arch Phys Med Rehabil* 91(5): 669–678.

17. Meaume S, et al (2009) Efficacy and safety of ornithine alpha-ketoglutarate in heel pressure ulcers in elderly patients: results of a randomized controlled trial. *J Nutr Health Aging* 13(7): 623–630.

18. Cereda E, Gini A, Pedrolli C, Vanotti A (2009) Disease-specific, versus standard, nutritional support for the treatment of pressure ulcers in institutionalized older adults: a randomized controlled trial. *J Am Geriatr Soc* 57(8): 1395–1402.

19. Moore-Zena EH, Cowman S (2009) Repositioning for treating pressure ulcers. *Cochrane Database Syst Rev* (2): CD006898.

20. Moore-Zena EH, Cowman S (2005) Wound cleansing.for pressure ulcers. *Cochrane Database Syst Rev* (4): CD004983.

21. Van Den Boogaard M, de Laat E, Spauwen P, Schoonhoven L (2008); The effectiveness of topical negative pressure in the treatment of pressure ulcers: a literature review. *Eur J Plast Surg* 31: 1–7.

22. Gardner SE, Hillis SL, Frantz RA (2009) Clinical signs of infection in diabetic foot ulcers with high microbial load. *Biol Res Nurs* 11: 119.

23. Serena TE, Hanft JR, Snyder R (2008) The lack of reliability of clinical examination in the diagnosis of wound infection: preliminary communication. *The Int J Low Extrem Wounds* 7(1): 32–35.

24. Gardner SE, et al (2006) Diagnostic validity of three swab techniques for identifying chronic wound infection. *Wound Rep Reg* 14: 548–557.

25. Neil JA, Munro CL (1997) A comparison of two culturing methods for chronic wounds. *Ostomy Wound Manage* 43(3): 20–30.

26. Ambrosch A, Lobmann R, Pott A, Preibler J (2008) Interleukin-6 concentrations in wound fluids rather than serological markers are useful in assessing bacterial triggers of ulcer inflammation. *Int Wound J* 5(1): 99–106.

27. Gardner SE, Frantz RA, Doebbeling BN (2001) The validity of the clinical signs and symptoms used to identify localized chronic wound infection. *Wound Rep Reg* 9: 178–186.

28. Bill TJ, et al (2001) Quantitative swab culture versus tissue biopsy: a comparison in chronic wounds. *Ostomy Wound Manage* 47(1): 34–37.

29. Ehrenkranz NJ, Alfonso B, Nerenberg D (1990) Irrigation-aspiration for culturing draining decubitus ulcers: correlation of bacteriological findings with a clinical inflammatory scoring index. *J Clin Microbiol* 28(11): 2389–2393.

30. Woo KY, Sibbald RG (2009) A cross-sectional validation study of using NERDS and STONEES to assess bacterial burden. *Ostomy Wound Manage* 55(8): 40–48.

31. Jeandrot A, et al (2008) Serum procalcitonin and C-reactive protein concentrations to distinguish mildly infected from non-infected diabetic foot ulcers: a pilot study. *Diabetologia* 51: 347–352.

32. Uzun G, et al (2007) Procalcitonin as a diagnostic aid in diabetic foot infections. *Tohoku J Exp Med* 213: 305–312.

33. Heym B, Rimareix F, Lortat-Jacob A, Nicolas-Chanoine MH (2004) Bacteriological investigation of infected pressure ulcers in spinal cord-injured patients and impact on antibiotic therapy. *Spinal Cord* 42: 230–234.

34. Slater RA, et al (2004) Swab cultures accurately identify bacterial pathogens in diabetic foot wounds not involving bone. *Diabet Med* 21: 705–709.

35. Ratliff CR, Rodeheaver GT (2002) Correlation of semi-quantitative swab cultures to quantitative swab cultures from chronic wounds. *Wounds* 14(9): 329–333.

36. Schmidt K, et al (2000) Bacterial population of chronic crural ulcers: is there a difference between the diabetic, the venous, and the arterial ulcer? *VASA* 29(1): 62–70.

37. Phillips B, Ball C, Sackett D, et al. (2010) Oxford Centre for Evidence-based Medicine – levels of evidence. http://www.cebm.net/index.aspx?o=1025 (accessed December 29, 2010).

38. National Pressure Ulcer Advisory Panel Support Standards Initiative. Terms and Definitions Related to Support Surfaces (2007) http://www.npuap.org/pdf/NPUAP_S3I_TD.pdf (accessed September 22, 2008).

39. Woodbury MG, Houghton PE (2004) Prevalence of pressure ulcers in Canadian healthcare settings. *Ostomy Wound Manage* 50(10): 22–24, 26, 28, 30, 32, 34, 36–38.

40. Schaum KD (2005) Special report: payment perspective: pressure-reducing support surfaces. *Ostomy Wound Manage* 51(2): 36–96.

41. Nixon J, et al (1998) A sequential randomised controlled trial comparing a dry visco-elastic polymer pad and standard operating table mattress in the prevention of post-operative pressure sores. *Int J Nurs Studies* 35: 193–203.

42. Vanderwee K, Grypdonck MH, DeFloor T (2005) Effectiveness of an alternating pressure air mattress for the prevention of pressure ulcers. *Age Ageing* 34: 261–267.

43. Nixon J, Cranny G, Iglesias C (2006) Randomised, controlled trial of alternating pressure mattresses compared with alternating pressure overlays for the prevention of pressure ulcers: PRESSURE (pressure relieving support surfaces) trial. *BMJ* 332: 1413–1415.

44. Iglesias C, et al (2006) Pressure relieving support surfaces (PRESSURE) trial: cost effectiveness analysis. *BMJ* 332: 1416–1418.

45. Bates-Jensen BM, Alessi CA, Al-Samarrai NR, Schnelle JF, (2003) The effects of an exercise and incontinence intervention on skin health outcomes in nursing home residents. *J Am Geriatr Soc* 51: 348–355.

46. Bourdel-Marchasson I, et al (2000) A multi-center trial of the effects of oral nutritional supplementation in critically ill older inpatients. GAGE group. groupe aquitain geriatrique d'Evaluation. *Nutrition* 16: 1–5.

47. Branom R (2001) "Constant force technology" versus low-air-loss therapy in the treatment of pressure ulcers. *Ostomy Wound Manage* 47(9): 38–46.

48. Day A, Leonard F (1993) Seeking quality care for patients with pressure ulcers. *Decubitus* 6(1): 32–43.

49. Ferrell BA, Osterweil D, Christenson P (1993) A randomized trial of low-air-loss beds for treatment of pressure ulcers. *JAMA* 269(4): 494–497.

50. Mulder GD, Taro N, Seeley JE, Andrews K (1994) A study of pressure ulcer response to low air loss beds vs. conventional treatment. *J Geriatr Dermatol* 2(3): 87–91.

51. Rosenthal MJ, Felton RM, Nastasi AE, Naliboff BD, Harker J, Navach JH (2003) Healing of advanced pressure ulcers by a generic total contact seat: 2 randomized comparisons with low air loss bed treatments. *Arch Phys Med Rehabil* 84(12): 1733–1742.

52. Russell L, Reynolds TM, Towns A, Worth W, Greenman A, Turner R (2003) Randomized comparison trial of the RIK and the nimbus 3 mattresses. *Br J Nurs* 12: 254–259.

53. Evans D, Land L, Geary A (2000) A clinical evaluation of the nimbus 3 alternating pressure mattress replacement system. *J Wound Care* 9(4): 181–186.

54. Nixon J, et al (2006) Randomised, controlled trial of alternating pressure mattresses compared with alternating pressure overlays for the prevention of pressure ulcers: PRESSURE (pressure relieving support surfaces) trial. *BMJ* 332(7555): 1413–1415.

55. Allman RM, Walker JM, Hart MK, Laprade CA, Noel LB, Smith CR (1987) Air-fluidized beds or conventional therapy for pressure sores. A randomized trial. *Ann Int Med* 107(5): 641–648.

56. Lee SK, Posthauer ME, Dorner B, Redovian V, Maloney MJ (2006) Pressure ulcer healing with a concentrated, fortified, collagen protein hydrolysate supplement: a randomized controlled trial. *Adv Skin Wound Care* 19(2): 92–96.

57. Thomas DR, et al (1997) Pressure ulcer scale for healing: derivation and validation of the PUSH tool. *Adv Skin Wound Care* 10(5): 96–101.

58. ter Riet G, Kessels AG, Knipschild PG (1995) Randomized clinical trial of ascorbic acid in the treatment of pressure ulcers. *J Clin Epidemiology* 48(12): 1453–1460.

59. Taylor TV, Rimmer S, Day B, Butcher J, Dymock IW (1974) Ascorbic acid supplementation in the treatment of pressure sores. *Lancet* 2(7880): 544–546.

60. Burgos A, et al (2000) Cost, efficacy, efficiency and tolerability of collagenase ointment versus hydrocolloid occlusive dressing in the treatment of pressure ulcers. A comparative, randomised, multicentre study. *Clin Drug Invest* 19(5): 357–365.

61. Pullen R, Popp R, Volkers P, Fusgen I (2002) Prospective randomized double-blind study of the wound-debriding effects of collagenase and fibrinolysin/deoxyribonuclease in pressure ulcers. *Age and Ageing* 31(2): 126–130.

62. Graumlich JF, et al (2003) Healing pressure ulcers with collagen or hydrocolloid: a randomized, controlled trial. *J Am Geriatr Soc* 51: 147–154.

63. Thomas DR, Diebold MR, Eggemeyer LM (2005) A controlled, randomized, comparative study of a radiant heat bandage on the healing of stage 3-4 pressure ulcers: a pilot study. *J Am Med Dir Assoc* 6(1): 46–49.

64. Subbanna PK, et al (2007) Topical phenytoin solution for treating pressure ulcers: a prospective, randomized, double-blind clinical trial. *Spinal Cord* 45: 739–743.

65. Muller E, van Leen MW, Bergemann R (2001) Economic evaluation of collagenase-containing ointment and hydrocolloid dressing in the treatment of pressure ulcers. *Pharmacoeconomics* 19(12): 1209–1216.

66. Alvarez OM, Fernandez-Obregon A, Rogers RS, Bergamo L, Masso J, Black M (2002) A prospective, randomized, comparative study of collagenase and papain-urea for pressure ulcer debridement. *Wounds* 14(8): 293–301.

67. Parish LC, Collins E (1979) Decubitus ulcers: a comparative study. *Cutis* 23(1): 106–110.

68. Sayag J, Meaume S, Bohbot S (1996) Healing properties of calcium alginate dressings. *J Wound Care* 5(8): 357–362.

69. Gerding GA, Browning JS (1992) Oxyquinoline-containing ointment vs. standard therapy for stage I and stage II skin lesions. *Dermatol Nurs* 4(5): 389–398.

70. Rees RS, Robson MC, Smiell JM, Perry BH (1999) Becaplermin gel in the treatment of pressure ulcers: a phase II randomized, double-blind, placebo-controlled study. *Wound Repair Regen* 7(3): 141–147.

71. Taly AB, Sivaraman Nair KP, Murali T, John A (2004) Efficacy of multiwavelength light therapy in the treatment of pressure ulcers in subjects with disorders of the spinal cord: A randomized double-blind controlled trial. *Arch Phys Med Rehabil* 85(10): 1657–1661.

72. ter Riet G, Kessels AG, Knipschild P (1995) Randomised clinical trial of ultrasound treatment for pressure ulcers. *BMJ* 310(6986): 1040–1041.

73. Gregor S, Maegele M, Sauerland S, Krahn JF, Peinemann F, Lange S (2008) Negative pressure wound therapy: a vacuum of evidence? *Arch Surg* 143(2): 189–196.

74. Kranke P, Bennett M, Roeckl-Wiedmann I, Debus S (2004) Hyperbaric oxygen therapy for chronic wounds. *Cochrane Database Syst Rev* 2: (CD004123).

75. Roeckl-Wiedmann I, Bennett M, Kranke P (2005) Systematic review of hyperbaric oxygen in the management of chronic wounds. *Br J Surg* 92(1): 24–32.

76. Ayello EA, Braden B (2002) How and why to do pressure ulcer risk assessment. *Adv Skin Wound Care.* 15(3): 125–131.

77. Landi F, et al (2003) Topical treatment of pressure ulcers with nerve growth factor: a randomized clinical trial. *Ann Int Med* 139(8): 635–641.

78. Nelson E, Bradley M (2007) Dressings and topical agents for arterial leg ulcers. *Cochrane Database Syst Rev* (1): CD001836.

79. Vermeulen H, Ubbink D, Goossens A, de Vos R, Legemate D (2004) Dressings and topical agents for surgical wounds healing by secondary intention. *Cochrane Database Syst Rev* (2): CD003554.

CHAPTER 13

Elder abuse

Erik J. Lindbloom, Landon D. Hough, & Karli R.E. Urban
Department of Family and Community Medicine, University of Missouri, Columbia, MO, USA

Introduction

Elder abuse, often more broadly referred to as elder mistreatment, has been a relatively recent topic of interest among clinicians and researchers. A letter regarding "granny-battering" was published in *BMJ* in 1975 [1]. In contrast to the attention paid by clinicians, researchers, and society to child abuse from the 1960s onward, elder abuse research did not begin in earnest until decades later [2–4]. It is likely that at least 4% of adults 65 years of age or older have suffered, or will suffer, some form of abuse in their later years, and this prevalence is significantly higher if one considers the broadest definition of elder mistreatment, including financial exploitation [5–8].

In its 2003 statement, the US National Research Council attempted to refine the definition of elder mistreatment [9]:

"Elder mistreatment" is defined in this report to refer to (a) intentional actions that cause harm or create a serious risk of harm (whether or not harm is intended) to a vulnerable elder by a caregiver or other person who stands in a trust relationship to the elder or (b) failure by a caregiver to satisfy the elder's basic needs or to protect the elder from harm. "Mistreatment" conveys two ideas: that some injury, deprivation or dangerous condition has occurred to the elder person and that someone else bears responsibility for causing the condition or failing to prevent it.

This definition differs from most legal statutes in that it excludes victimization of elders by strangers. The Research Council considered self-neglect as a separate domain of elder protection, and it did not specifically address resident-to-resident mistreatment. Both of these areas have been receiving increased research attention lately [10, 11].

Researchers have established the detrimental health effects of elder abuse and neglect, such as frequent emergency department visits and a threefold increase in mortality [12, 13]. Much of the original research on long-term care (LTC) facility mistreatment is cited outside the medical literature, in such places as nursing and social work databases [14].

Older adults are potential victims in a variety of living environments and care situations, including private residences and LTC. LTC residents may be particularly vulnerable to abuse and neglect because most suffer from cognitive impairment, behavioral abnormalities, or physical limitations that have been reported as risk factors for abuse and neglect [3, 4, 14–22]. Many residents are unable to report abuse or neglect, or they are fearful that reporting may lead to retaliation, or otherwise negatively affect their lives [23, 24].

Evidence-Based Geriatric Medicine: A Practical Clinical Guide, First Edition. Edited by Jayna M. Holroyd-Leduc and Madhuri Reddy.
© 2012 Blackwell Publishing Ltd. Published 2012 by Blackwell Publishing Ltd.

Witnessed mistreatment is common in LTC. A 1987 survey of 577 LTC staff members from 31 facilities found that more than one-third (36%) had witnessed at least one incident of physical abuse during the preceding 12 months, and 10% reported they had committed such acts themselves [25]. Psychological or verbal abuse was even more common, with 81% of the staff reporting they had observed, and 40% reporting they had committed, at least one incident of psychological or verbal abuse during that 12-month time period. A follow-up study reported similar findings [26]. An analysis report of the US Online Survey Certification and Reporting System (OSCAR) data system in 2001 by the Special Investigations Division of the US House Committee on Government Reform asserts that abuse of residents is a significant issue in the United States LTC facilities [27]. The report concluded that during a 2-year period, nearly one-third of all certified facilities had been cited for some type of abuse violation that had the potential to cause harm or had actually caused harm to a resident.

In some respects, elder mistreatment in LTC may be more apparent than in other settings due to the ever-increasing oversight and scrutiny that LTC providers receive. In private residences, isolation and financial exploitation by the caregiver often hinder the timely recognition of dangerous care situations [4]. Additionally, the rapid expansion of alternatives to skilled LTC facilities has increased the number and variety of environments in which older adults are potentially dependent on others and vulnerable to mistreatment.

At the core is a vulnerable or dependent older adult suffering at the hands of a perpetrator who could be opportunistic, sociopathic, or simply overwhelmed by the burden of care. Because of its complexity and frequent ambiguity (as with a victim who may be unable or unwilling to seek help) elder abuse is underreported, particularly by physicians. Physicians constituted only 1.3% of the reports to the US ombudsmen programs in the late 1990s, despite it being mandatory for US physicians to report elder abuse [28]. A survey of 122 Canadian physicians found that there is widespread uncertainty about the definition and clinical signs of abuse, with 72% citing a lack of knowledge about where to call for help, and 56% reporting difficulty in determining what constitutes elder abuse [29].

In this chapter, we address: (1) the types of elder abuse, (2) how to identify whether an older adult is a victim of abuse, and (3) how to prevent or reduce elder abuse.

Search strategy

We conducted a literature search with the assistance of two medical librarians. The search strategy, covering the years 1980 through mid-2010 and limited to English language, retrieved citations from the following bibliographic databases: MEDLINE, MEDLINE In-Process, CINAHL, Current Contents, Scopus, Sociological Abstracts, Social Services Abstracts, Social Work Database and Ageline. The following grouped concepts were combined accordingly, and searched as subject headings and/or truncated text words (indicated by "$") across all databases: "elder abuse or abus$ or mistreat$ or maltreat$ or assault$ or neglect$ or violen$ or exploit$ or batter$ or intimidate$," and "elder$ or older or geriatri$ or gerontolog$ or senior$ or aged or frail elderly." For mistreatment specific to institutional care, an additional keyword search included: "nursing home$ or intermediate care facilit$ or skilled nursing facilit$ or assisted living facilit$ or homes for the aged." A total of 416 citations were retrieved from this search. Abstracts and titles were reviewed for evidence of original research or systematic review. For this chapter, we graded relevant clinical studies using the Oxford Centre for Evidence-based Medicine Levels of Evidence.

What are the types of elder abuse?

The first standardized definitions of elder mistreatment were published by a consensus panel in 1993, and these classifications have remained the foundation of elder mistreatment investigations ever since (Table 13.1) [30].

Physical abuse

Physical abuse includes acts of violence that may result in pain, injury, impairment, or disease. An often cited scenario is staff retaliation against a physically aggressive or antagonistic resident. In one Swedish study involving 848 staff interviews, LTC staff members' most common reaction to resident violence was aggression (32%) [31]. In another study from Florida involving extensive semistructured interviews of 21 LTC staff members and Adult Protective Services investigators,

Table 13.1 Types of elder abuse

Physical abuse

Physical neglect

Psychological abuse

Financial or material mistreatment

Violation of personal rights

Sexual abuse

Source: [30, 73].

direct care staff reported aggressive behavior from residents almost daily, ranging from verbal threats to physical assault [32]. When staffing was low, care was rushed and aggression in either direction sometimes resulted. Upset staff members sometimes needed time and space to distance themselves from aggressive residents, and if this was not possible abuse of residents could sometimes result.

The same author's earlier work with the same population differentiated between "reactive" and "sadistic" abusers, and discussed the concept of "immunity" to aggressive resident behavior [33]. Immunity is defined as the ability to protect oneself from the impact of abuse by residents, resisting responses that are detrimental to oneself or residents. If a staff member was able to maintain immunity, then retaliation for the aggressive behavior did not occur. The reactive abuser temporarily loses this immunity and lashes out, while the sadistic abuser is incapable of ever developing immunity in the first place. Factors related to the ability to maintain immunity included job satisfaction, stress or violence at home, fatigue, and substance abuse issues. Job satisfaction and burnout were also associated with deliberate abusive behavior in another study [25]. Workload and burnout issues have also been well documented in several other studies [34–37]. A nurse's perception of abuse as a significant problem may be related to the amount of direct patient care. In one qualitative study of ten registered nurses in Canadian LTC facilities, administrative nurses felt abuse was not common in their facilities, whereas those involved in direct patient care felt it was common [38].

Several case series have explored the circumstances around accidental deaths due to physical restraint use and bed rails, occasionally involving an attempt to conceal the cause of death [39–44].

Physical neglect

Physical neglect is the failure to provide the goods or services necessary for optimal functioning or to avoid harm. Neglect in LTC may certainly overlap with concepts of psychological abuse (e.g., social isolation) and disparities in quality of care [45, 46]. In many cases, particularly those involving pressure ulcers, malnutrition, and dehydration, care providers and researchers may have difficulty making a distinction between neglect and poor care quality. Based on the definition of physical neglect as "the failure to provide the goods or services necessary for optimal functioning or to avoid harm," it is clear that these are in fact the same thing.

New residents presenting to LTC often have preexisting pressure sores, and such sores may represent a type of organ failure at the end of life [47, 48]. Differing opinions exist about whether all new pressure sores should be considered evidence for neglect [49–51]. The degree of variation in incidence rates between institutions, as well as the ability to significantly alter pressure sore incidence with systematic care changes, suggests that facility and staff factors play a major role in the development of pressure sores [52–55]. Individual resident risk factors also clearly exist, such as impaired mobility and dependence on others for activities of daily living; increased attention to skin care in these residents may lower the incidence of pressure sores [48, 56].

Malnutrition and dehydration are common in LTC, with prevalence rates of 80% or higher for both combined [57, 58]. Eating, chewing, and swallowing problems are common, and may be subtle enough to be underappreciated by LTC staff [59, 60]. Residents with comparably lower calorie intake have a higher mortality rate, even adjusting for comorbid conditions [58, 61]. Withholding nutrition or hydration, particularly at the time of consideration of feeding tube placement, may often be an appropriate end-of-life decision agreed upon by the care team and the resident or his/her representatives. However, qualitative reports cite that staff sometimes deliberately withhold food and fluids from residents who wish to eat or drink because of the additional effort involved [59, 62]. In a review of qualitative studies, patterns were observed where poor oral health, dysphagia, and inadequate staffing led to weight loss, use of pureed diets, and decreased appetite for regular food in a facility [59]. A lack of food preference available in the facility (e.g., an exclusively western diet offered to a Chinese resident) also led to a resident's significant weight loss. It was observed that when a family member assisted a resident with meals, the resident did not lose weight. Fluid intake was inadequate in almost all the residents observed, often due to fluids being out of reach or not having straws easily accessible. A case series from two US public hospitals showed clusters of cases of hypernatremic dehydration that suggested fluid deprivation and poor care quality in both institutional and private home settings [63].

Psychological abuse

Psychological abuse is conduct causing mental anguish in an older person, or the failure to provide a dependent older individual with social stimulation. Psychological abuse, including intimidation and isolation, is probably more prevalent than physical abuse in LTC, but is difficult to definitely ascertain because of a lack of clear markers [21, 25, 31, 64–66]. Aggressive LTC residents (sometimes labeled by staff as "bad") and a stressful work environment have been shown to be associated with a higher likelihood of psychological abuse [21, 64]. Work stress may be more closely related to psychological abuse than it is to physical abuse [25]. An interview with experts from a state medical society in the United States discussed the concept of "polite abuse," including actions such as residents sleeping in their wheel chair rather than a bed, or always being taken last to an event or meal [67].

Financial or material mistreatment

Financial or material mistreatment includes misuse of an older adult's income or resources for the financial or personal gain of the perpetrator, or failure to use available fund and resources necessary to sustain or restore the health and well-being of the older adult. According to the US National Research Council, elder financial abuse differs from elder physical abuse and neglect in that, "financial abuse is more likely to occur with the tacit acknowledgement and consent of the elder person and can be more difficult to detect and establish" [9]. A recent validation study surveyed experts about a theoretical model and investigative framework for this type of mistreatment [68, 69]. This model includes a vulnerable, often isolated older person and a person exerting undue influence or exploiting a new or long-term relationship. Furthermore, assets may be transferred without appropriate documentation or proper disclosure that the victim understood the arrangement. That arrangement is disproportionately beneficial to the perpetrator without consideration given to the effect on others, particularly the victim.

Material theft is a common concern among family members of LTC residents, with one US survey reporting that 47% of LTC residents' family members noted missing items and 1.5% of LTC staff members self-reported theft [70]. Six percent of staff members reported seeing coworkers steal and almost 20% suspected that coworkers had stolen from residents.

Violation of personal rights

Violation of personal rights encompasses any disregard of the older adult's rights and capability to make decisions for him or herself. In LTC, the balance between personal autonomy and the provision of adequate care for residents is an ever-present issue. One report quoted staff members admitting that they were more likely to withhold personal choices from particularly aggressive residents [64].

Sexual abuse

Although not explicitly listed in the definitions above, sexual abuse may span several of these categories, and have unique forensic markers and risk factors, such as sexually transmitted infections, anogenital trauma, and a past history of sex offenses by the perpetrator [15, 71, 72]. It was listed as a separate subcategory of vulnerable adult abuse by the UK Department of Health in 2000 [73].

Clinical bottom line

The definition of elder abuse includes a variety of physical, psychological, and material mistreatment.

How do you identify a victim of elder abuse?

Physical and psychological abuse

Clinical scenario

An 83-year-old male resident of a LTC facility is evaluated during monthly rounds. He has a history of advanced Alzheimer's disease, which has progressed rapidly over the last several months. His ambulation with a two-wheel walker has increasingly raised concern for wandering, since the LTC facility does not have a locked dementia unit. Recently, two of the nurse assistants transferred to another facility, and have not yet been replaced. The remaining staff members are feeling overworked and find it difficult to care for the number of residents in their unit.

On review of nurse charting, there are several instances mentioned of aggressive behavior from this patient. He is noted to have become more combative during bathing and dressing, physically striking nursing staff on several occasions. An injury report was filed by a staff member, who the resident bit while she was assisting him with dressing 2 weeks ago. Staff members present today report that he is a very difficult resident to care for and have avoided attempts to bathe him in the last week. One nurse refers to him as "the problem child."

On exam you find the resident in bed attempting to climb over a raised bedrail, and you note abrasions to both wrists. Physical (wrist) restraints are on the nightstand although there has not been an order for any restraints on this patient. There are other areas of excoriation on his face and trunk at various stages of healing, and poor hygiene is evident. When nursing staff are asked about the nature of his injuries, the response is "We can't be with all the residents all the time."

Until recently, there has been little study into pathognomonic signs of elder abuse. Some findings that are highly suspicious of child abuse, such as certain types of long bone fractures, have been documented as spontaneous occurrences in LTC residents [74]. Recently published studies on bruising in older adults have helped to distinguish accidental trauma from more suspicious injuries. Large bruises (>5 cm), and any size bruises on the face and posterior torso, are more associated with physical abuse in older adults [75, 76]. Bruises on the extremities are most often accidental,

Table 13.2 Historical and physical exam findings suggestive of elder mistreatment

Historical

Functional dependence

Depression

Dementia (particularly a recent rapid decline in cognitive function)

History of violence or aggression by either the victim or perpetrator

Behavioral change

Inadequate explanation or documentation of any injury

Physical Exam

Injuries to the trunk, head, and/or anogenital regions

Evasive or defensive responses

Weight loss

Pressure ulcers

Genital infections

Poor hygiene

Source: [2, 16, 20, 78–80].

although the lateral aspect of the right arm may still be considered suspicious for an inflicted or defensive injury, particularly when large. These and other findings during the history and physical exam that may suggest mistreatment are listed in Table 13.2. Environmental characteristics (such as unclean living conditions) or caregiving dynamics, in addition to any physical signs, may offer other clues to the presence of elder abuse, particularly if the victim suffers from dementia [77]. Several abuse-screening instruments exist that assess historical risk factors and physical findings [78–80].

Neglect and poor care quality

Clinical scenario

A 78-year old female LTC resident is seen for a scheduled follow-up visit. She suffered a stroke 1 year ago with resulting aphasia and right-sided hemiparesis. Since admission 12 months ago she has lost 10 kg and has become increasingly bedridden, with less time spent in her wheel chair. She requires assistance with all meals and is on a pureed diet as recommended from a recent swallowing evaluation. While no pressure ulcers were noted on her admission exam, she is currently being treated for a stage 2 sacral pressure ulcer and bilateral stage 1 heel ulcers. Nursing records indicate she finishes about 25% of each meal and requires a great deal of assistance with meals. Her only next of kin is a son who lives several hours away. He has visited twice in the past year and occasionally telephones to check in with nursing staff and talk to his mother.

The resident is examined in her room today with her eyeglasses on. She has a full pitcher of water resting on the bedside table well out of her reach. She is easily fatigued with transfer to the chair and is less interactive than on previous visits. The physical exam is notable for a cachectic female with dry oral mucosa, aphasia, right-sided hemiparesis, and a progressing stage 2 sacral pressure ulcer despite treatment with a protective barrier film and orders to turn patient every 2 hours while in bed. Recent labs are notable for hypernatremia, and an elevated BUN and creatinine from baseline.

This scenario illustrates the often blurry distinction between physical neglect and poor care quality. The difference may be largely semantic, but the responsibility for this poor care can sometimes be clarified through a careful review of the records. An appropriate plan of care may be present, but it may be difficult to follow without adequate staffing or simply ignored by an irresponsible caregiver.

Violation of personal rights and financial/material issues

Clinical scenario

A 71-year-old woman, well known to you, presents for a scheduled 3-month follow-up of her chronic medical problems. She has a past medical history of hypertension, hyperlipidemia, and coronary artery disease. Prior to entering the examination room, you review her vital signs and note her blood pressure is 168/112 (previously 128/85) and her weight is 112 pounds (previously 125 pounds). You enter the room and note that she appears slightly unkempt, although she is usually well-groomed, and her clothes appear stained. Your physical examination, including a cognitive assessment, is otherwise unchanged. You discuss your concern regarding her elevated blood pressure and weight loss. She admits that over the past month she has been not taking her medications, stating, "You know how much things cost these days." She tells you that her grandson, who controls the finances in the household and picks up her medicine, has needed her social security income to settle outstanding debts after being laid off. He has also been withdrawing large amounts from her savings account.

Victims of financial mistreatment may often be aware of the malfeasance, and they may be reluctant or unwilling to disclose the activity [9]. The physician's role in such a scenario is reporting of the suspicion, which then allows further investigation by individuals experienced in detecting such exploitation [68, 69].

Clinical bottom line

Suspicion or identification of elder abuse often requires the synthesis of historical, social, environmental, and physical factors. Findings during the history and physical exam that may suggest mistreatment are listed in Table 13.2.

How can elder abuse be prevented or reduced?

Physical and psychological abuse may be a result of temporary caregiver decompensation, institutional understaffing, poor training, or overt acts, and all may be preventable. However, a recent systematic review of interventions for elder abuse did not find enough high-quality studies of similar interventions to allow generalizable conclusions about efficacy [81]. Evidence for prevention or reduction in abuse primarily comes from individual studies with unique interventions or educational programs. One report from three large LTC facilities in the United States documented a decrease in physical restraint use after the US Omnibus Budget Reconciliation Act of 1990, but continued bed rail use despite a lack of evidence for fall prevention [82]. A case-control study of specialized dementia units in the United States documented a significant decrease in physical restraint use without a corresponding increase in pharmacologic restraints (Level 3b evidence) [83]. Educational programs focusing on care of cognitively impaired adults has been shown to improve attitudes among LTC staff (Level 1b evidence) [84]. Conflict resolution and stress management training have cut abuse reports 24%–55% and improved job satisfaction in several studies (Level 2b evidence) [26, 85, 86]. Improved job satisfaction and attitudes would presumably result in lower job turnover and more successful hiring for open positions, which in turn would improve care. Higher job turnover rates in LTC have been shown to be associated with worse quality of care, including higher rates of pressure sores, psychoactive drug use, and restraint use (Level 2b evidence) [87–89]. Less staff may similarly diminish care quality, although that may depend on the specific type of staff member (Level 2b evidence) [89, 90].

Clinical bottom line

Elder abuse may be preventable. Proper staff training and increased job satisfaction may contribute to the reduction in abuse.

Summary

The complexity of defining elder abuse is due in large part to the broad variety of situations that constitute mistreatment. With the rising percentage of older adults throughout the world, and the ever-expanding variety of care arrangements to accommodate this aging population, conditions conducive to mistreatment will continue to manifest. The evidence base is steadily growing in this field, and further details about all aspects of elder abuse are available for healthcare providers and the public at several online resources [91–93].

Acknowledgment

Assistance with literature searching was provided by Susan Meadows, MLS and Susan Elliott, MLS. Dr. Lindbloom has received funding for elder mistreatment research from the US Department of Justice (National Institute of Justice), the Robert Wood Johnson Foundation, the American Federation for Aging Research, and the John A. Hartford Foundation. Dr. Lindbloom mentored Dr. Hough through a medical student research program sponsored by the Missouri Academy of Family Physicians.

References

1. Burston GR (1975) Granny-battering. *BMJ* 3: 592.
2. Fulmer TT, Cahill VM (1984) Assessing elder abuse: a study. *J Gerontol Nurs* 10: 16–20.
3. Pillemer K, Finkelhor D (1988) The prevalence of elder abuse: a random sample survey. *Gerontologist* 28: 51–57.
4. Lachs MS, Pillemer K (1995) Abuse and neglect of elderly persons. *N Engl J Med* 332: 437–443.
5. United States Congress House Select Committee on Aging, Subcommittee on Human Services (1991) Elder abuse: what can be done? Hearing before the Subcommittee on Human Services of the Select Committee on Aging, House of Representatives, One Hundred Second Congress. First session, May 15, 1991. Washington, DC: US Government Printing Office.
6. Rosenblatt DE, Cho KH, Durance PW (1996) Reporting mistreatment of older adults: the role of physicians. *J Am Geriatr Soc* 44: 65–70.
7. Cooper C, Selwood A, Livingston G (2008) The prevalence of elder abuse and neglect: a systematic review. *Age Ageing* 37: 151–160.
8. Mouton CP, et al (2004) Prevalence and 3-year incidence of abuse among postmenopausal women. *Am J Public Health* 94: 605–612.
9. National Research Council (2003) *Elder Mistreatment: Abuse, Neglect, and Exploitation in an Aging America*. Washington, DC: National Academies Press.
10. Dyer CB, Goodwin JS, Pickens-Pace S, Burnett J, Kelly PA (2007) Self-neglect among the elderly: a model based on more than 500 patients seen by a geriatric medicine team. *Am J Public Health* 97: 1671–1676.
11. Lachs M, et al (2007) Resident-to-resident elder mistreatment and police contact in nursing homes: findings from a population-based cohort. *J Am Geriatr Soc* 55: 840–845.
12. Lachs MS, et al (1997) ED use by older victims of family violence. *Ann Emerg Med* 30: 448–454.
13. Lachs MS, Williams CS, O'Brien S, Pillemer KA, Charlson ME (1998) The mortality of elder mistreatment. *JAMA* 280: 428–432.
14. Lindbloom EJ, Brandt J, Hough LD, Meadows SE (2007) Elder mistreatment in the nursing home: a systematic review. *J Am Med Dir Assoc* 8: 610–6.
15. Burgess AW, Dowdell EB, Prentky RA (2000) Sexual abuse of nursing home residents. *J Psychosoc Nurs Ment Health Serv* 38: 10–18.
16. Dyer CB, Pavlik VN, Murphy KP, Hyman DJ (2000) The high prevalence of depression and dementia in elder abuse or neglect. *J Am Geriatr Soc* 48: 205–208.
17. Lachs MS, Berkman L, Fulmer T, Horwitz RI (1994) A prospective community-based pilot study of risk factors for the investigation of elder mistreatment. *J Am Geriatr Soc* 42: 169–173.
18. Lachs MS, Williams C, O'Brien S, Hurst L, Horwitz R (1996) Older adults. An 11-year longitudinal study of adult protective service use. *Arch Intern Med* 156: 449–453.

19. Lachs MS, Williams C, O'Brien S, Hurst L, Horwitz R (1997) Risk factors for reported elder abuse and neglect: a nine-year observational cohort study. *Gerontologist* 37: 469–474.

20. Paveza GJ, et al (1992) Severe family violence and Alzheimer's disease: prevalence and risk factors. *Gerontologist* 32: 493–497.

21. Pillemer K, Bachman-Prehn R (1991) Helping and hurting: predictors of maltreatment of patients in nursing homes. *Res Aging* 13: 74–95.

22. Wolf RS, Pillemer KA (1989) *Helping Elderly Victims: the Reality of Elder Abuse.* New York: Columbia University Press.

23. Atlanta Long Term Care Ombudsman Program (2001) *The Silenced Voice Speaks Out: a Study of Abuse and Neglect of Nursing Home Residents.* Atlanta, GA: Atlanta Legal Aid Society.

24. Hayley DC, Cassel CK, Snyder L., Rudberg MA (1996) Ethical and legal issues in nursing home care. *Arch Intern Med* 156: 249–256.

25. Pillemer K, Moore DW (1989) Abuse of patients in nursing homes: findings from a survey of staff. *Gerontologist* 29: 314–320.

26. Pillemer K, Hudson B (1993) A model abuse prevention program for nursing assistants. *Gerontologist* 33: 128–131.

27. U.S. House of Representatives (2004) Abuse of residents is a major problem in U.S. nursing homes prepared for Rep. Henry A. Waxman. July 31, 2001. Washington, DC, U.S. House of Representatives, Committee on Government Reform, Special Investigations Division, Minority Staff.

28. Administration on Aging (U.S.) (2005) Long-term care ombudsman report: FY 1998 with comparisons of national data for FY 1996–1998. September 9, 2004. Washington, DC, U.S. Department of Health and Human Services, Administration on Aging.

29. Krueger P, Patterson C (1997) Detecting and managing elder abuse: challenges in primary care. The Research Subcommittee of the Elder Abuse and Self-Neglect Task Force of Hamilton–Wentworth. *CMAJ* 157: 1095–1100.

30. Aravanis SC, et al (1993) Diagnostic and treatment guidelines on elder abuse and neglect. *Arch Fam Med* 2: 371–388.

31. Astrom S, et al (2004) Staff's experience of and the management of violent incidents in elderly care. *Scand J Caring Sci* 18: 410–416.

32. Shaw MMC (2004) Aggression toward staff by nursing home residents: findings from a grounded theory study. *J Gerontol Nurs* 30: 43–54.

33. Shaw MMC (1998) Nursing home resident abuse by staff: exploring the dynamics. *J Elder Abuse Neglect* 9: 1–21.

34. Foner N (1994) Nursing home aides: saints or monsters? *Gerontologist* 34: 245–250.

35. Hare J, Pratt CC (1988) Burnout: differences between professional and paraprofessional nursing staff in acute care and long-term care health facilities. *J Appl Gerontol* 7: 60–72.

36. Mercer SO, Heacock P, Beck C (1993) Nurses' aides in nursing homes: perceptions of training, work loads, racism, and abuse issues. *J Gerontol Soc Work* 21: 95–112.

37. Waxman HM, Carner EA, Berkenstock G (1984) Job turnover and job satisfaction among nursing home aides. *Gerontologist* 24: 503–509.

38. Hirst SP (2002) Defining resident abuse within the culture of long-term care institutions. *Clin Nurs Res* 11: 267–284.

39. Dube AH, Mitchell EK (1986) Accidental strangulation from vest restraints. *JAMA* 256: 2725–2726.

40. Miles SH (2002) Deaths between bedrails and air pressure mattresses. *J Am Geriatr Soc* 50: 1124–1125.

41. Miles SH, Irvine P (1992) Deaths caused by physical restraints. *Gerontologist* 32: 762–766.

42. Miles SH (2002) Concealing accidental nursing home deaths. *HEC Forum* 14: 224–234.

43. Parker K, Miles SH (1997) Deaths caused by bedrails. *J Am Geriatr Soc* 45: 797–802.

44. Corey TS, Weakley-Jones B, Nichols GR, Theuer HH (1992) Unnatural deaths in nursing home patients. *J Forensic Sci* 37: 222–227.

45. Bravo G, Dubois MF, De Wals P, Hebert R, Messier L (2002) Relationship between regulatory status, quality of care, and three-year mortality in Canadian residential care facilities: a longitudinal study. *Health Serv Res* 37: 1181–1196.

46. Mor V, Zinn J, Angelelli J, Teno JM, Miller SC (2004) Driven to tiers: socioeconomic and racial disparities in the quality of nursing home care. *Milbank Q* 82: 227–256.

47. Brandeis GH, Morris JN, Nash DJ, Lipsitz LA (1990) The epidemiology and natural history of pressure ulcers in elderly nursing home residents. *JAMA* 264: 2905–2909.

48. Sternberg J, Spector WD, Kapp MC, Tucker RJ (1988) Decubitus ulcers on admission to nursing homes: prevalence and residents' characteristics. *Decubitus* 1: 14–20.

49. Thomas DR (2001) Are all pressure ulcers avoidable? *J Am Med Dir Assoc* 2: 297–301.

50. Tsokos M, Heinemann A, Puschel K (2000) Pressure sores: epidemiology, medico-legal implications and forensic argumentation concerning causality. *Int J Legal Med* 113: 283–287.

51. Brandeis GH, Berlowitz DR, Katz P (2001) Are pressure ulcers preventable? A survey of experts. *Adv Skin Wound Care* 14: 244–248.

52. Rudman D, Slater EJ, Richardson TJ, Mattson DE (1993) The occurrence of pressure ulcers in three nursing homes. *J Gen Intern Med* 8: 653–658.

53. Rudman D, Mattson DE, Alverno L, Richardson TJ, Rudman IW (1993) Comparison of clinical indicators in two nursing homes. *J Am Geriatr Soc* 41: 1317–1325.

54. Berlowitz DR, Bezerra HQ, Brandeis GH, Kader B, Anderson JJ (2000) Are we improving the quality of nursing home care: the case of pressure ulcers. *J Am Geriatr Soc* 48: 59–62.

55. Berlowitz DR, Young GJ, Brandeis GH, Kader B, Anderson JJ (2001) Health care reorganization and quality of care: unintended effects on pressure ulcer prevention. *Med Care* 39: 138–146.

56. Brandeis GH, Ooi WL, Hossain M, Morris JN, Lipsitz LA (1994) A longitudinal study of risk factors associated with the formation of pressure ulcers in nursing homes. *J Am Geriatr Soc* 42: 388–393.

57. Aziz SJ, Campbell-Taylor I (1999) Neglect and abuse associated with undernutrition in long-term care in North America: causes and solutions. *J Elder Abuse Neglect* 10: 91–117.

58. Elmstahl S, Persson M, Andren M, Blabolil V (1997) Malnutrition in geriatric patients: a neglected problem? *J Adv Nurs* 26: 851–855.

59. Kayser-Jones J (2002) Malnutrition, dehydration, and starvation in the midst of plenty: the political impact of qualitative inquiry. *Qual Health Res* 12: 1391–1405.

60. Kayser-Jones J, Schell E, Lyons W, Kris AE, Chan J, Beard RL (2003) Factors that influence end-of-life care in nursing homes: the physical environment, inadequate staffing, and lack of supervision. *Gerontologist* 43(Special Issue 2): 76–84.

61. Ryan C, Bryant E, Eleazer P, Rhodes A, Guest K (1995) Unintentional weight loss in long-term care: predictor of mortality in the elderly. *South Med J* 88: 721–724.

62. Kayser-Jones J (2000) A case study of the death of an older woman in a nursing home: are nursing care practices in compliance with ethical guidelines? *J Gerontol Nurs* 26: 48–54.

63. Himmelstein DU, Jones AA, Woolhandler S (1983) Hypernatremic dehydration in nursing home patients: an indicator of neglect. *J Am Geriatr Soc* 31: 466–471.

64. Meddaugh DI (1993) Covert elder abuse in the nursing home. *J Elder Abuse Neglect* 5: 21–37.

65. Tarbox AR (1983) The elderly in nursing homes: psychological aspects of neglect. *Clin Gerontol* 1: 39–52.

66. Weatherall M (2001) Elder abuse: a survey of managers of residential care facilities in Wellington, New Zealand. *J Elder Abuse Neglect* 13: 91–99.

67. Kennedy M (2000) The subtle and the overt: identifying elder abuse. *WMJ* 99: 10–14.

68. Kemp BJ, Mosqueda LA (2005) Elder financial abuse: an evaluation framework and supporting evidence. *J Am Geriatr Soc* 53: 1123–1127.

69. Wilber KH, Reynolds SL (1996) Introducing a framework for defining financial abuse of the elderly. *J Elder Abuse Neglect* 8: 61–80.

70. Harris DK, Benson ML (1999) Theft in nursing homes: an overlooked form of elder abuse. *J Elder Abuse Neglect* 11: 73–90.

71. Burgess AW, Hanrahan NP (2004) Issues in elder sexual abuse in nursing homes. *Nurs Health Pol Rev* 3: 5–17.

72. Teaster PB, Roberto KA (2004) Sexual abuse of older adults: APS cases and outcomes. *Gerontologist* 44: 788–796.

73. UK Department of Health (2000) No secrets: guidance on developing and implementing multi-agency policies and procedures to protect vulnerable adults from abuse http://www.dh.gov.uk/en/Publicationsandstatistics/Publications/PublicationsPolicyAndGuidance/DH_4008486 (accessed November 22, 2011).

74. Kane RS, Goodwin JS (1991) Spontaneous fractures of the long bones in nursing home patients. *Am J Med* 90: 263–266.

75. Mosqueda L, Burnight K, Liao S (2005) The life cycle of bruises in older adults. *J Am Geriatr Soc* 53: 1339–1343.

76. Wiglesworth A, Austin R, Corona M, Schneider D, Liao S, Gibbs L, Mosqueda L (2009) Bruising as a marker of physical elder abuse. *J Am Geriatr Soc* 57: 1191–1196.

77. Wiglesworth A, Mosqueda L, Mulnard R, Liao S, Gibbs L, Fitzgerald W (2010) Screening for abuse and neglect of people with dementia. *J Am Geriatr Soc* 58: 493–500.

78. Fulmer T, Street S, Carr K (1984) Abuse of the elderly: screening and detection. *J Emerg Nurs* 10: 131–140.

79. Reis M, Nahmiash D (1998) Validation of the indicators of abuse (IOA) screen. *Gerontologist* 38: 471–480.

80. Yaffe MJ, Wolfson C, Lithwick M, Weiss D (2008) Development and validation of a tool to improve physician identification of elder abuse: the Elder Abuse Suspicion Index (EASI). *J Elder Abuse Neglect* 20: 276–300.

81. Ploeg J, Fear J, Hutchison B, MacMillan H, Bolan G (2009) A systematic review of interventions for elder abuse. *J Elder Abuse Neglect* 21: 187–210.

82. Capezuti E, Maislin G, Strumpf N, Evans LK (2002) Side rail use and bed-related fall outcomes among nursing home residents. *J Am Geriatr Soc* 50: 90–96.

83. Sloane PD, Mathew LJ, Scarborough M, Desai JR, Koch GG, Tangen C (1991) Physical and pharmacologic restraint of nursing home patients with dementia. Impact of specialized units. *JAMA* 265: 1278–1282.

84. Richardson B, Kitchen G, Livingston G (2002) The effect of education on knowledge and management of elder abuse: a randomized controlled trial. *Age Ageing* 31: 335–341.

85. Braun KL, Suzuki KM, Cusick CE, Howard-Carhart K (1997) Developing and testing training materials on elder abuse and neglect for nurse aides. *J Elder Abuse Neglect* 9: 1–15.

86. Menio D, Keller BH (2000) CARIE: a multifaceted approach to abuse prevention in nursing homes. *Generations* 24: 28–32.

87. Castle NG, Engberg J (2005) Staff turnover and quality of care in nursing homes. *Med Care* 43: 616–626.

88. Castle NG (2001) Administrator turnover and quality of care in nursing homes. *Gerontologist* 41: 757–767.

89. Zimmerman S, Gruber-Baldini AL, Hebel JR, Sloane PD, Magaziner J (2002) Nursing home facility risk factors for infection and hospitalization: importance of registered nurse turnover, administration, and social factors. *J Am Geriatr Soc* 50: 1987–1995.

90. Harrington C, Zimmerman D, Karon SL, Robinson J, Beutel P (2000) Nursing home staffing and its relationship to deficiencies. *J Gerontol B Psychol Sci Soc Sci* 55: S278–S287.

91. National Center on Elder Abuse. http://www.ncea.aoa.gov/ (accessed November 22, 2011).

92. Clearinghouse on Abuse and Neglect of the Elderly. http://www.cane.udel.edu/ (accessed November 22, 2011).

93. Center of Excellence on Elder Abuse and Neglect. http://www.centeronelderabuse.org/ (accessed November 22, 2011).

CHAPTER 14

A good death: appropriate end-of-life care

Cari Levy[1,2] *& Jean S. Kutner*[3]

[1]University of Colorado Denver School of Medicine, Denver, CO, USA
[2]Denver VA Medical Center, Denver, CO, USA
[3]University of Colorado, Denver School of Medicine, Aurora, CO, USA

Introduction

The definition of a "good death" depends on a person's values and is therefore, a highly individualized concept. Some individuals value "life at all costs," while others value comfort measures over life-extending measures. Despite very different definitions regarding what constitutes life-sustaining interventions, common themes emerge from studies describing preferences for care at the end of life.

This chapter focuses on appropriate end-of-life care for older adults. Four clinical topics and the evidence base for each topic are described as follows:

1 What is a good death?
2 How is managing pain in the older adult unique?
3 What evidence exists for treatment of dyspnea at the end of life?
4 What role do advance directives play at the end of life for older adults?

Search strategy

We searched PubMed that comprises citations for biomedical literature from MEDLINE, life science journals, and online books beginning January 1, 1995 through June 30, 2010. We restricted to the English language and age over 65 years. For the same time period, we searched the Cochrane Database of Systematic Reviews. The general search strategy was to identify systematic reviews and meta-analyses of randomized controlled clinical trials for each topic. Consensus statements, when available, were also reviewed for each topic. Medical Subject Heading (MeSH) search terms included: "end-of-life," "quality of death," "pain," "medication," "treatment," "dyspnea," and "advance directives." For this chapter, we graded relevant clinical studies using the Oxford Centre for Evidence-based Medicine Levels of Evidence.

What is a good death?

We identified 47 articles combining the following MeSH terms: "end-of-life," "death," and "quality." We excluded articles focused on one disease state in order to focus on general characteristics of death rather than those associated with specific disease states. Nine studies were included in this review and focused on exploration of patient and family caregiver, as well as healthcare provider, perspectives regarding the components of a "good death." These studies are exploratory, using qualitative methodology (Level 4 evidence).

A Canadian study in which focus groups were conducted with chronically ill, long-term care residents delineated five dimensions of a good death: (1) pain and symptom management, (2) avoiding prolongation of dying, (3) achieving a sense of control, (4) relieving burden on others, and (5) strengthening relationships with others [1]. Similar domains were described in a

Evidence-Based Geriatric Medicine: A Practical Clinical Guide, First Edition. Edited by Jayna M. Holroyd-Leduc and Madhuri Reddy.
© 2012 Blackwell Publishing Ltd. Published 2012 by Blackwell Publishing Ltd.

focus group study among chronically ill patients, bereaved family members, and health professionals in the Southeast United States. These individuals defined a good death as entailing: pain and symptom management, preparation for death, achieving a sense of completion, contributing to others, affirmation of the whole person, and clear decision-making [2].

A prospective cohort study conducted in the Northwest United States included three groups ($N = 670$): (1) patients with chronic obstructive pulmonary disease (COPD) and their family members, (2) hospice patients and family members, and (3) patients and family members who had participated in trials of complementary and alternative therapies at the end of life [3]. Participants rated the importance of 28 items (e.g., pain control, finding meaning and purpose in life, having healthcare costs taken care of) plus place of death, presence of others at death, and state of consciousness just prior to death, then selected and ranked their five most important. The investigators then differentiated between high (defined as the top five priorities for at least 25% of the participants), medium (the top five priorities for 10%–20%), and low priority (mentioned by less than 10%) areas. High-priority items included spending time with family and friends, pain control, breathing comfort, maintaining dignity and self-respect, being at peace with dying, avoiding strain on loved ones, and avoiding life support. There were only two statistically significant associations between participant characteristics and priority scores. As level of education increased, participants placed higher priority on having available means to hasten death, and racial/ethnic minorities placed higher priority on having funeral arrangements in order, than White non-Hispanic respondents [3].

In another prospective cohort study of 988 terminally ill patients and 893 caregivers in six randomly selected cities in the United States (Worchester, MA; St. Louis, MO; Tucson, AZ; Birmingham, AL; Brooklyn, NY; Mesa County, CO) interviews were used to develop a model of the mechanism by which terminally ill patients and their families experience economic, psychosocial, and other burdens. This model suggests that terminally ill patients with physical symptoms experience substantial care requirements and, in turn, economic and other burdens. The underlying factors that are associated with significant care needs and eco-

nomic burdens—older age, lower income, poor physical function, and incontinence—are not readily modifiable or amenable to medical interventions. Therefore the only interventions that may be able to reduce burdens will probably be directed at attending to patients' care needs. A patient's fear of being a burden appears to be a primary motivation for inquiries about euthanasia or physician-assisted suicide [4].

A prospective longitudinal multicenter cohort study of patient preferences among individuals aged 60 years old or older ($N = 414$) with limited life expectancy due to cancer, congestive heart failure, or chronic obstructive pulmonary disease found that 99% would choose to undergo a treatment that was low burden and restored health. In contrast, 27% would choose a treatment that afforded survival but with severe functional impairment, and only 11% would choose a treatment that afforded survival but with severe cognitive impairment [5]. In another study conducted among 414 hospitalized patients aged 80 years or older, older patients were able to assess their health values using the time-trade-off technique, reflecting preferences for current health relative to a shorter but healthier life. Most patients were unwilling to trade much time for excellent health, but preferences varied greatly. Proxies were not able to gauge the health values of this population, arguing that health values should be elicited directly from the patient [6].

Patients tend to judge medical interventions as desirable if they have the potential to return the individual to his or her most valued life activities [6]. The outcomes of interventions, including cognitive and physical functioning, self-care, productivity, and emotional or care-taking burden on loved ones, rather than the interventions themselves, inform treatment decisions [6]. Patients prefer to weigh facts and realities, talk with loved ones about decisions, consider all available choices, and postpone decisions until their condition warrants making more decisions [6]. Advanced age has been found to be relevant to treatment decision-making, taking into account personal losses experienced and fear of future losses, the perception that serious illness in old age carries a poor prognosis, and a relative emphasis on maintaining function rather than on longevity per se [7, 8].

Focus groups conducted in the Northwest United Sates among patients with advanced illness, bereaved family members, nurses, and physicians who participated in end-of-life care identified the following physician attributes as important at the end of life: communication with patients, emotional support, accessibility and continuity, competence, respect and humility, team communication and coordination, patient education, personalization, pain and symptom management, inclusion and recognition of family, attention to patient's values, and support of patient decision-making [9].

Clinical bottom line

Appropriate end-of-life care includes adherence to patient values and preferences, expert symptom management, continuity and coordination of care, care for the whole person, including emotional and spiritual well-being, and family support.

Despite considerable agreement about the highest priorities during the end-of-life period, the process of dying and death is highly individualized, making it essential that we ask, and listen to our patients to ascertain their priorities as we work with them around end-of-life decision-making.

How is pain management unique in the older adult?

We identified 86 articles using the following MeSH terms: "pain" AND "medication" AND "treatment" AND "geriatric." Because of differences in medication availability across different countries, we elected to focus on articles conducted in the United States, and medications available for prescription in the United States. We excluded articles focused on location or disease-specific pain management. This resulted in review of 32 articles.

Relief of physical pain is one of the most common patient needs at the end of life [10]. Pain, when unrecognized and untreated, can result in depression, insomnia, falls, decreased socialization, and loss of function. The prevalence of pain in community-dwelling older adults ranges from 25% to 50% [11]. The American Geriatrics Society (AGS) panel on persistent pain in older persons states that up to 80% of long-term care residents have substantial pain, and 25% of those have received neither analgesic medication nor non-pharmacological treatment for their pain [11–13].

Pain management

Pain management can be challenging in older adults because of the difficulty in assessing pain due to cognitive or other impairments (e.g., auditory, visual, motor). In addition, symptoms of pain in older individuals may manifest as delirium, disturbances in mood, and/or functional decline [14]. Although opioids are often cited as a causative factor in delirium, proper pain management has been shown to actually decrease the incidence of delirium in older adults [15, 16]. Symptom assessment scales should match the cognitive and functional abilities of each patient [17, 18].

Alterations in opiate pharmacokinetics, due to decreases in creatinine clearance, gastrointestinal (GI) transit time, and lean body mass that accompany aging, present another challenge in pain management for older adults. The rate at which certain drugs are absorbed can be altered in the elderly because of decreased GI transit time and increased gastric pH, secondary to use of proton pump inhibitors, H_2 receptor antagonists, or antacids. With aging, there are also changes in body composition including loss of lean body mass, an increase in adipose tissue, and decrease in total body water. These changes can affect drug distribution. For example, lipophilic drugs have a greater volume of distribution and take longer to be eliminated from the body [19].

Pharmacodynamics are also altered by physiologic changes such as decreased renal and hepatic blood flow, which decrease metabolism of drugs in older adults [11, 20, 21]. Morphine, hydromorphone, and gabapentin are primarily cleared through the kidneys and are more apt to accumulate in the setting of reduced renal function than opioids such as fentanyl and methadone [22, 23]. For older patients with renal and/or hepatic dysfunction, dose escalation percentages should be reduced according to the half-life of the medications [24]. Short-acting oral single agent opioids can be safely escalated every 2 hours, while sustained release oral opioids should not be escalated sooner than every 24 hours. In the case of the fentanyl patch, methadone, or levorphanol, no adjustment should be made earlier than 72 hours [25–27] (Level 3 evidence). Additional impairments in drug metabolism include a reduction of first pass metabolism of opiates in older adults due to impaired Phase I reactions (i.e., oxidation, hydroxylation, and dealkylation) [20]. This and other alterations in drug metabolism in the older adult generally cause drugs used to be more potent and have a longer duration of action than predicted.

Because of pharmacokinetic and pharmacodynamic changes with aging, opioids should be started at the lower dose, approximately 25%–50% of the dose given to younger patients. Meperidine and propoxyphene should be avoided in the older patients [28]. Meperidine has active metabolites that can cause neuroexcitation, nervousness, and seizures. Propoxyphene has not been shown to be more effective than placebo [29] (Level 2c evidence). Tramadol is not recommended in patients who are taking serotonergic medications or in those with underlying seizure disorders, and dose reductions are required in the setting of hepatic dysfunction [11]. Partial opioid agonists (i.e., pentazocine, butorphenol, buprenorphine, and nalbuphine) are not recommended due to analgesic ceiling effects, hallucinations, dysphoria, and risk of precipitating withdrawal in opioid-dependent patients [28]. If codeine is administered, one must recognize that its effectiveness depends on metabolism into its seven active metabolites, yet as many as 30% of the population are poor hydroxylators of debrisoquine required for this activation resulting in unpredictable levels of the final metabolite, morphine [23].

Other common problems that should be taken into consideration when caring for older adults include polypharmacy, multiple comorbidities, and the potential of more side effects or treatment failures when compared to younger adults. Strategies for treating pain safely in the older patient include: simplifying the pain regimen, reducing the number of medications prescribed, and beginning drugs at lower dosages and titrating upward as needed (i.e., "start low and go slow.") [11]. In general, doses can be initiated at 25%–50% of the starting dose for younger adults.

Because of risks of GI bleeding and renal failure with use of nonselective nonsteroidal anti-inflammatory drugs (NSAIDs), these medications are rarely the most appropriate first choice for pain management in older adults. Opiates may be appropriate in severe pain with careful monitoring [11]. Older adults may fear becoming addicted to opioids and often need education about differences between tolerance, physical dependence, and addiction [30]. Side effects such as constipation and urinary retention are common in older adults and require careful monitoring especially in cognitively impaired or nonverbal patients [31].

Common reasons that pain medications are required for older adults

Osteoarthritis

Osteoarthritis is common in elderly [32]. NSAIDs are frequently used to treat osteoarthritis, but potentially can cause heart failure or renal failure. Furthermore, NSAIDs may be contraindicated in the elderly because of concomitant medication use or because of previous peptic ulcer disease. In a systematic review and meta-analysis of randomized placebo controlled trials, 23 trials including 10,845 patients, median age of 62.5 years, followed for 8 years, NSAIDs reduced short-term pain in osteoarthritis of the knee slightly better than placebo, but the evidence did not support long-term use of NSAIDs for this condition because of serious adverse effects associated with oral NSAIDs (Level 1a evidence) [33]. The risk of upper GI bleeding with NSAIDs varies 20-fold depending on the drug, and by three- to sevenfold depending on the dose chosen. Risk is maximal during the first week and decreases thereafter.

Acetaminophen is not associated with upper GI bleeding at any dose and is recommended as the first-line analgesic wherever possible (Level 1a evidence) [34]. In an analysis of NSAIDs compared to acetaminophen in osteoarthritis, NSAIDs were statistically superior in reducing rest and walking pain compared with acetaminophen yet safety, measured by discontinuation due to adverse events, was not statistically different between NSAID- and acetaminophen-treated groups (Level 1a evidence) [35]. Short-term use (2–3 weeks) of topical NSAIDS can produce marked reduction in inflammation and pain with acceptable side effect profiles (Level 1a evidence) [36–39].

Neuropathic pain

Tricyclics and carbamazepine are efficacious for treatment of neuropathic pain (number needed to treat (NNT) of 3.5 for 50% pain relief in diabetic neuropathy and 2.1 for 50% pain relief in postherpetic neuralgia) (Level 1a evidence) [40]. These medications are limited by side effects and the potential for drug–drug

Table 14.1 Treatments for pain

Preferred Agents for Elderly Patients	Acceptable in Elderly with Careful Monitoring	Not Recommended in Elderly
Aminophenol: acetaminophen	Nonsteroidal anti-inflammatory: ibuprofen, meloxicam, naproxen, diclofenac, etodolac, fenoprofen, ketoprofen, sulindac, celecoxib,	Nonsteroidal anti-inflammatory: indomethacin, ketorolac
Opioid analgesics: morphine, oxycodone, hydrocodone + acetaminophen, hydromorphone, fentanyl, oxymorphone	Opioid analgesics: methadone, codeine, buprenorphine	Opioid analgesics: butorphenol, meperidine, pentazocine, propoxyphene
Salicylates (nonacetylated): Salsalate	Salicylate: aspirin	Nonsteroidal anti-inflammatory mixed COX-1 and COX-2 inhibitors: piroxicam, oxaprozin
Miscellaneous: tramadol	Miscellaneous: topical capsaicin, diclofenac gel, duloxetine, diclofenac patch, lidocaine patch, serotonin reuptake inhibitors, and mixed reuptake inhibitors	
	Anticonvulsants: carbamazepine, gabapentin, pregabalin	

interactions in older adults [41]. Antiepileptic drugs, such as gabapentin, have side effects of somnolence and ataxia, but have a better overall side effect profile and provide similar efficacy (Level 1a evidence) [40]. When using gabapentin for treatment of neuropathic pain in older adults, recommendations are to begin with a dose of 100 mg at bedtime and increase the dose as tolerated to achieve relief from pain while monitoring for falls and somnolence. Safer alternatives in the older patient include serotonin reuptake inhibitors and mixed reuptake inhibitors (i.e., citalopram, duloxetine, sertraline, venlafaxine) (Level 1a evidence) [42, 43].

Clinical bottom line

Pain is often neither recognized nor adequately treated in older adults.

Pharmacokinetic and pharmacodynamics necessitate careful selection of appropriate medications and initial doses that are lower than starting doses for younger persons.

Given the high prevalence of pain in older adults and challenges associated with treatment, it is imperative to assess, evaluate, treat, and recognize side effects associated with the pharmacologic management of pain,

with specific consideration of barriers to doing so in older adults (Table 14.1).

What evidence exists for treatment of dyspnea at the end of life?

We identified 79 articles by combining the following MeSH terms: "dyspnea," "end-of-life," and "treatment." We included only articles specifically focused on dyspnea, excluding those focused on general symptom burden. This resulted in review of 29 articles.

While many studies on dyspnea include older adults, few focus exclusively on the older population. Until data are available that specifically focus on older patients, currently available data must be extrapolated to the older population.

Breathlessness is one of the most common symptoms experienced in the advanced stages of nonmalignant disease and affects as many as 70% of patients with advanced cancer [44–46]. The American Thoracic Society defines dyspnea as a subjective experience of breathing discomfort that consists of qualitatively distinct sensations that vary in intensity; dyspnea is a very personal experience [47]. The experience of dyspnea can be affected by tumor growth, pleural effusion, progressive comorbid disease, cancer cachexia, and any number of other conditions affecting functional and/or lung capacity [44–46]. Twenty percent of cancer patients report psychological distress attributed to dyspnea, which is a strong determinant of quality of life and health status [46, 48–50]. Furthermore, physician and patient assessments of dyspnea do not correlate indicating that physician assessment is not a reliable indicator of the experience of dyspnea [51].

The first step in managing dyspnea is treating the underlying cause. At the end of life, when treatment of the underlying cause is not the goal of care, the focus should be on symptom control in an effort to decrease the sensation of dyspnea. A three-step ladder for treatment of dyspnea recommends first optimizing bronchodilators, exercise training, and supplemental oxygen in accordance with COPD guidelines. The second step, if dyspnea persists or worsens in the ladder, is using nonpharmacological therapies including pulmonary rehabilitation, pursed-lip breathing, a fan, relaxation techniques, and paced activities. The third step is use of palliative pharmacological interventions such as morphine and anxiolytics (Level 3b evidence) (Table 14.2) [52, 53].

Patients often report symptomatic improvement with inhaled short-acting beta-agonist bronchodila-

tors in the management of both stable and acute exacerbations of COPD. In a meta-analysis of patients with COPD, a significant improvement in daily breathlessness score was observed during treatment with a beta-agonist when compared to placebo (Standardized Mean Difference (SMD) 1.33; 95% confidence interval (CI) 1.01–1.65) (Level 1a evidence) [54]. One study that used a validated questionnaire for "quality of life" assessment, found highly significant improvements in the scores for dyspnea ($p = 0.003$) and fatigue ($p = 0.0003$) during treatment with salbutamol (Level 1a evidence) [54, 55].

A series of randomized controlled trials have consistently demonstrated the effectiveness of opioids for treatment of dyspnea and as a result, these medications are considered the drugs of choice for dyspnea [56–58]. In the opioid naïve patient, low doses of oral (10–15 mg) or parenteral morphine (2–5 mg) are recommended, but in opioid-tolerant patients, higher doses may be required [59]. In a meta-analysis of nebulized opioids the evidence supporting efficacy is weak, but benefit has been reported in uncontrolled case reports [60].

While a systematic review of 103 studies provides evidence to support the use of physical exercise in COPD training to improve health-related quality of life and functional exercise capacity, [61] this did not specifically target patients in the final months of life. In a meta-analysis of pulmonary rehabilitation, improvement in dyspnea, fatigue, emotional function, and an enhancement of patients' control over their condition occurred during the rehabilitation program [62]. In contrast, in a meta-analysis of breathing control (relaxed basal, diaphragmatic, or abdominal breathing) as the sole intervention, breathing control had a detrimental effect on the work of breathing (SMD 1.06; 95% CI 0.52–1.60) and dyspnea (SMD 1.47; 95% CI 0.88–2.05) among patients with severe respiratory disease [63].

The use of palliative oxygen to relieve breathlessness toward the end of life is a common practice, and is supported by consensus guidelines published by the American College of Chest Physicians and the Scientific Committee of the Association of Palliative Medicine [64, 65]. However, the effect of oxygen therapy over breathing room air on relief of dyspnea due to end-stage cancer or cardiac failure failed to demonstrate a consistent beneficial effect of oxygen

Table 14.2 Treatments for dyspnea

Evidence-Based— Supported by Clinical Trial Data	Supported by Case Reports and/or Observational Data
Treat the underlying cause	Theophylline combined with beta agonist (COPD patients)
Beta-agonist bronchodilators	Supplemental oxygen
Opioids (oral or parenteral)	Nebulized furosemide
Exercise training	Nebulized opioids
Pulmonary rehabilitation (pursed-lip breathing, fan, relaxation, paced activities)	Benzodiazepines
Steroids for COPD exacerbations	

COPD, chronic obstructive pulmonary disease.

inhalation over inhalation of room air (Level 1b evidence) [66]. The failure to demonstrate a beneficial effect for oxygen inhalation is limited by the small volume of well-conducted research studies available and there is a subset of cancer patients that appeared to feel better during oxygen inhalation [67]. Thus, despite lack of evidence, one will not know if benefit will be realized without a therapeutic trial (based on symptom relief not pulse oximetry). Administration of oxygen using a nasal cannula is generally preferred over an oxygen mask. Oxygen delivery in excess of 4–6 L/min tends to increase discomfort and there is no evidence that rates higher than this are of benefit for the actively dying patient [68].

A systematic review and meta-analysis of the effect of theophylline in combination with short-acting or long-acting inhaled beta2-agonists on dyspnea in patients with COPD demonstrated significant relief of dyspnea (Level 1b evidence). The effect of theophylline combined with beta2-agonists to that of a placebo, was a statistically significant improvement in mean dyspnea (–0.78; 95% CI –1.26 to –0.29). An improvement in dyspnea was also observed with the administration of theophylline combined with beta2-agonists, compared to that of theophylline alone (–0.19; 95% CI –0.34 to 0.04) [69]. While these studies only included patients with stable COPD, one could argue that due to the unpredictable risk of mortality among COPD patients, the studies are also relevant to the end-of-life population [70, 71].

Nebulized furosemide may relieve the sense of dyspnea and improve some physiological measurements, but the studies included in a systematic review of this therapy are small clinical trials or observational (Level 3a evidence) [72].

In a systematic review of steroids for acute exacerbations of dyspnea, there was a significant improvement in breathlessness and no significant effect on mortality. However, the optimal dose and length of treatment regime needs to be better defined (Level 1b evidence) [73].

In a meta-analysis of benzodiazepine use for treatment of dyspnea, seven studies were identified, including 200 analyzed participants with advanced cancer and COPD (Level 3a evidence) [74]. These studies did not show a beneficial effect of benzodiazepines for the relief of breathlessness in patients with advanced cancer or COPD. Benzodiazepines were associated with more sedation than placebo but less than with opioids.

Clinical bottom line

Evidence-based treatments for dyspnea includes: treatment of the underlying condition, beta-agonists, opioids, exercise, pulmonary rehabilitation, and steroids in acute exacerbations of COPD.

Use of theophylline when combined with a beta-agonist, oxygen, nebulized morphine or furosemide, and benzodiazepines are less evidence-based practices and supported only by case reports or observational data.

What role do advance directives play at the end of life for older adults?

We identified 359 articles by combining the following MeSH terms: "advance directives" and "end-of-life." We excluded articles that were location or disease-specific and those not focused specifically on the influence of advance directives on end-of-life care, resulting in review of 15 articles.

Advance directives are documented for only 5%–30% of the general population in the United States. In a study of resuscitation preference documentation across the United States, Canada, Australia, and Sweden, preferences were documented at the time of hospital admission for 11% of patients [75]. This is despite evidence that patients value the ability to plan in advance of illness and physicians consider advance directives helpful in clinical decision-making [76]. Evidence exists indicating that advance directives do not influence care decisions (Level 1a evidence); [77] however, knowledge of advance care planning has increased in recent years with 29% of Americans in 2006 reporting knowledge of advance directives compared to only 12% in 1990 [78]. In addition, research focused on the effects of advance care documentation among patients at high risk of death, rather than the population as a whole, demonstrates that advance care planning strongly influences care delivery at the end of life by increasing the likelihood that a patient's wishes will be carried through.

Both patient and physician-level barriers account for suboptimal advance directive documentation among older adults. Patient-level barriers include:

(1) deferring decisions to others, (2) the topic is too distressing to discuss, (3) lack of knowledge about advance directives, (4) difficulty understanding advance care planning documents, and (5) planning to complete the documents at a later time. Physician-level barriers include: (1) lack of skills to discuss advance care planning, (2) lack of time to discuss advance care planning, (3) lack of perceived patient literacy, (4) lack of privacy, and (5) a belief that the patient is not ill enough to need advance directives [79]. In a study of resident physicians, cardiopulmonary resuscitation (CPR) was discussed with 71% of patients at the time of admission to the hospital, but more in-depth discussions about values and goals of care were only reported for 32% of patients [80]. The resident physician's attributed this to time pressures, unfamiliarity with the patient, uncertainty about documentation procedures, and a belief that peers and their supervising physicians valued CPR discussions more than discussions of values and goals [80].

Executing an advance directive is important for several reasons. First, the majority of older persons experience significant disability in the year preceding death that renders them unable to make decisions on their own behalf [81, 82]. In the absence of discussions about or documentation of preferences for care, surrogates are inaccurate in their predictions of what type of care a loved one would want [83]. In addition, it is difficult to predict when to initiate discussions of advance directives based on illness trajectory. Among adults older than 70 years of age enrolled in a study about illness trajectory who did not have a disability at study enrollment, the following five trajectories occurred in the decade preceding death: (1) catastrophic (20%), (2) accelerated (18%), (3) progressive (24%), (4) persistently severe (22%), and (5) none (17%) [84]. Only a diagnosis of dementia was associated with a predictable trajectory of progressive illness. The variability observed in these trajectories illustrates that the course of illness among older adults is unpredictable, making it difficult to accurately time discussions about advance directives. These data together with the knowledge that capacity often suffers at the end of life and surrogate decision-making is frequently inaccurate, suggests that advance directive discussions should occur with all older adults regardless of current medical condition or illness trajectory.

Care preferences among older adults in the months preceding death vary. Illness awareness and discussion of advance directives improve the chances that care preferences are honored. Among patients for whom treatment preferences were assessed in the 3–6 months before death, 72% preferred symptom-focused care, while 28% preferred life-extending care. Of note, those who received life-extending therapy did not live any longer than those who did not receive care aimed at extending life. The 39% of patients who recognized the terminal nature of their disease were more likely to prefer symptom-directed care (odds ratio (OR) 2.4; 95% CI 1.4–4.2). Awareness of terminal illness and a discussion about goals of care with a physician were also associated with receipt of care consistent with preferences [85]. In a study of advance directives, 34% of decedents who lost decision-making capacity had neither a living will nor a designated Durable Medical Power of Attorney (DMPOA). Persons with a DMPOA were less likely to receive "all care possible" (OR 0.54; 95% CI 0.34–0.86) [86] and less likely to die in a hospital (OR 0.72; 95% CI 0.55–0.93) [87]. Among those aged 81 years who died between 2000 and 2006, those with living wills were more likely to place limits on care (93%) or to select a plan focused on comfort care (96%), as opposed to requesting "all care possible" (2%). Of those requesting comfort care, 97% of received care as requested. In a longitudinal, multi-institutional cohort study of patients with metastatic cancer, only 37% reported having end-of-life discussions with their physician. For those who did have discussions about their preferences for care at the end of life, these discussions were associated with: (1) patient acceptance that the illness was terminal (OR 2.2; 95% CI 1.4–3.4), (2) having a do not resuscitate (DNR) order (OR 3.1; 95% CI 2.0–4.0), (3) valuing comfort over life extension (OR 2.6; 1.5–4.5), and (4) completion of an advance directive (OR 1.9; 95% CI 1.3–3.0). In a study of quality of life at the end of life, deaths among patients who received fewer aggressive interventions and who were enrolled in hospice for a longer period of time before death were associated with a higher quality of life [88].

Older adults' preferences for care are most likely to be respected when a known and respected clinician guides them through the advance care planning process. Among older adults who were engaged in the

"Respecting Choices" program ($N = 309$) facilitated by a trained medical staff, 81% ($N = 125$) completed advance directives in the intervention group, in contrast to 1% ($N = 1$) in the control group. Preferences for end-of-life care were respected for 86% of subjects in the intervention versus 30% of subjects in the control group ($p < 0.001$). Family satisfaction with end-of-life care in the intervention group was 76% versus 16% in the control group ($p < 0.001$) [89].

Clinical bottom line

While a body of research indicates that living wills do not influence care [77] in the general population, more recent data focused specifically on populations at higher risk of mortality demonstrates that advance directives do influence care among older adults by increasing the likelihood that the patient's wishes will be carried through.

All older adults should be offered the opportunity to document advance care plans because trajectory of illness is often unpredictable, and many lose the capacity to make decisions at the end of life.

There is a tendency among older adults to choose limited or comfort care when asked specifically about aggressiveness of care, and care is more likely to be consistent with stated preferences when advance directives are in place.

Summary

While the process of dying and death is highly individualized, appropriate end-of-life care includes adherence to patient values and preferences, expert symptom management, coordination of care, and care for the whole person with attention to supporting both the emotional and spiritual needs of patients and family. Pain is a commonly reported symptom at end of life and treatment of pain among older adults requires special attention to pharmacodynamics due to lower lean body mass and decreases in renal clearance. The evidence base for treatment of dyspnea, also a commonly reported symptom at the end of life, supports first treating the underlying cause and then use of beta-agonists, opioids, exercise, pulmonary rehabilitation, and steroids in acute exacerbations of COPD. Other treatments are commonly used but the evidence base is less well-established for these treatments. Finally,

while a body of research indicates that living wills do not influence care in the general population, more recent data focused specifically on populations at higher risk of mortality demonstrates that advance directives do influence care among older adults, and that care is more likely to be consistent with stated preferences when advance directives are in place.

References

1. Singer PA, Martin DK, Merrijoy K (1999) Quality end-of-life-care: patients' perspectives. *JAMA* 281: 163–168.
2. Steinhauser KE, Clipp EC, McNeilly M, Christakis NA, McIntyre LM, Tulsky JA (2000) In search of a good death: observations of patients, families, and providers. *Ann Intern Med* 132: 825–832.
3. Downey L, Engelberg RA, Curtis JR, Lafferty WE, Patrick DL (2009) Shared priorities for the end-of-life period. *J Pain Symptom Manage* 37: 175–188.
4. Emanuel EJ, Fairclough DL, Slutsman J, Emanuel LL (2000) Understanding economic and other burdens of terminal illness: the experience of patients and their caregivers. *Ann Intern Med* 132: 451–459.
5. Fried TR, Bradley EH, Towle VR, Phil P, Allore H (2002) Understanding the treatment preferences of seriously ill patients. *N Engl J Med* 346: 1061–1066.
6. Tsevat J, Dawson NV, Wu AW, et al (1998) Health values of hospitalized patients 80 years and older. *JAMA* 279: 371–375.
7. Steinhauser KE, Alexander SC, Byock IR, George LK, Tulsky JA (2009) Seriously ill patients' discussions of preparation and life completion: an intervention to assist with transition at the end of life. *Palliat Support Care* 7: 393–404.
8. Rosenfeld KE, Wenger NS, Kagawa-Singer M (2000) End-of-life decision making: a qualitative study of elderly individuals. *J Gen Intern Med* 15: 620–625.
9. Curtis JR, Wenrich MD, Carline JD, Shannon SE, Ambrozy DM, Ramsey PG (2001) Understanding physicians' skills at providing end-of-life care: perspectives of patients, families, and health care workers. *J Gen Intern Med* 16: 41–49.
10. Wijk H, Grimby A (2008) Needs of elderly patients in palliative care. *Am J Hosp Palliat Care* 25: 106–111.
11. American Geriatrics Society Panel on Pharmacological Management of Persistent Pain in Older Persons (2009) Pharmacological management of persistent pain in older persons. *J Am Geriatr Soc* 57: 1331–1346.
12. Won AB, Lapane KL, Vallow S, Schein J, Morris JN, Lipsitz LA (2004) Persistent nonmalignant pain and analgesic prescribing patterns in elderly nursing home residents. *J Am Geriatr Soc* 52: 867–874.
13. AGS Panel on Persistent Pain in Older Persons (2002) The management of persistent pain in older persons. *J Am Geriatr Soc* 50: S205–S224.
14. Ferrell BA (1995) Pain evaluation and management in the nursing home. *Ann Intern Med* 123: 681–687.

15. Morrison RS, et al (2003) Relationship between pain and opioid analgesics on the development of delirium following hip fracture. *J Gerontol A Biol Sci Med Sci* 58: 76–81.

16. Morrison RS, et al (2003) The impact of post-operative pain on outcomes following hip fracture. *Pain* 103: 303–311.

17. Ferrell BA, Ferrell BR, Rivera L (1995) Pain in cognitively impaired nursing home patients. *J Pain Symptom Manage* 10: 591–598.

18. Morrison LJ, Morrison RS (2006) Palliative care and pain management. *Med Clin North Am* 90: 983–1004.

19. Goldstein NE, Morrison RS (2005) Treatment of pain in older patients. *Crit Rev Oncol Hematol* 54: 157–164.

20. Tegeder I, Lotsch J, Geisslinger G (1999) Pharmacokinetics of opioids in liver disease. *Clin Pharmacokinet* 37: 17–40.

21. Murphy EJ (2005) Acute pain management pharmacology for the patient with concurrent renal or hepatic disease. *Anaesth Intensive Care* 33: 311–322.

22. Davison SN (2003) Pain in hemodialysis patients: prevalence, cause, severity, and management. *Am J Kidney Dis* 42: 1239–1247.

23. Dean M (2004) Opioids in renal failure and dialysis patients. *J Pain Symptom Manage* 28: 497–504.

24. Hanks GW, Reid C (2005) Contribution to variability in response to opioids. *Support Care Cancer* 13: 145–152.

25. Hanks GW, Reid C, Forbes K (2005) Re: use of strong opioids in advanced cancer pain. *J Pain Symptom Manage* 29: 113–114.

26. Weissman DE (1996) Hospital care for dying patients. *N Engl J Med* 335: 1765–1766.

27. Weissman DE, et al (1999) Recommendations for incorporating palliative care education into the acute care hospital setting. *Acad Med* 74: 871–877.

28. Hanlon JT, et al (2009) Consensus guidelines for oral dosing of primarily renally cleared medications in older adults. *J Am Geriatr Soc* 57: 335–340.

29. Barkin RL, Barkin SJ, Barkin DS (2006) Propoxyphene (dextropropoxyphene): a critical review of a weak opioid analgesic that should remain in antiquity. *Am J Ther* 13: 534–542.

30. Reid CM, Gooberman-Hill R, Hanks GW (2008) Opioid analgesics for cancer pain: symptom control for the living or comfort for the dying? A qualitative study to investigate the factors influencing the decision to accept morphine for pain caused by cancer. *Ann Oncol* 19: 44–48.

31. Verhamme KM, Sturkenboom MC, Stricker BH, Bosch R (2008) Drug-induced urinary retention: incidence, management and prevention. *Drug Saf* 31: 373–388.

32. Seed SM, Dunican KC, Lynch AM (2009) Osteoarthritis: a review of treatment options. *Geriatrics* 64: 20–29.

33. Bjordal JM, Ljunggren AE, Klovning A, Slordal L (2004) Non-steroidal anti-inflammatory drugs, including cyclooxygenase-2 inhibitors, in osteoarthritic knee pain: meta-analysis of randomised placebo controlled trials. *BMJ* 329: 1317.

34. Lewis SC, Langman MJ, Laporte JR, Matthews JN, Rawlins MD, Wiholm BE (2002) Dose-response relationships between individual nonaspirin nonsteroidal antiinflammatory drugs (NANSAIDs) and serious upper gastrointestinal bleeding: a meta-analysis based on individual patient data. *Br J Clin Pharmacol* 54: 320–326.

35. Lee C, Straus WL, Balshaw R, Barlas S, Vogel S, Schnitzer TJ (2004) A comparison of the efficacy and safety of nonsteroidal antiinflammatory agents versus acetaminophen in the treatment of osteoarthritis: a meta-analysis. *Arthritis Rheum* 51: 746–754.

36. Biswal S, Medhi B, Pandhi P (2006) Longterm efficacy of topical nonsteroidal antiinflammatory drugs in knee osteoarthritis: metaanalysis of randomized placebo controlled clinical trials. *J Rheumatol* 33: 1841–1844.

37. Mason L, Moore RA, Edwards JE, Derry S, McQuay HJ (2004) Topical NSAIDs for chronic musculoskeletal pain: systematic review and meta-analysis. *BMC Musculoskelet Disord* 5: 28.

38. McCleane G (2007) Topical analgesics. *Anesthesiol Clin* 25: 825–39, vii.

39. McCleane G (2007) Topical analgesics. *Med Clin North Am* 91: 125–139.

40. Ahmad M, Goucke CR (2002) Management strategies for the treatment of neuropathic pain in the elderly. *Drugs Aging* 19: 929–945.

41. McCleane G (2007) Pharmacological pain management in the elderly patient. *Clin Interv Aging* 2: 637–643.

42. Lee YC, Chen PP (2010) A review of SSRIs and SNRIs in neuropathic pain. *Expert Opin Pharmacother* 11: 2813–2825.

43. Eardley W, Toth C (2010) An open-label, non-randomized comparison of venlafaxine and gabapentin as monotherapy or adjuvant therapy in the management of neuropathic pain in patients with peripheral neuropathy. *J Pain Res* 3: 33–49.

44. Reuben DB, Mor V (1986) Dyspnea in terminally ill cancer patients. *Chest* 89: 234–236.

45. Ripamonti C (1999) Management of dyspnea in advanced cancer patients. *Support Care Cancer* 7: 233–243.

46. Bruera E, Schmitz B, Pither J, Neumann CM, Hanson J (2000) The frequency and correlates of dyspnea in patients with advanced cancer. *J Pain Symptom Manage* 19: 357–362.

47. Lanken PN, et al (2008) An official American Thoracic Society clinical policy statement: palliative care for patients with respiratory diseases and critical illnesses. *Am J Respir Crit Care Med* 177: 912–927.

48. Bekelman DB, Hutt E, Masoudi FA, Kutner JS, Rumsfeld JS (2008) Defining the role of palliative care in older adults with heart failure. *Int J Cardiol* 125: 183–190.

49. Tanaka K, Akechi T, Okuyama T, Nishiwaki Y, Uchitomi Y (2002) Prevalence and screening of dyspnea interfering with daily life activities in ambulatory patients with advanced lung cancer. *J Pain Symptom Manage* 23: 484–489.

50. Tanaka K, Akechi T, Okuyama T, Nishiwaki Y, Uchitomi Y (2002) Impact of dyspnea, pain, and fatigue on daily life activities in ambulatory patients with advanced lung cancer. *J Pain Symptom Manage* 23: 417–423.

51. Shumway NM, Wilson RL, Howard RS, Parker JM, Eliasson AH (2008) Presence and treatment of air hunger in severely ill patients. *Respir Med* 102: 27–31.

52. Rocker G, Horton R, Currow D, Goodridge D, Young J, Booth S (2009) Palliation of dyspnoea in advanced COPD: revisiting a role for opioids. *Thorax* 64: 910–915.

53. Tranmer JE, Heyland D, Dudgeon D, Groll D, Squires-Graham M, Coulson K (2003) Measuring the symptom experience of seriously ill cancer and noncancer hospitalized patients near the end of life with the memorial symptom assessment scale. *J Pain Symptom Manage* 25: 420–429.

54. Ram FS, Sestini P (2003) Regular inhaled short acting beta2 agonists for the management of stable chronic obstructive pulmonary disease: Cochrane systematic review and meta-analysis. *Thorax* 58: 580–584.

55. Sestini P, Renzoni E, Robinson S, Poole P, Ram FS (2002) Short-acting beta 2 agonists for stable chronic obstructive pulmonary disease. *Cochrane Database Syst Rev* (4): CD001495.

56. Abernethy AP, Currow DC, Frith P, Fazekas BS, McHugh A, Bui C (2003) Randomised, double blind, placebo controlled crossover trial of sustained release morphine for the management of refractory dyspnoea. *BMJ* 327: 523–528.

57. Johnson MJ, McDonagh TA, Harkness A, McKay SE, Dargie HJ (2002) Morphine for the relief of breathlessness in patients with chronic heart failure–a pilot study. *Eur J Heart Fail* 4: 753–756.

58. Mazzocato C, Buclin T, Rapin CH (1999) The effects of morphine on dyspnea and ventilatory function in elderly patients with advanced cancer: a randomized double-blind controlled trial. *Ann Oncol* 10: 1511–1514.

59. Allard P, Lamontagne C, Bernard P, Tremblay C (1999) How effective are supplementary doses of opioids for dyspnea in terminally ill cancer patients? A randomized continuous sequential clinical trial. *J Pain Symptom Manage* 17: 256–265.

60. Jennings AL, Davies AN, Higgins JP, Gibbs JS, Broadley KE (2002) A systematic review of the use of opioids in the management of dyspnoea. *Thorax* 57: 939–944.

61. Langer D, Hendriks E, Burtin C et al (2009) A clinical practice guideline for physiotherapists treating patients with chronic obstructive pulmonary disease based on a systematic review of available evidence. *Clin Rehabil* 23: 445–462.

62. Lacasse Y, Martin S, Lasserson TJ, Goldstein RS (2007) Meta-analysis of respiratory rehabilitation in chronic obstructive pulmonary disease. A Cochrane systematic review. *Eura Medicophys* 43: 475–485.

63. Lewis LK, Williams MT, Olds T (2007) Short-term effects on outcomes related to the mechanism of intervention and physiological outcomes but insufficient evidence of clinical benefits for breathing control: a systematic review. *Aust J Physiother* 53: 219–227.

64. Mahler DA, et al (2010) American College of Chest Physicians consensus statement on the management of dyspnea in patients with advanced lung or heart disease. *Chest* 137: 674–691.

65. Booth S, Wade R, Johnson M, Kite S, Swannick M, Anderson H (2004) The use of oxygen in the palliation of breathlessness. A report of the expert working group of the Scientific Committee of the Association of Palliative Medicine. *Respir Med* 98: 66–77.

66. Abernethy AP, et al (2010) Effect of palliative oxygen versus room air in relief of breathlessness in patients with refractory dyspnoea: a double-blind, randomised controlled trial. *Lancet* 376: 784–793.

67. Cranston JM, Crockett A, Currow D (2008) Oxygen therapy for dyspnoea in adults. *Cochrane Database Syst Rev* (3) CD004769.

68. Bruera E, Sweeny C, Ripamonti C (2002) Dyspnea in patients with advanced cancer. In: Berger AK, Portenoy R, Weissman DE (eds) Principles and Practice of Palliative Care and Supportive Oncology, Second Edition. New York: Lippincott-Raven.

69. Zacarias EC, Castro AA, Cendon S (2007) Effect of theophylline associated with short-acting or long-acting inhaled beta2-agonists in patients with stable chronic obstructive pulmonary disease: a systematic review. *J Bras Pneumol* 33: 152–160.

70. Fox E, Landrum-McNiff K, Zhong Z, Dawson NV, Wu AW, Lynn J (1999) Evaluation of prognostic criteria for determining hospice eligibility in patients with advanced lung, heart, or liver disease. SUPPORT Investigators. Study to Understand Prognoses and Preferences for Outcomes and Risks of Treatments. *JAMA* 282: 1638–1645.

71. Seneff MG, Wagner DP, Wagner RP, Zimmerman JE, Knaus WA (1995) Hospital and 1-year survival of patients admitted to intensive care units with acute exacerbation of chronic obstructive pulmonary disease. *JAMA* 274: 1852–1857.

72. Newton PJ, Davidson PM, Macdonald P, Ollerton R, Krum H. (2008) Nebulized furosemide for the management of dyspnea: does the evidence support its use? *J Pain Symptom Manage* 36: 424–441.

73. Walters JA, Gibson PG, Wood-Baker R, Hannay M, Walters EH (2009) Systemic corticosteroids for acute exacerbations of chronic obstructive pulmonary disease. *Cochrane Database Syst Rev* (1): CD001288.

74. Simon ST, Higginson IJ, Booth S, Harding R, Bausewein C (2010) Benzodiazepines for the relief of breathlessness in advanced malignant and non-malignant diseases in adults. *Cochrane Database Syst Rev* (1): CD007354.

75. Cook DJ, et al (2001) Cardiopulmonary resuscitation directives on admission to intensive-care unit: an international observational study. *Lancet* 358: 1941–1945.

76. Torke AM, Moloney R, Siegler M, Abalos A, Alexander GC (2010) Physicians' views on the importance of patient preferences in surrogate decision-making. *J Am Geriatr Soc* 58: 533–538.

77. Fagerlin A, Schneider CE (2006) Enough. The failure of the living will. *Hastings Cent Rep* 34: 30–42.

78. Parker K (2009) Coping with end-of-life decisions. http://pewresearch.org/pubs/1320/opinion-end-of-life-care-right-to-die-living-will.

79. Ramsaroop SD, Reid MC, Adelman RD (2007) Completing an advance directive in the primary care setting: what do we need for success? *J Am Geriatr Soc* 55: 277–283.

80. Smith AK, Ries AP, Zhang B, Tulsky JA, Prigerson HG, Block SD (2006) Resident approaches to advance care planning on the day of hospital admission. *Arch Intern Med* 166: 1597–1602.

81. Liao Y, McGee DL, Cao G, Cooper RS (1999) Black-white differences in disability and morbidity in the last years of life. *Am J Epidemiol* 149: 1097–1103.

82. Guralnik JM, LaCroix AZ, Branch LG, Kasl SV, Wallace RB (1991) Morbidity and disability in older persons in the years prior to death. *Am J Public Health* 81: 443–447.

83. Shalowitz DI, Garrett-Mayer E, Wendler D (2006) The accuracy of surrogate decision makers: a systematic review. *Arch Intern Med* 166: 493–497.

84. Gill TM, Gahbauer EA, Han L, Allore HG (2010) Trajectories of disability in the last year of life. *N Engl J Med* 362: 1173–1180.

85. Mack JW, Weeks JC, Wright AA, Block SD, Prigerson HG (2010) End-of-life discussions, goal attainment, and dis-tress at the end of life: predictors and outcomes of receipt of care consistent with preferences. *J Clin Oncol* 28: 1203–1208.

86. Silveira MJ, Kim SY, Langa KM (2010) Advance directives and outcomes of surrogate decision making before death. *N Engl J Med* 362: 1211–1218.

87. Teno JM, Gruneir A, Schwartz Z, Nanda A, Wetle T (2007) Association between advance directives and quality of end-of-life care: a national study. *J Am Geriatr Soc* 55: 189–194.

88. Wright AA, et al (2008) Associations between end-of-life discussions, patient mental health, medical care near death, and caregiver bereavement adjustment. *JAMA* 300: 1665–1673.

89. Detering KM, Hancock AD, Reade MC, Silvester W (2010) The impact of advance care planning on end of life care in elderly patients: randomised controlled trial. *BMJ* 340: c1345.

Index

Evidence-Based Geriatric Medicine: A Practical Clinical Guide, First Edition. Edited by Jayna M. Holroyd-Leduc and Madhuri Reddy.
© 2012 Blackwell Publishing Ltd. Published 2012 by Blackwell Publishing Ltd.

Printed and bound by CPI Group (UK) Ltd, Croydon, CR0 4YY